Molecular Aspects of Toxicology

Molecular Aspects of Toxicology

By

D. E. Hathway

D.Sc., Ph.D. (Lond.), F.I.Biol., F.R.C.Path., C.Chem., F.R.S.C.

formerly Company Research Associate,
Imperial Chemical Industries PLC,
Central Toxicology Laboratory

The Royal Society of Chemistry
Burlington House, London W1V 0BN

British Library Cataloguing in Publication Data

Hathway, D. E.
Molecular aspects of toxicology.
1. Toxicology
I. Title
615.9′001 RA1195

ISBN 0-85186-068-0

Typeset by Bath Typesetting Ltd., Bath,
and printed by J. W. Arrowsmith Ltd., Bristol

Made in Great Britain

Introduction

Toxicology covers a wide field, which comprises chemical toxicology, cosmetics toxicology, environmental toxicology, food and drugs toxicology, industrial toxicology, pesticide toxicology, and the toxicology of atmospheric pollution, and which involves acute and long-term testing as well as special tests for carcinogenicity, irritation, mutagenicity, and teratogenicity. In the testing phase, diagnoses are reached through the disciplines of chemical pathology, clinical medicine, and pathology, and, in the experimental one, explanation is sought through chemical/biochemical and pharmacological methods.

My impression from a long period of fundamental research in relation to current toxicological problems is that this field tends to be fragmented and that a critical judgement of toxicological matters is difficult to evoke. It was for these reasons that I thought I should like to write a book that would stress the structure and continuity of this subject.

In practice, the problem of diversity in toxicology is dealt with to some extent by judicious recruitment of young scientists, at varying stages of specialization, into a multi-disciplinary team. This is all very well as far as it goes but leaves something to be desired, (i) as a basic understanding of the subject is important to all of its practitioners and (ii) as it is to be hoped that there is still plenty of room for wide research, particularly on problems at the molecular level. It was felt that the fundamental basis of toxicology might be represented by a least common multiple derived from the various specialisms (*v. supra*) and that essentially the structure and continuity of its molecular aspects were involved.

Apart from the question of seeing the subject as a whole, there is that of seeing it with critical judgement. Toxicology is more difficult than is generally supposed, perhaps on account of its inherent complexity, and clarity about fundamental terms is essential. That this is not as straightforward as would seem to be the case is apparent from some working ideas, which are expressed in a way that acquires a more descriptive form and, as a result, one tends to believe that one understands things, which in fact one does not. Similarly, with simple mathematical equations that play a significant scientific role, the scope and limitations tend to be overlooked, and their precise meaning is lost. Critical judgement is especially important to the experimental toxicologist, whose professional opinion might be sought about a sudden crisis in which the health and safety of human beings may be at risk.

The subject matter of this book is organized into chapters that deal with separate subjects and, whilst this treatment reveals the structure of molecular aspects of toxicology, it inevitably incurs slight reiteration of ideas about some of the individual intoxicants, but any such overlapping material is treated from rather different points of view in the various contexts concerned.

The present book does not claim to replace the primary sources of toxicological information, upon which it largely depends itself, but attempts to draw a thread through the subject matter in a way that seeks to unify the subject as a whole and to chart a course through the main arguments. I hope that it will be useful to chemists engaged in molecular biology and workers concerned with toxicology and cancer research in particular, as well as to pharmacologists and specialists in drug development and occupational hygiene and medicine in general.

The author is greatly indebted to Dr. Frank L. Rose, C.B.E., F.R.S., for going through the entire manuscript and eliminating a number of errors. He would like to thank Dr. Rudolf Süss, Deutsches Krebsforschungszentrum, Heidelberg, for contributing Chapter 12 on 'Host Factors and Cellular Aspects', Dr. P. G. Gardam, Manager of Books, and his colleagues of The Royal Society of Chemistry for their professional help and interest, and Dr. I. F. H. Purchase and the staff of I.C.I.'s Central Toxicology Laboratory for their continuing support. Finally, it is a real pleasure to record my gratitude to Mrs. Marjory J. Purser for her invaluable help in preparing the typescript.

November 1982 D. E. HATHWAY

Contents

Part I Toxicity of Foreign Compounds

Part II Relation between Dose and Effect and Time

Chapter 4 Biological Action

Chapter 5 Extension of Simple Theory to Toxicology

Part III Metabolism

Chapter 6 Metabolic Pathways for Industrial Chemicals and Pesticides

Chapter 7 Kinetic Considerations

Part IV Pharmacogenetics

Chapter 8 Species Differences in Metabolism and Toxicity

Part V Biochemical Lesions

Chapter 9 Mode of Action Studies

Part VI Chemical Carcinogenesis

Chapter 10 Importance of Chemical Non-enzymic Reactions *in Vivo*

Chapter 11 Possible Mechanisms of Carcinogenesis and their Biological Significance

Abbreviations

c.n.s.	central nervous system
ED_{50}	the effective dose in 50% of a group of animals
i.g.	intragastric
i.m.	intramuscular
i.p.	intraperitoneal
i.v.	intravenous
LD_{50}	the dose which kills one-half of a group of animals
mol. wt.	molecular weight (molecular weights are ratios, and it is incorrect to add the word 'daltons')
p.o.	by mouth
s.c.	subcutaneous
$t_{0\cdot5}$	biological half-life, *e.g.* of a drug
ATP	adenosine 5′-triphosphate
CoA and acyl-CoA	co-enzyme A and its acyl derivative
FAD	flavin-adenine dinucleotide
GSH	glutathione
NAD	nicotinamide-adenine dinucleotide
NAD^+	nicotinamide-adenine dinucleotide, oxidized (preferred)
NADH	nicotinamide-adenine dinucleotide, reduced (preferred)
NADP	nicotinamide-adenine dinucleotide phosphate
$NADP^+$	nicotinamide-adenine dinucleotide phosphate, oxidized (preferred)
NADPH	nicotinamide-adenine dinucleotide phosphate, reduced (preferred)
PAPS	3′-phosphoadenosine 5′-phosphosulphate
UDP	uridine 5-pyrophosphate

Part I

Toxicity of Foreign Compounds

Chapter 1 Assessment of Toxic Risk

1 Introduction

This chapter discusses the dawn of man's awareness of the toxicity of foreign compounds in his environment, some concepts of toxicology, the toxicity of compounds, and the risk entailed, especially in connection with industrial processes. The narrative is slanted towards industrial and pesticide toxicology, because the continuing use of toxic substances makes it important to understand their effects in depth, *viz.* at the molecular level.

2 The Toxicity of Natural Products

The recognition of what to eat with impunity from amongst the profusion of plant products that were available was one of man's earliest achievements, and there followed the cultivation of crops and husbandry of livestock for food. Records show that rodent control has been practised for over 5000 years, and man's practical experience of animal behaviour made him suspicious of any human food that rodents avoided, and which may have become contaminated through storage.

Later, on account of the unpalatability of his diet, medieval man sought flavouring principles beyond the narrow range of acidulants (apples), bitters (hops and lemon and orange peels), and sweetening agents (like honey and some roots) that were near to hand. For this purpose, he began to use bay leaves (*Umbellularia* spp.), brown mustard (*Brassica juncea*), calamus oil (*Acorus calamus*), gentian root, liquorice (*Glycyrrhiza glabra*), nutmeg and mace (both from *Myristica fragans*), peppers, oil of peppermint (*Mentha piperita*), quassia, safrole (*Sassafras* and *Cinnamonum* spp.), woodruff (*Asperula odorata*), wormwood (*Artemisia absinthum*) and yarrow (*Achillea millefolium*), and many others. We know now that these plant products contain well-defined organic compounds, which are responsible for the flavours that the crude mixtures afford. Such a range of spices were safe to use for the purpose concerned, but other natural products were not. There might be mentioned snake and toad venoms and the fish poisons in *Derris elliptica* (rotenone) and *Menispermum cocculus* (picrotoxin).

The selection of these culinary ingredients must have necessitated much trial and error, and the same method would have guided man's search for medicinal principles. Thus, the idea of fertility attaches to the venereal properties attributed to extracts derived from crushed yohimbé bark (containing yohimbine) and that of longevity to the action on the heart, which is caused by the leaves of the ordinary purple foxglove (*Digitalis pupurea*). Digitalis glycosides restore an elderly person's auricular fibrillation to a normal rhythm. According to Egyptian records, castor oil has been used as a purgative and squills (*Scilla*) as an expectorant since 1550 BC. Ipecacuanha (*emetine*) was used for the same purpose by the natives of Brazil before 1600. For centuries, pain has been alleviated by recourse to opium and by the chewing and/or smoking of hashish (*Cannabis sativa*). Reserpine, in extracts of the climbing shrub *Rauwolfia serpentina* is a major tranquillizer, which has been used for centuries by the poor people of Bihar to calm the insane and to quieten children. Mescal buttons (containing mescaline) from the Mexican cactus have been known for a long time to produce hallucinations.[1–4]

This brief outline shows that, with the passage of time, man has become increasingly aware of the toxicity of foreign compounds in his environment and that, sometimes, he has been able to benefit from these effects. It ought to be stated clearly that the foregoing results were achieved by empirical means and that the evidence, which is cumulative, was obtained from observations in man.

3 Concepts of Toxicology

Toxicology is the study of the injurious effects of chemical substances on living organisms, usually mammals, and as we have seen (see Preface), there are several sub-specialisms. Thus, food and drugs toxicology involves essentially different criteria and thinking from industrial and pesticide toxicology. For the most part, food and drugs are ingested, and the absolute safety of the products to consumer and patient alike is a pre-requisite. Indeed, a minor side-effect, which may result from trial use of a candidate drug, is a sufficiently damaging feature to mitigate against its further development. In the case of food additives, regulations need to be even more stringent as, unlike drugs, food is taken throughout the entire life-span (and in the 1960s, some faulty biological testing caused an

[1] K. Beringer, 'Meskalinrausch', Springer, Berlin, 1927.
[2] H. Klüver, 'Mescal', Kegan Paul, London, 1928.
[3] A. Huxley, 'The Doors of Perception', 1954.
[4] D. H. Lawrence, 'The Woman Who Rode Away', in *The Dial*, July/August 1925.

established product to be banned for several years). On the other hand, industrial chemicals and pesticides are not eaten, and the Factory Acts' requirements forbid workmen to eat, where fumes and dusts may contaminate their food. Industrial chemicals and pesticides gain access to the body through percutaneous absorption and by inhalation. Thus, industrial and pesticide toxicology is concerned with the safety-in-use of substances, which may be toxic *per se*. In fact, industrial toxicology has been defined as 'the study of chemicals (including pesticides), which are used in industrial processes, in respect of their liability to produce adverse effects upon the health or efficiency of workers, under industrial conditions of exposure.' It follows that industrial and pesticide toxicology ought to have an investigative component, for in our affluent/industrial society, mankind is learning to live in proximity to the manufacture and use of chemicals, which cannot always be replaced by more harmless ones. In this context, molecular explanation for toxicity is of paramount importance because of the continuing use of chemical substances that may be toxic. But, the prime objective of food and drugs toxicology is screening, and candidate products on which suspicion rests are discarded and they never enter the human environment. Experiments in animals make up the common ground of these diverse aspects of toxicology.

In the fifteenth century, Paracelsus postulated that '*Alle Dinge sind Gifte*'. Oxygen toxicity is a well-known phenomenon (see Chapter 5), and if either common salt or sodium bicarbonate, the ions of which contribute to the electrolyte balance in the body, is administered in sufficient quantity, it would afford toxic effects. Thus industrial and pesticide toxicology is concerned not only with the nature of the toxic effects that a particular substance would exert, which would be found from experiments in animals, but with the amounts that are necessary to produce them, and also with those factors that influence the extent to which the substance will enter the operative's body in the working place. Experiments in which chemicals are administered to or injected into animals do not parallel realistically the conditions relating to human exposure.

The routes of entry into the body have been mentioned previously, and here it is necessary to refer only to the sort of substances that are absorbed into the body percutaneously and by inhalation, and to their physicochemical properties. Aniline, nitrobenzene, and other aromatic amino- and nitro-derivatives, phenol and the cresols, diethylstilboestrol, dichlorvos and parathion, *etc*., as well as HCN are absorbed readily through the skin. The lipophilicity of these compounds is important to this transport process, but the membrane excludes very large lipid-soluble molecules. Ionox 330 is a good example of a substance that is lipid-soluble and water-insoluble, does not form mixed micelles, and that is not transported across essential membranes.[5,6] However, the commonest route of entry into the body in industrial poisoning is by inhalation, and for example CO, HCN, H_2S, benzene, chloroform, methanol, methyl chloride, methylene chloride, Pb vapour, *etc*. are readily absorbed in this way. This implies that these substances are gases or that they are highly volatile or that they are suspended in the atmosphere in the form of a dust, fume, or mist. When

[5] A. S. Wright, R. S. Crowne, and D. E. Hathway, *Biochem. J.*, 1965, **95**, 98.
[6] D. E. Hathway, *Adv. Food Res.*, 1966, **15**, 1.

substances are taken-up by inhalation, they may exert a local effect on the respiratory tract, and this applies, for example, to $COCl_2$, HCl, and SO_2. Some may be readily absorbed and exert a systemic effect, for example CO, HCN, H_2S (Chapter 5).

4 The Toxicity of a Compound

The toxicity of a compound is something that can be measured by experiments in animals. Acute oral toxicity provides: (i) a measure (of toxicity) to a first approximation for a particular substance: (ii) some idea as to its mode of action in the body: (iii) some indication of similarities or differences amongst species in response to that substance. The objective would seem to be the determination of the nature of the toxic effect and the order of magnitude of the dose that will produce it. Estimation of acute toxicity, for example of the LD_{50} (*i.e.* the dose which kills one-half of a group of animals), does not give any indication whatever of the response of animals to repeated, small, sub-lethal doses. Yet industrial and pesticide intoxications follow repeated exposure to a toxic substance, and chronic lead poisoning is by far the most common form of intoxication that there is. The value of acute toxicity testing amounts to the useful information (*v. supra*) that it provides for sub-acute and/or chronic toxicity testing.

Chronic toxicity testing, which takes account of the long-term effects of small doses, is of much greater value than acute testing *per se*. The lowest level of exposure, in terms of weight kg^{-1}, ought to be chosen so as to exceed the anticipated human exposure, and it should not cause harmful effects. On the other hand, it is customary to select as the highest dose level one, which will produce harmful effects, but which will allow a considerable proportion of the animals to survive the long period of exposure. This procedure is said to give some idea of the severity of effects to be expected from excessive exposure and to afford severe conditions (consistent with tumour induction if the substance is carcinogenic), as the test is conducted throughout the greater part of an animal's lifetime. Too much attention should not be given to qualitative descriptions of harmful effects, which need to be put into perspective and, for example, the long-term effects of aspirin would sound alarming, if considered on their own.

Dogma and uncritical thinking threaten to incarcerate the testing phase in toxicology and impede its ready comprehension. Thus, the real objective of acute toxicity testing (*v. supra*) is sometimes misunderstood, and the idea that an LD_{50} value will go some of the way towards an understanding of chronic poisoning is a tacit assumption made in the Robens Report (1973). Utter inertia seems to surround the way in which the very simple tests[7–9] have been made. Yet it would be hard to justify on rational grounds high dose-level long-term testing, in which the metabolizing capacity of the animal for foreign compounds is grossly over-loaded, the metabolic pathways become saturated, and the resulting data are suspect. Moreover, the conditions imposed by these high dose-levels

[7] E. M. K. Geiling and P. R. Cannon, *J. Am. Med. Assoc.*, 1938, **111**, 919.
[8] J. M. Barnes and F. A. Denz, *Pharmacol. Rev.*, 1954, **6**, 191.
[9] J. H. Gaddum, 'Pharmacology', Oxford University Press, London, 3rd edn., 1948.

would never be encountered in the human situation, and their supposed objectives (*v. supra*) would not stand close scrutiny.

Other terminology, which is used in the testing phase of toxicology, refers to 'no-effect levels': TLV (threshold limit values) or MAC (maximum allowable concentrations). These values are identical only at ceiling TLVs, where atmospheric concentrations oscillate permissibly on either side of a time-weighted average. Unlike physical constants, such values have no real scientific value, and are often based on limited evidence. At best, they represent an informed opinion about safe conditions, but they have no statutory significance. It is not surprising that these values get changed from time to time; usually in a downward direction. What is confusing is that TLVs are incommensurate with the risk involved. Thus, in 1981, benzene has a TLV of 10 p.p.m. (in 1975, 25 p.p.m.) and phenol of 5 p.p.m. (in 1975, 5 p.p.m.), but benzene presents a greater risk than phenol. It is fairly difficult to maintain an atmospheric concentration below the TLV in the case of benzene, but this does not apply to the less volatile phenol. In connection with this implied criticism, reference is made to a paper,[10] in which it is concluded that the toxicities of unspecific toxicants (Chapters 4 and 5) might be compared by the values of their chemical potentials. The order of the insect toxicities,[10] which includes benzene and phenol, is relevant.

5 The Toxic Risk from that Compound

The toxic risk of a compound is a function both of its toxicity and of the factors facilitating its absorption into the body (*v. supra*). Thus, compounds that are readily taken up percutaneously present more risk than ones which are not, and similarly with volatile compounds that are readily inhaled as opposed to involatile ones. Hydrogen and sodium cyanides provide a good example of this. Their toxicities, which depend on the dissociation of CN^- *in vivo*, are almost identical, but they present different toxic risks. Thus, spillage of hydrogen cyanide is followed by volatilization, and inhalation of the vapour, if it is present in more than a very low atmospheric concentration, will kill the recipient. Similarly, a small splash on the skin will be absorbed very rapidly, and the operator will die. On the other hand, sodium cyanide is used commonly in various industries with much less caution than hydrogen cyanide. It is involatile, there is little if any airborne dust, and it is not absorbed percutaneously to any appreciable extent. Thus, although sodium cyanide has a very high acute toxicity, it is unabsorbed by the body and does not cause poisoning.

6 The Toxic Risk from an Industrial Process

The toxic risk of an industrial process depends on the toxic risk of the compound concerned and the operating conditions. Thus, the nickel carbonyl process (Mond) for refining nickel from nickel-rich ores and matte used to be associated with a damaging incidence of lung and nasal cancer in its work-force, but now that the process is conducted continuously in special chemical plant, which remains sealed, the operators are no longer poisoned by $Ni(CO)_4$. The incidence

[10] J. Ferguson, *Proc. R. Soc. London, Ser. B*, 1939, **127**, 387.

of associated cancer has been eradicated. This illustrates the necessity of inspecting an industrial operation before attempting to assess the risk that may be involved. Wet processes are usually less hazardous than dry ones, and for example, the preparation of supported nickel catalysts by the reduction in hydrogen of a slurry of the support material impregnated with nickel salts is relatively, if not entirely, free from risk. But, the melting of cupro-nickel alloys at high temperature, unless there is adequate ventilation to cope with the nickel vapour, will produce conditions, if they are repeated often enough, conducive (*via* inhalation) to the induction of nickel cancer. Similarly, whilst the handling of lead ingots is free from toxic risk, the melting of lead which is integral (i) to the preparation of the much used $PbCrO_4$ and $PbMoO_4$ pigments, (ii) to the cupellation of silver from argentiferous lead, and (iii) to the 'wiping' of lead joints is a potential source of lead poisoning. In a particular case, it is therefore important that the the hygienist be aware of what may be involved in the various procedures of, for example, bagging (a product), blending, distillation, evaporation, filtration, grinding, precipitation, spray drying, *etc.*

7 Perspectives in Carcinogenicity

During the last decade, public awareness of carcinogenesis has grown as a result of:

(i) increased epidemiology, which has exposed occupational risks from cancer:
(ii) the publicity from litigation:
(iii) increased experiments in animals, which have shown many industrial chemicals and pesticides to be carcinogens:
(iv) sophisticated chemical/biochemical instrumentation that has revealed the presence of carcinogenic impurities in products not normally considered to be carcinogenic *per se*.

A large number of chemical substances may be involved. Thus, the United States National Institute for Occupational Safety and Health 1972 List of Toxic Substances described 645 entries as carcinogenic or neoplastic. The size of the problem becomes obvious, when it is recognized, for example, that α-naphthylamine, which responsible chemical munufacturers have long suspected as being carcinogenic and have ceased to make, is not described as either carcinogenic or neoplastic by the NIOSH List. This rather suggests that other carcinogens may have escaped notice.

N-Phenyl-2-naphthylamine (PBN), which has been used in the rubber industry as an antioxidant for many years, illustrates the problem of impurities. PBN is not a carcinogen *per se*,[11] but g.c. analysis showed that in the past, commercial material in the UK had contained 15–50 mg kg^{-1} of 2-naphthylamine. In recent years, levels of < 1 mg kg^{-1} have been reported.[12] Despite the widespread use of PBN (*v. supra*), no excess incidence of tumours has been attributed to it in workers

[11] P. L. Batten and D. E. Hathway, *Br. J. Cancer*, 1977, **35**, 342.
[12] C. A. Veys, A Study of the Incidence of Bladder Tumours in Rubber Workers, MD Thesis, University of Liverpool, 1973.

who joined the rubber industry after Nonox S had been abandoned in 1949.[12–14] (Nonox S was the antioxidant which caused an occupational risk of bladder tumours in workmen who joined the industry before 1950.[15–17]) In fact, an expert committee (1973) has recommended that rubber workers, exposed to such materials as PBN with carcinogenic impurities, ought not to be subject to urinary screening, in comparison with workers known to be at risk of chemically induced bladder cancer. This apparent absence of risk from PBN, which during the period of epidemiological surveys[12–14] contained up to 50 p.p.m. of 2-naphthylamine, is a result which may have implications for other materials with carcinogenic impurities.

Perhaps something ought to be said about the evidence from animal studies. It follows from the account of the toxic risk of industrial processes (Section 6) that despite the fact that a substance may be carcinogenic to animals, it need not necessarily produce tumours in workers exposed occupationally. Thus, CCl_4 is carcinogenic in hamsters, mice, and rats, and chloroform produces kidney tumours in mice, but despite the very considerable exposures in man, there is no evidence at all to suggest that these solvents are human carcinogens. Whilst tannic acid and various tanning extracts cause liver tumours in rats, epidemiological surveys do not reveal any incidence of tannin-induced tumours amongst leather tanners, who may have had a lifetime's exposure to vegetable tannins.[18] Although these substances may present a risk, which on present evidence seems to be unlikely, all new evidence ought to be critically appraised.

For all carcinogens that have ever been identified, a dose level can be found that will not cause tumours in a small population of animals. A 'safe' dose for operatives, who are exposed occupationally to small amounts of identifiable carcinogens, is one that does not produce a significant increase in tumours above those in a population of unexposed individuals. In industrial toxicology, the emphasis shifts from the possible carcinogenicity of substances to that of industrial processes. The continuation of an industrial process that does not harm the workforce, compared with abandoning ones that do, must depend on various criteria:

(i) critical evaluation of the qualitative and quantitative evidence for carcinogenic risk:

(ii) epidemiological evidence of risk to man:

(iii) the physico-chemical properties of the compound in question in as much as they influence absorption under occupational conditions:

(iv) structural relationship of the compound in question to known carcinogens, for example of 1,1,2-trichloroethylene and vinylidene chloride to vinyl

[13] A. J. Fox, D. C. Lindars, and R. Owen, *Br. J. Ind. Med.*, 1974, **31**, 140

[14] H. G. Parkes, *J. Nat. Cancer Inst.*, 1969, **43**, 249.

[15] R. A. M. Case, M. E. Hosker, D. B. McDonald, and J. T. Pearson, *Br. J. Ind. Med.*, 1954, **11**, 75.

[16] R. A. M. Case and J. T. Pearson, *Br. J. Ind. Med.*, 1954, **11**, 213.

[17] R. A. M. Case and M. E. Hosker, *Br. J. Prev. Soc. Med.*, 1954, **8**, 39.

[18] IARC Monographs on the Evaluation of the Carcinogenic Risk of Chemicals to Man, Volume 25, 'Wood, Leather and Some Associated Industries', IARC, Lyon, France, 1981, 201–247.

chloride and of methylene-bis-(*o*-chloroaniline) [MOCA] to 4-aminobiphenyl and benzidine.

In this connection, moreover, the risk from a process involving a frank carcinogen can be greatly diminished. There might be cited:

(i) the new technology, which was introduced into the Mond process for refining nickel, and its contribution to the obliteration of associated lung and nasal cancer (*v. supra*):

(ii) the manufacture of PBN that is virtually free from the dangerous 2-naphthylamine impurity, by incorporating into the preparative method a condensation reaction to trap primary amine, and thus to prevent risk of bladder cancer:

(iii) controlled reaction conditions have wiped out the risk of paranasal sinus and laryngeal cancer[19] from by-product in propan-2-ol manufacture:

(iv) improved technology has facilitated the 'safe' manufacture of vinyl chloride, by reducing the atmospheric concentrations in the vicinity of the virtually sealed chemical plant to below a carcinogenic dose, and thereby safeguarding the workforce from liver angiosarcomas:

(v) it has proved possible, by reducing the exposure and preventing scatter, to use carcinogenic *X*-rays for medical diagnosis:

(vi) by maintenance of adequate precaution, highly dangerous radio-isotopes can be used safely for industrial processes.

[19] IARC Monographs on the Evaluation of the Carcinogenic Risk of Chemicals to Man, Volume 15, 'Some Fumigants, the Herbicides 2,4-D and 2,4,5-T, Chlorinated Dibenzodioxins and Miscellaneous Industrial Chemicals', IARC, Lyon, France, 1977, pp. 223–243.

Chapter 2 Structure–Activity Considerations

1 Introduction

In connection with structure–activity relationships, much attention has been paid to the lipophilicity of biologically active compounds, and a very important contribution to these problems was made by the impressive work on 'the parabolic dependence of drug action (for relevant series of compounds) upon lipophilic character'[1] and substituent constants.[2] These findings are especially relevant to the discovery of the most active member of a series of homologues,[3] as well as to the prediction of the activity of other, similarly related compounds. However, the importance of ionization to the biological activity of sulphonamides was established[4,5] over forty years ago and this fact, although largely ignored, has widespread implications for other classes of compound. From another standpoint, the fact that the relationships between structure and activity for many drugs and pesticides is represented conventionally by single-peak curves, such as parabolas, strongly suggests that such unimodal curves might be explicable in terms of the joint effect of two inversely related parameters, such as ionization and lipophilicity, which are molecular properties, and which are quadratic with respect to molecular size (M). This concept has not been explicitly stated before. A simple graphical approach, like the one which has been mentioned might be useful, as it may be extended so as to afford the possibility of separating, within an homologous series, the effects of structure on biocidal and mammalian toxicity. Selective toxicity is important and, for example, a candidate pesticide for development is chosen from amongst a small number of homologues with promising biocidal properties by its selectivity towards different organisms. From another point of view, a parabolic relationship describes the specificity of vertebrate sensory receptors to heat, light, and sound, and draws attention to the widespread occurrence of this sort of quadratic relationship. This raises the possibility that receptor specificity may contribute, in some cases, to unimodal structure–activity curves. Arguments like the foregoing ones probe the con-

[1] C. Hansch, A. R. Steward, S. M. Anderson, and D. Bentley, *J. Med. Chem.*, 1968, **11**, 1.
[2] C. Hansch and A. J. Leo, 'Substituent Constants for Correlation Analysis in Chemistry and Biology,' John Wiley and Sons, New York, 1979.
[3] M. H. Miller, H. L. Howes, R. V. Kasubick, and A. R. English, *J. Med. Chem.*, 1970, **13**, 849.
[4] P. H. Bell and R. O. Roblin, *J. Am. Chem. Soc.*, 1942, **64**, 2905.
[5] P. B. Cowles, *Yale J. Biol. Med.*, 1942, **14**, 599.

temporary approach to structure–activity and suggest that some reappraisal may be worthwhile: a preliminary communication* has been made.

* *Chem.-Biol. Interact.*, 1982, **42**(1), 1.
Additional Abbreviations have been used in this Chapter: C_r, molar concentration of a drug to produce a standard biological response; LDL_0, the lowest dose of a substance, introduced by any route over any period of time in one or more portions, which is reported to have caused death in animals; MED, the lowest oral dose of the test substance or drug that clears 100% of the infected mice of infection when administered daily on 3 consecutive days; MIC, minimum concentration causing complete inhibition of growth *in vitro*; *P*, the partition coefficient; pK_a, minus log of the dissociation constant of an acid; R_M equals log $(1/R_F - 1)$, where R_F is the relative band speed (partition chromatography).

2 Structure–Activity Plots

Unimodal Curves through the Joint Effect of Two Inversely Related Parameters.— Much experimental evidence (*v. infra*) supports the contention that ionization (*I*) and lipophilicity (*L*) are the physico-chemical factors that are most likely to be involved, as micellar and surface properties, which affect the transport of foreign compounds within the cell and the organism, are complex functions *per se*. In the general case where, for example, *I* and *L* contribute strongly to the $(1/LD_{50})$ function, the assumption is made that $(1/LD_{50})$ represents the sum of the two parameters (Figure 1). Sulphonamide drugs afford an outstanding example of the phenomenon considered here (*v. infra*). It is relevant that the new parabolic curves (Figures 2 and 3), which have now been constructed from

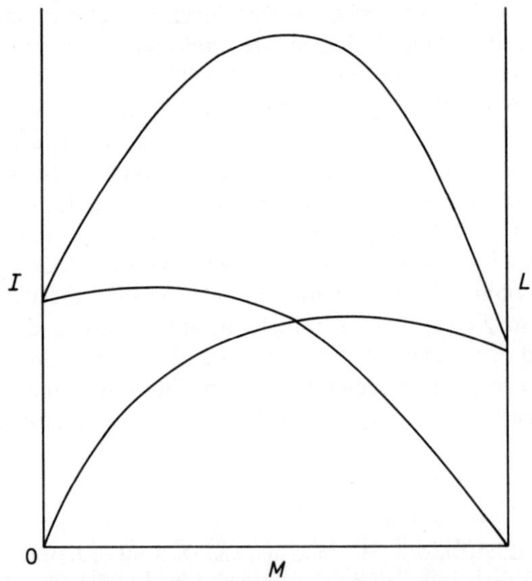

Figure 1 *Mammalian toxicity* $(1/LD_{50})$ *curve constructed from those for ionisation* (*I*) *and lipophilicity* (*L*) *respectively* versus *the molecular weight* (*M*) *of the homologues. The smooth curve representing electrolytic dissociation relates to the left-hand ordinate and that for lipophilicity to the right-hand ordinate.*

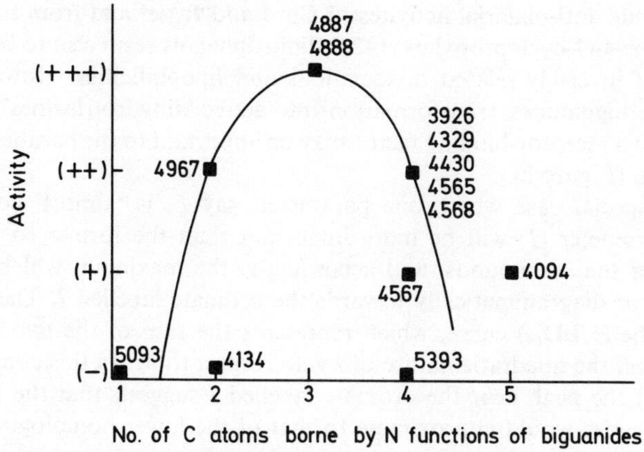

Figure 2 *Activity of some chlorophenylbiguanide anti-malarials against* Plasmodium gallinaceum *in chicks* versus *the number of* C *atoms* (R + R′ + R″) *borne by the* N *functions.*[6]

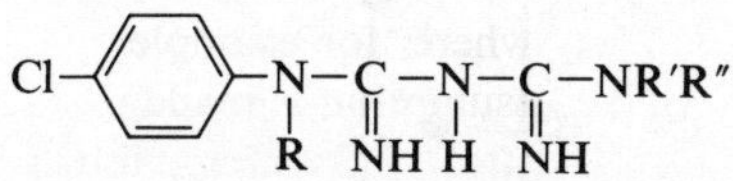

Numbering refers to the compounds in the Curd and Rose paper.[6] *The activity after a standard dosing procedure is indicated either as inactive* (−), *slight* (+), *marked* (++), *or very high* (+++).

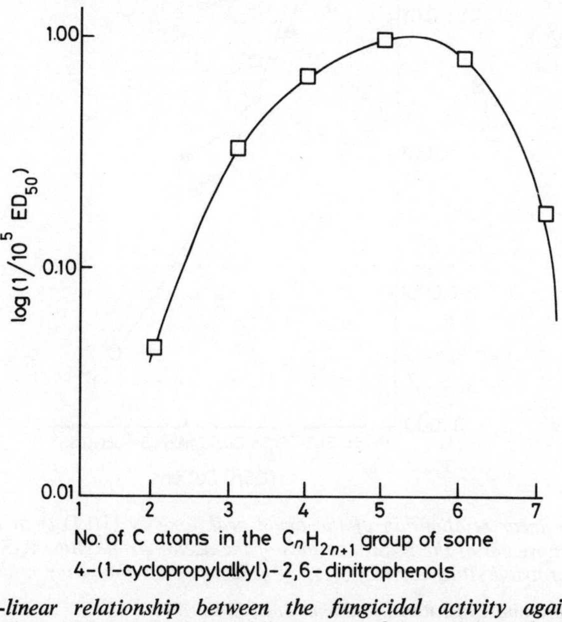

Figure 3 *Log-linear relationship between the fungicidal activity against Cucumber powdery mildew caused by* Oidium *spp. of some* 4-(1-*cyclopropylalkyl*)-2,6-*dinitrophenols and the number of C atoms in the* C_nH_{2n+1} *alkyl grouping.*

the biguanide anti-malarial activites of Curd and Rose[6] and from the fungicide data[7] for the 4-(1-cyclopropylalkyl)-2,6-dinitrophenols seem also to be explicable in terms of inversely related dissociations and lipophilicities. However, in the case of the biguanides, transformation into active 'dihydrotriazines' (chapter 6) occurs, and a receptor-binding factor may be important to the parabolic relationship shown (Figure 2).

In the special case where one parameter, say L, is 'almost' constant, the second parameter (I) will be more important than the former to the toxicity ($1/LD_{50}$) of the compounds, and accordingly, the maximum will be displaced to low M or diagrammatically towards the ordinate labelled I. The downward trend of the ($1/LD_{50}$) curve, which represents the sum of the two parameters, would reflect the quadratic nature of I with respect to M. In this connection, the position of the peak near the ordinate labelled I suggests that the lipophilicity of such a series would approximate to that of the lower homologues, and that

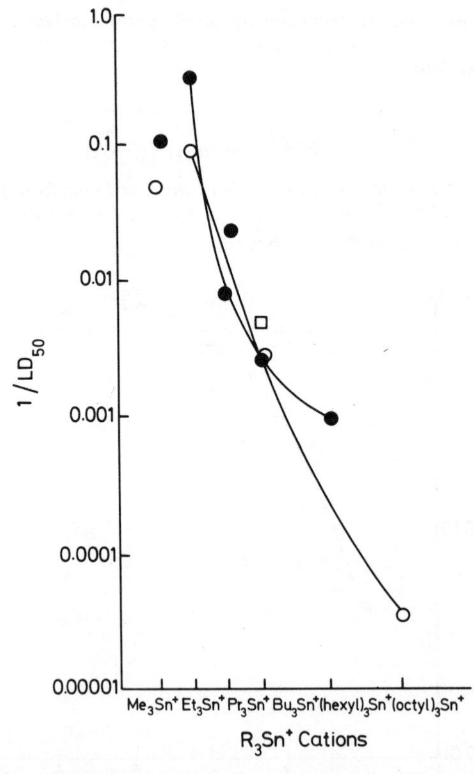

Figure 4 *Log-linear relationship of the acute oral toxicity* ($1/LD_{50}$) *in rats* versus *the ionic weight of the* R_3Sn^+ *cations of the acetoxytrialkyltins* R_3SnOAc (●) *and chlorotrialkyltins* R_3SnCl (○). □ *Refers to bis(tributyltin) oxide.*

[6] F. H. S. Curd and F. L. Rose, *J. Chem. Soc.*, 1946, 729.

[7] D. R. Clifford, D. M. Fieldgate, D. A. M. Watkins, and D. Woodcock, *Proc. 2nd Int. Congr. Pestic. Chem.*, 1971, **5**, 281.

this value is sufficient for these agents to penetrate biological membranes. The acetoxy- and chloro-trialkyltins exemplify the special case. Thus, the near collinearity of the log-linear plots of acute toxicity in rats ($1/LD_{50}$) *versus* the ionic weight of the R_3Sn^+ cations belonging to the acetoxy- and chloro-trialkyltins in Figure 4, which is now constructed from the work of Barnes and Stoner,[8] shows acute toxicity to be largely independent of group X, but to be influenced profoundly by the R substituent in both homologous series, R_3SnX. The downward trend of the curves and the possibility of a smooth peak between the methyl and ethyl members of these series is supported by the similar trend of points on a scatter diagram (Figure 5), which might be constructed with the same axes as the ones in Figure 4, and which uses all of the data[9] for every trialkyltin compound that has been tested for acute toxicity, including three commercial biocides, bis(tributyltin) oxide, Fenbutatin oxide, and Cyhexatin.

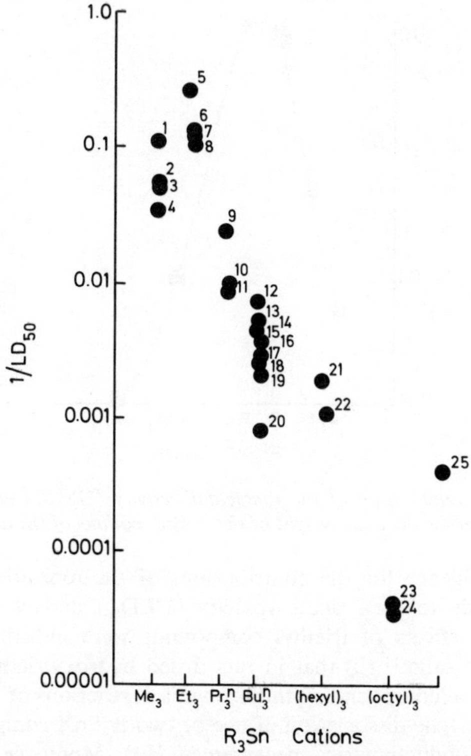

Figure 5 *Scatter diagram of the acute oral toxicities* ($1/LD_{50}$) *in rats* versus *the ionic weight of the* R_3Sn^+ *cations belonging to the trialkyltin compounds* 1—25.

[8] J. M. Barnes and H. B. Stoner, *Br. J. Ind. Med.*, 1958, **15**, 15.
[9] P. J. Smith, 'Toxicological Data on Organotin Compounds,' International Tin Research Institute, London, 1979, pp. 1—20.

The fact that this broad trend of values for the trialkyltin compounds parallels the shape of the foregoing curves (Figure 4) for the two homologous series, and that this array of compounds included acetoxy-, benzoyloxy-, chloro-, fluoro-, hydroxy-, iso-octylacetoxymercapto- and oleyloxy-trialkyltins and their oxides, sulphides *etc.* can be interpreted only on the assumption that the ionization of these compounds occurs under the physiological conditions (pH 0—8) found in animals. In addition, the log-linear plot of fungicidal activity (1/MIC) of the acetoxy-trialkyltins, R_3Sn^+ cations (Figure 6), which is constructed out of the work of van der Kerk and Luijten[10]) like that (Figure 4) for the ($1/LD_{50}$) function, is quadratic in form. The more clearly established peak in Figure 6 gives stronger support to the interpretation of both Figures 4 and 6 in terms of a joint effect of two inversely related parameters.

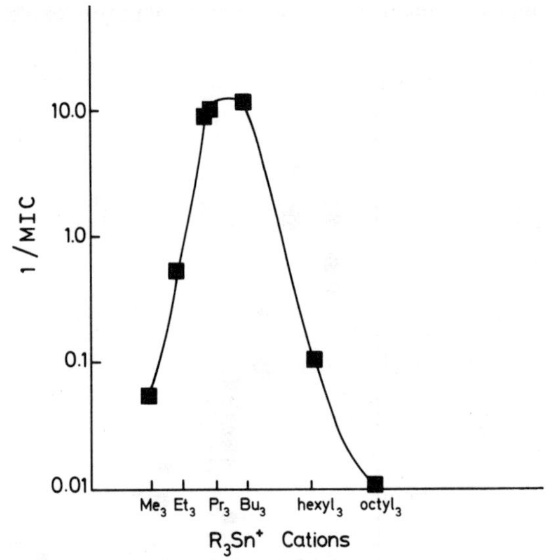

Figure 6 *Log-linear relationship of the fungicidal activity* (1/MIC) *against* Penicillium italicum versus *the ionic weight of the* R_3Sn^+ *cations of the acetoxytrialkyltins.*

Independent evidence for the contributions of the ionization of trialkyltin R_3SnX compounds to their acute toxicity ($1/LD_{50}$) derives from the facts: (i) that the toxic effects of triethyl compounds were indistinguishable from those of inorganic salts:[11] (ii) that in rats dosed hydroxytriethyltin, there was tissue retention of a 'compound' with the chemical reactions of Et_3Sn^+ cation:[12] (iii) that the electrolytic dissociation of one or two R_3SnX compounds has been established by conductimetric measurement.[13,14] Moreover, a connection

[10] G. J. M. van der Kerk and J. G. A. Luijten, *J. Appl. Chem.*, 1954, **4**, 314.
[11] T. P. White, *Arch. exp. Pathol. Pharmakol.*, 1881, **13**, 53.
[12] J. E. Cremer, *Biochem. J.*, 1957, **67**, 87.
[13] A. B. Thomas and E. G. Rochow, *J. Inorg. Nucl. Chem.*, 1957, **4**, 205.
[14] R. S. Tobias and M. Yasunda, *J. Phys. Chem.*, 1964, **68**, 1820, and unpublished work by R. S. Tobias, B. A. Nevett, H. N. Farrar, M. Hughes, and I. Ogrins mentioned in this reference.

between acute toxicity and the dissociation of R_3SnX compounds to give R_3Sn^+ cations (*v. supra*) implicates in turn the lipophilicity of the undissociated forms, which assists the transport of these substances throughout the mammal and which leads to the well-authenticated c.n.s. effects observed.[11,15] The lack of dissociation data for a range of R_3SnX compounds prevents the construction of curves from calculated points (*cf.* Figure 4 and 6) to test the foregoing hypothesis, and this constraint applies to nearly all of the groups of compounds discussed in this article.

It is relevant that ionization may make the greatest contribution to the biological activity of the old alkyl quaternary ammonium plant-growth substances, and in this connection the new parabolic curve (Figure 7), which has

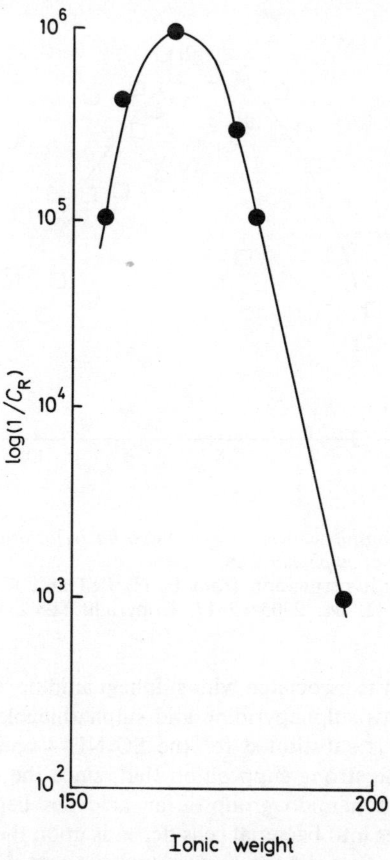

Figure 7 *Log-linear relationship between plant-growth activity* ($1/C_R$), *concerned with the lowest concentration of some bromoalkyltrimethylammonium bromides which caused a shortening in the stem of* (*Thatcher*) *wheat plants, and the ionic weights.*

[15] H. B. Stoner, J. M. Barnes, and J. I. Duff, *Br. J. Pharmacol.*, 1955, **10**, 16.

now been constructed from Tolbert's[16] log $(1/C_R)$ data, closely resembles Figure 6 for the organo-tins, for which ionization is very important.

Dependence of Activity on Ionization and Lipophilicity.—Bell and Roblin[4] found that for forty-six sulphonamides, the plot of pK_a *versus* bacteriostatic activity, log $(1/C_R)$, afforded a parabolic curve (Figure 8), such that the bacteriostatic activity was maximal where the pK_a of the agent was close to the pH of the culture medium, and decreased progressively as the pK_a values departed in either direction from this pH value. It had been found independently that decreased

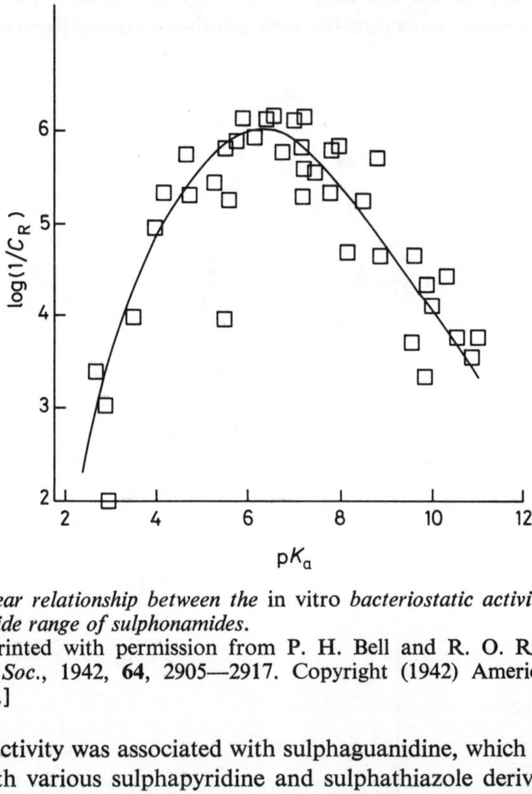

Figure 8 *Log-linear relationship between the* in vitro *bacteriostatic activity and acidity for a wide range of sulphonamides.*

[Reprinted with permission from P. H. Bell and R. O. Roblin, *J. Am. Chem. Soc.*, 1942, **64**, 2905—2917. Copyright (1942) American Chemical Society.]

anti-bacterial activity was associated with sulphaguanidine, which has no acidic group, and with various sulphapyridine and sulphathiazole derivatives, where the SO_2NMe— group is substituted for the SO_2NH— one, so that no anion might be formed.[17] The strong supposition that, since the optimal pK for the ionization of the sulphonamido group as an acid lies between 6 and 8, the penetration of the drugs into bacterial cells depends upon the un-ionized forms,[5] seems to have been confirmed[18] by the fact that the rate-determining steps for sulphonamide action in a cell-free system and an whole cell system have similar substituent dependencies. This makes a common reaction probable. Comparison

[16] N. E. Tolbert, *J. Biol. Chem.*, 1960, **235**, 475.
[17] R. G. Shepherd, A. C. Bratton, and K. C. Blanchard, *J. Am. Chem. Soc.*, 1942, **64**, 2532.
[18] G. H. Miller, P. H. Doukas, and J. K. Seydel, *J. Med. Chem.*, 1972, **15**, 700.

of the linear free-energy relationships obtained for the two systems indicates that a common parabolic dependency of sulphonamide anti-bacterial activity on pK_a (Figure 4) or on molecular size (M) is consistent with Cowles' theory.[5] Permeability of the intact bacteria to these drugs was unimportant unless they were present in $>90\%$ as the ionized form. Anti-bacterial performance was somewhat improved if slightly hydrophilic sulphonamides were made a little more lipophilic, but it declined with further increases, and this would be expected where lipophilicity is not a major contributive factor. An alternative explanation to the foregoing might involve receptor binding, as sulphonamides are known to be incorporated into modified folic acid syntheses.

Seventy years after Meyer[19] and Overton[20] had correlated the hypnotic action of structurally unrelated drugs with their olive oil–water partition, Hansch *et al.*[1] found that the hypnotic action of groups of barbiturates depended to a great extent on their relative lipophilic characteristics,[21] as defined by their octan-1-ol water P values. Hansch and co-workers'[1] model is formulated by equation 1, where k,k',k'' are constants and where C is used[1] with the same meaning as C_R in the list of abbreviations (*q.v.*).

$$\log(1/C) = -k(\log P)^2 + k'(\log P) + k'' \qquad (1)$$

This expression makes a good fitting equation for the voluminous data of Hansch *et al.*;[1] the constants permitting of considerable adjustment. The parabolic relationship ensured by the squared term agreed with Ferguson's[22] observation that when a certain degree of lipophilicity had been built into the parent structure of a series of homologues, further increases diminished biological activity *pro rata*. The working hypothesis of Hansch *et al.*[1] was 'that such fall-off in activity was the decrease in mobility of drug movement through biological material, when one departed in either direction from lipophilic character.' Thus, for an homologous series of drugs to participate in a particular biological action, a favoured balance between lipophilic and hydrophilic properties was envisaged,[1] so that those with an ideal balance would reach the target organ(s) in minimal time. This agrees with results for sulphonamides, obtained by investigation of their ionization, and with results for barbiturates, obtained by investigation of their lipophilicity.

In further support of the dependence of a parabolic relationship upon lipophilicity, the case of the 2-methyl-5-nitroimidazole anti-protozoal agents and of the *N*-n-alkyltritylamine molluscicides might be mentioned. Where, for example, (1/MED) was plotted against the P values without recourse to the theoretical treatment of Hansch *et al.*,[1] an imperfect parabolic relationship resulted (Figure 9) for some 2-methyl-5-nitroimidazole anti-protozoal agents with aliphatic sulphone-containing side-chains in the 1-position:[3] octan-1-ol water P-values were used. In this figure, a parabolic relationship held over a narrow range of structure and compounds bearing, for example, acetylenic

19 H. H. Meyer, *Arch. exp. Pathol. Pharmakol.*, 1899, **42**, 109.
20 E. Overton, 'Studien uber die Narkosen,' Gustav Fischer, Jena, 1901.
21 K. Meyer and H. Hemmi, *Biochem. Z.*, 1935, **277**, 39.
22 J. Ferguson, Colloques internationaux du Centre nationale de la recherche scientifique, Paris, No. 26: Mécanisme de la Narcose, 1951, p. 25.

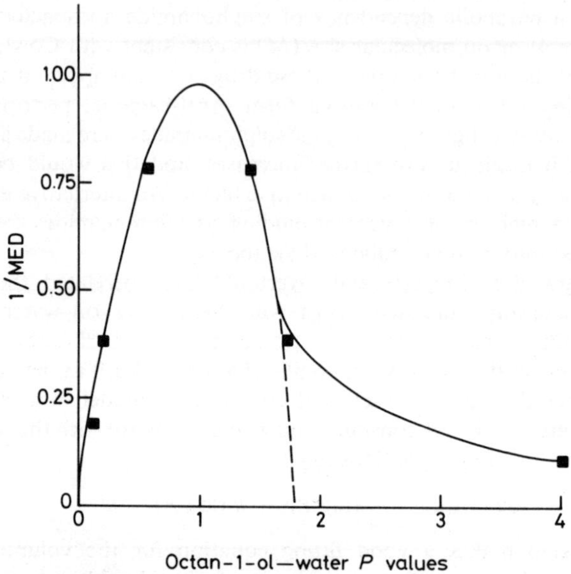

Figure 9 *Relationship between the efficiency of 2-methyl-5-nitroimidazole drugs with aliphatic sulphone-containing side-chains, expressed in terms of* (1/MED), *to clear protozoa in mammals and the octan-1-ol–water* P *values.*

[Reprinted with permission from M. W. Miller, H. L. Howes, R. V. Kasubick, and A. R. English, *J. Med. Chem.*, 1970, **13**, 849—852. Copyright (1970) American Chemical Society.]

side-chains could not be included without departing from the relationship. By maintaining the principal σ-contributing residues (the nitroimidazole and sulphone groups) constant, and varying the π contribution (*v. infra*), a smooth parabola was obtained until π contribution reached 'a certain level', beyond which considerable tailing occurred. However, the neat parabola (Figure 9) was useful for establishing near maximum potency within the limitations previously defined, and in this way, the favourable agent tinidazole (1) was apparent. A complete parabolic curve (Figure 10) resulted[23] when the molluscicidal activities of the *N*-n-alkyltritylamines were plotted against the corresponding R_M[24] values.

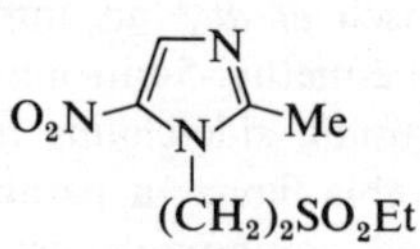

(1)

[23] C. B. C. Boyce and B. V. Milborrow, *Nature*, 1965, **208**, 537.
[24] E. C. Bate-Smith and R. G. Westall, *Biochim. Biophys. Acta.*, 1950, **4**, 427.

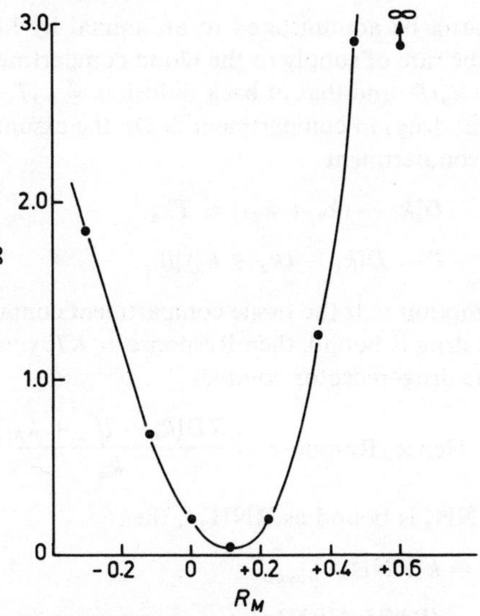

Figure 10 *Relationship between* LD_{50} ($\log_{10}$ molar concentration $\times 10^7$) *and* R_M *for the* N-*n-alkyltritylamine series.*

[Reprinted with permission from C. B. C. Boyce and B. V. Milborrow, *Nature*, 1965, **208**, 537—539. Copyright (1965) Macmillan Journals, London.]

Application of Kinetics to the Problem of Structure–Activity.—In another approach to structure–activity problems, a two-compartmental model might be used to simulate drug distribution in the organism. The characteristics of the model are shown in Figure 11, and the rate constants for renal and metabolic elimination are k_2 and k_5; penetration into tissues and the back-diffusion into blood are represented by k_3 and k_4.

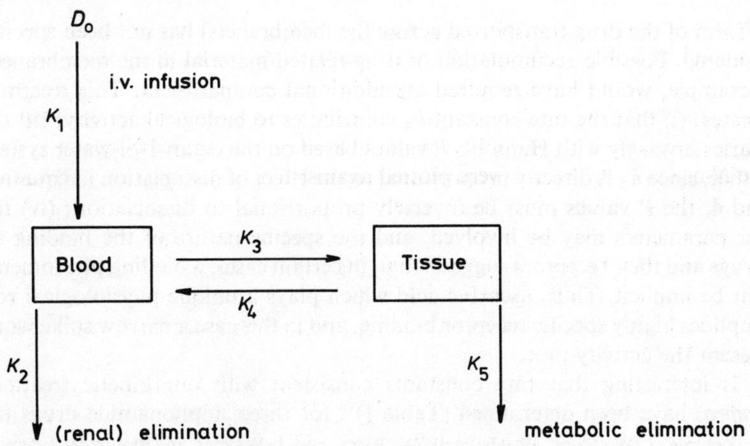

Figure 11 *Two-compartment model simulating drug distribution.*

If dose D_0 of a drug be administered to an animal by i.v. infusion at concentration D, then the rate of supply to the blood compartment $= k_1 D$, the rate of removal $= (k_2 + k_3)D$, and that of back diffusion $= k_4 T$, where T represents the steady state (total drug) in compartment 2. On the assumption that $k_1 > k_2 + k_3$, in the blood compartment

$$D[k_1 - (k_2 + k_3)] = Tk_4$$

Whence,
$$T = D[k_1 - (k_2 + k_3)]/k_4$$

On the further assumption that the tissue compartment contains drug receptors, and that unchanged drug is bound, then Response $= KT$, where K is the dissociation constant of the drug–receptor complex.

$$\text{Hence, Response} = \frac{KD[k_1 - (k_2 + k_3)]}{k_4} \qquad (2)$$

However, if drug RNH_2 is bound as RNH_3^+, then

$$\text{Response} = k[RNH_3^+]_{\text{local}},$$

where
$$k_b = \frac{[RNH_3^+][OH^-]}{[RNH_3OH]} \text{ and } T = [RNH_3OH] + [RNH_3^+],$$

$$\text{and the Response} = \frac{KD[k_1 - (k_2 + k_3)]}{k_4} \cdot \left[\frac{1}{1 + \frac{[OH^-]}{k_b}}\right] \qquad (3)$$

Similarly, if the drug RCO_2H is bound as RCO_2^-, then

$$\text{Response} = \frac{KD[k_1 - (k_2 + k_3)]}{k_4} \cdot \left[\frac{1}{1 + \frac{[H^+]}{k_a}}\right] \qquad (4)$$

The form of the drug transported across the membrane(s) has not been specially considered. Possible accumulation of drug-related material in the membrane(s), for example, would have required an additional compartment. This treatment indicates: (i) that the rate constant k_3 contributes to biological activity; (ii) that k_3 varies inversely with Hansch's P values based on the octan-1-ol-water system; (iii) that, since k_3 is directly proportional to the effect of dissociation in equations 3 and 4, the P values must be inversely proportional to dissociation; (iv) that other parameters may be involved, and the specific nature of the binding (K) of drugs and their receptors suggests that, in certain cases, a binding phenomenon might be implicit. Thus, ascorbic acid which plays a unique physiological role, exemplifies highly specific receptor binding, and in this case a narrow spike would represent the activity plot.

It is interesting that rate constants consistent with our kinetic treatment (*v. supra*) have been determined (Table 1)[25] for three sulphonamide drugs that

[25] H. Keberle, J. W. Faigle, P. Hedwall, W. Riess, and J. Wagner, in 'Biological Effects of Drugs in Relation to the Plasma Concentrations,' ed. D. S. Davies and B. N. C. Prichard, Macmillan, London, for the British Pharmacological Society, 1973, pp. 13—24.

had not been investigated previously.[4] The hydrophilic, inactive sulphonamide (line 1) was characterized by its rapid renal elimination and slow penetration into and diffusion out of the tissue compartment, whereas the most active drug (line 2) penetrates rapidly into the tissue, and is slowly eliminated and metabolized. The only apparent difference between the semi-lipophilic (line 2) and lipophilic (line 3) drugs is that the latter one diffuses more rapidly out of the tissues, $k_4 < k_3$. This situation holds where the drug shows marked affinity for tissue macromolecules and accumulates in that compartment. High tissue concentration seems to be disadvantageous to sulphonamide activity, and some receptor-binding phenomenon might be implicated.

Table 1

Sulphonamide type	*Rate*		*constants*	
	k_2	k_3	k_4	k_5
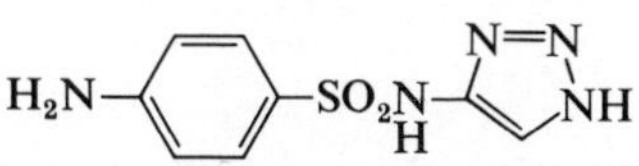	1.0	0.2	0.2	0.1
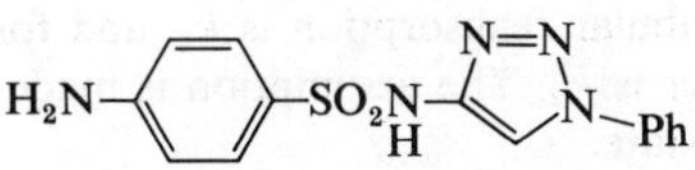	0.05	1.0	1.0	0.1
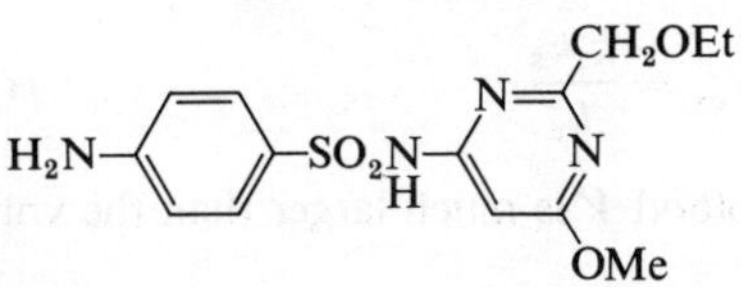	0.01	1.0	0.2	0.1

It follows from another simple model for hepatic acetylation[26] that, if k_{Ac} be the rate constant,

then
$$k_{\mathrm{Ac}} = \left[\frac{K_1 K_2}{K_1 + K_2}\right] k_3 \tag{5}$$

where K_1 and K_2 are binding constants for penetration into the liver and back-diffusion into blood; k_3 refers to a critical rate-determining step after the drug is bound to liver tissue. In order to obtain the logarithmic value of k_{Ac}, equation 6 was formulated, where α, ρ, and c are free energy-related substituent constants, such that log k_3 can be described by a linear combination of them. $[\mathrm{H}^+]$ is the hydrogen ion concentration of the blood. The proviso is made that the second term on the left-hand side of equation 6, which concerns the dissociation effect

[26] T. Fujita, in 'Biological Correlations—the Hansch Approach,' ed. W. van Valkenburg, American Chemical Society, Washington D.C., 1972, pp. 80—97.

of the free drug, is not meant to imply that the neutral form alone is responsible for metabolism.

$$\log k_{Ac} + \frac{\log [H^+] + K_a}{[H^+]} = \alpha\pi + \rho\Delta pK_a + c, \qquad (6)$$

where K_a is the dissociation constant of the sulphonamide, and ΔpK_a, the electronegativity parameter of the N^1 substituent in the sulphonamide molecule.

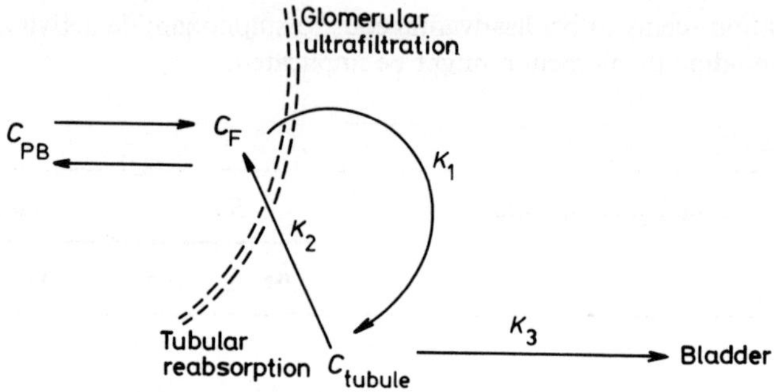

Figure 12 *Model for renal excretion.*

Consideration of the model for renal excretion (Figure 12)[26] shows that the rate constant for the decrease in drug concentration in the blood through glomerular ultrafiltration is k_1, for the tubular reabsorption is k_2, and for the movement of drug from tubule to bladder is k_3. The assumption is made that $k_2 > k_3$, and that (C_{tubule}) is in a steady state.

Hence,

$$k_{ex} = \frac{k_1 k_3}{k_2} \qquad (7)$$

It is assumed that the total volume of blood V is much larger than the volume dV, filtered in unit time.

The rate of decrease for the amount of free drug *via* glomerular ultrafiltration is $C_f \mathrm{d}V$ at any time, so that the rate of decrease for the concentration in blood $-\left(\frac{C_f}{\mathrm{dt}}\right)_g$ is given by equation 8.

$$-\left(\frac{\mathrm{d}C_f}{\mathrm{dt}}\right) = C_f \cdot \frac{\mathrm{d}V}{V} \qquad (8)$$

Hence, the rate of decrease for the C_{total} by the same route is described by equation 9.

$$-\left(\frac{\mathrm{d}C_f}{\mathrm{dt}}\right)_g = -\left(\frac{\mathrm{d}C_{pb}}{\mathrm{dt}} + \frac{\mathrm{d}C_f}{\mathrm{dt}}\right)_g = -\left(\frac{1 + k_1k_2}{k_1 + k_2}\right)\left(\frac{\mathrm{d}C_f}{\mathrm{dt}}\right)_g$$

$$= \left(1 + \frac{k_1k_2}{k_1 + k_2}\right) C_f \cdot \frac{\mathrm{d}V}{V} = C \cdot \frac{\mathrm{d}V}{V} \qquad (9)$$

Thus, the rate constant k_1 is described as dV/V, which is constant through a series of compounds, unless the test organism be changed.

Since the ratio of k_2 to k_3 would be proportional to the concentration of the neutral drug in the tubule and to its permeability through the tubular membrane, the logarithm of k_2/k_3 is described by equation 10, where $[H^+]$ is that of the urine in the tubule.

$$\log\frac{k_2}{k_3} = \log\frac{[H^+]}{K_a + [H^+]} + \log \text{permeability} + \text{constant} \qquad (10)$$

Log permeability can be related to the so-called free-energy related parameters. Thus, the value of $\log k_{ex}$ can be expressed by equation 11, which can be further modified to give equation 12, where α, ρ, and *c* are constants (*v. supra*).

$$\log k_{ex} = \log k_1 - \log\frac{k_2}{k_3} = \frac{\log K_a + [H^+]}{[H^+]} + \alpha\pi + \rho\Delta pK_a + c \qquad (11)$$

$$\log k_{ex} - \frac{\log K_a + [H^+]}{[H^+]} = \alpha\pi + \rho\Delta pK_a + c \qquad (12)$$

By means of equation 6 and equation 12, Fujita[26] analysed the data obtained for the rates of metabolism (acetylation) and excretion of a number of sulphonamide drugs.

It will be seen that by taking the effect of dissociation into consideration the logarithmic values of the rate constants for the acetylation and excretion of sulphonamide drugs (and on account of them the biological activity) correlate with the sum of 'the hydrophobicity constant' π and the electronegativity parameter ΔpK_a of the N^1 substituent in the sulphonamide molecule. Thus, whilst physico-chemical considerations open up the possibility of other parameters contributing to biological activity, the interaction of ionization and lipophilicity is important, at any rate for the sulphonamides.

Before closing this sub-section, a number of points are worth mentioning. First, *prima facie* consideration of the work of Hansch *et al.*[1] may suggest that a complete symmetrical parabola would result whenever $\log(1/C_r)$ is plotted against $\log P$ for lipid-soluble drugs (equation 1), provided that steric and electronic factors are kept constant. However, in the majority of studies by Hansch *et al.*, observations of increasing lipophilicity were made only for compounds with up to or slightly beyond the optimal P_0 value, where $\log P_0$ was obtained by putting the derivative $\frac{d\log(1/C)}{d\log P}$ equal to zero and solving the equation for log *P*. These workers[1] stated that neat parabolic relationships were not obtained from every set of raw data. Whilst this chapter provides evidence (Figures 2, 3, 7, 10, 13, and 14) of complete parabolic curves for structure–activity relationships, they may be rare, and such a possibility would be utterly consistent with the contribution of several rate processes to the kinetic models that have been considered. Secondly, the sort of receptor phenomenon that is suggested by the kinetic treatment (*v. supra*) is undoubtedly involved in the case of the plant-growth hormones,[27] since the peak corresponding to the physiological hormone indol-3-ylacetic acid is a narrow one, rather like that for ascorbic acid (*v. supra*). The peak for the synthetic 1-naphthylacetic acid, which mimics the physiological hormone in every way, envelopes the one for indol-3-lyacetic acid, but is three times as wide (Figure 13). (The fact that the powerful action of indol-3-ylacetic acid is abolished by the substitution of a methyl group in 2-position is consistent with the receptor specificity argument.) Unlike the previously mentioned plant hormones, which promote growth, 2,4,6-trichlorophenoxyacetic acid inhibits it[27] and acts probably at another receptor. Thirdly, whilst the particularly fine curves (Figure 14) for the various acaricidal activities of a series of n-alkylthiocyanate homologues[28] might be interpreted in terms of receptor specificity, there is no real evidence for this supposition and, in much the same way that the mollusci-cidal properties of the *N*-n-alkyltritylamine homologues[23] have been found to depend on their lipophilicity, the same may also be true for the acaricides.

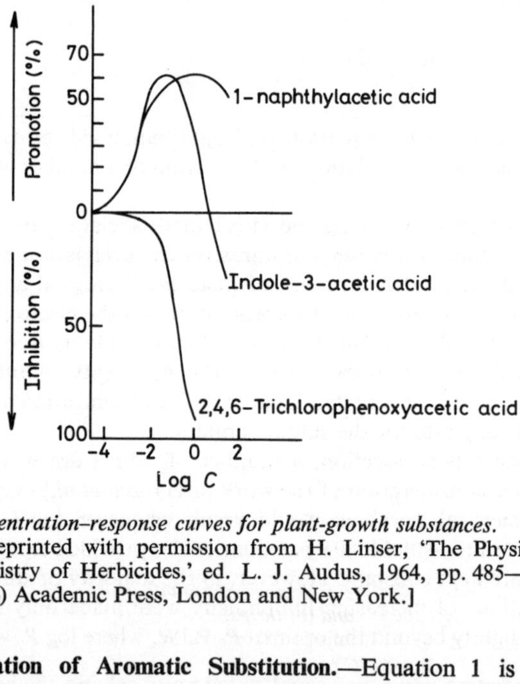

Figure 13 *Concentration–response curves for plant-growth substances.*
[Reprinted with permission from H. Linser, 'The Physiology and Biochemistry of Herbicides,' ed. L. J. Audus, 1964, pp. 485—505. Copyright (1964) Academic Press, London and New York.]

The Complication of Aromatic Substitution.—Equation 1 is unsatisfactory for lipid-soluble aromatics, as values of P depend on molecular size, and various biological activities associated with *ortho-*, *meta-*, and *para*-positional isomers cannot be accommodated. By comparison, the treatment of Lien *et al.*[29] accounts

[27] H. Linser, in 'The Physiology and Biochemistry of Herbicides,' ed. L. J. Audus, Academic Press, London and New York, 1964, pp. 485—505.
[28] E. W. Bousquet, P. L. Salzberg, and H. F. Dietz, *Ind. Eng. Chem.*, 1935, **27**, 1342.
[29] E. J. Lien, C. Hansch, and S. M. Anderson, *J. Med. Chem.*, 1968, **11**, 430.

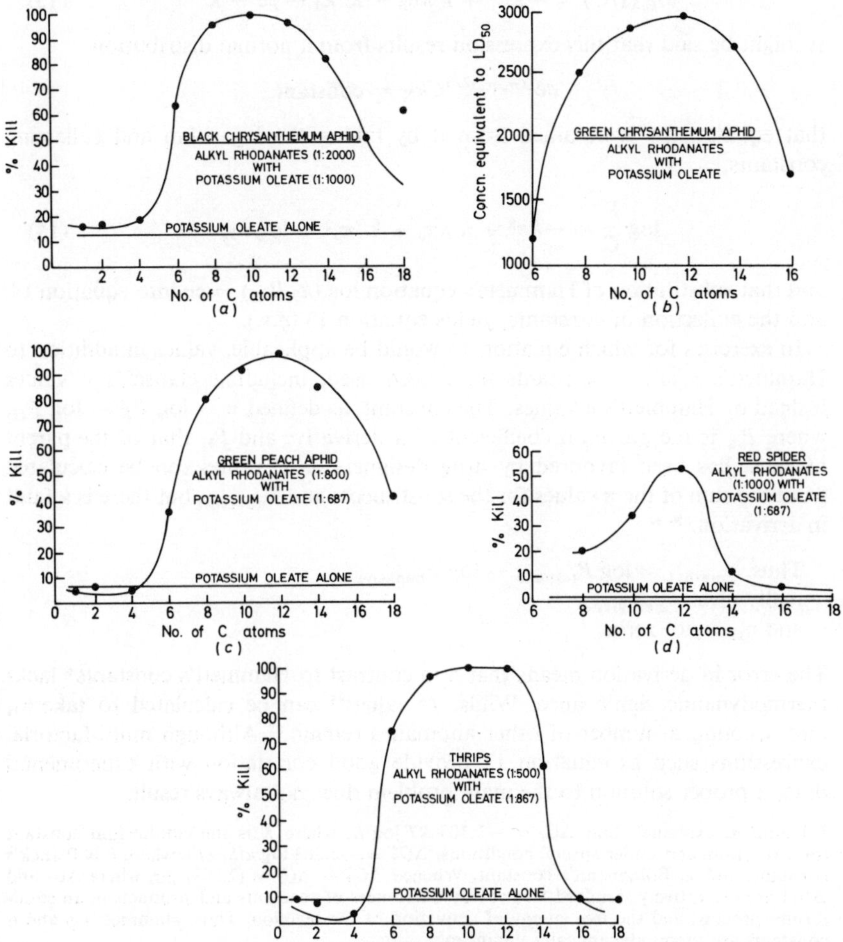

Figure 14 *Relative efficiency of n-alkylthiocyanate homologues against: (a) black chrysanthemum aphids; (b) green chrysanthemum aphids; (c) green peach aphids; (d) red spider; and (e) thrips.*

[Reprinted with permission from E. W. Bousquet, P. L. Salzberg, and H. F. Dietz, *Ind. Eng. Chem.*, 1935, 1342—1344. Copyright (1935) American Chemical Society.]

for this matter properly, and their use of equation 13[30] correlates various variables and Hammett's[31] ρ and σ constants, which arise from consideration of aromatic substitution and linear free energy.

[30] C. Hansch and T. Fujita, *J. Am. Chem. Soc.*, 1964, **86**, 1616.
[31] L. P. Hammett, 'Physical Organic Chemistry. Reaction Rates, Equilibria and Mechanisms,' 2nd edn., McGraw-Hill Book Company, New York, 1970, pp. 347—390.

$$\log (1/C) = -k\pi^2 + k'\pi\pi_0 - k''\pi_0 + \rho\sigma + k'''' \quad (13)$$

It might be said that this expression results from a normal distribution

$$ae^{-(\pi-\pi_0)^2/b}Ck_X = \text{constant},$$

that equation 14 is obtained from it by taking the logarithm and collecting constants,

$$\log \frac{1}{C} = -k\pi^2 + k'\pi\pi_0 - k''\pi_0^2 + \log k_X + k''' \quad (14)$$

and that substitution of Hammett's equation $\log (k_X/k_H) = \rho\sigma$ into equation 14, and the collection of constants, yields equation 13 (*q.v.*).

In exercises for which equation 13 would be applicable, values in addition to Hammett's ρ and σ constants have been used, including Hansch's π values instead of Hammett's σ values. The constant, as defined $\pi = \log P_X - \log P_H$, where P_X is the partition coefficient of a derivative and P_H that of the parent nucleus, has been favoured by drug designers as P values can be calculated from the sum of the π values for the substituents and $P_{nucleus}$, but there is a fault in derivation.[32–34]

Thus, $\pi_{methyl} = \log P_{toluene} - \log P_{benzene}$
really gives $\pi_{methylene}$,
and π_H is not zero.

The error in derivation means that π in contrast to Hammett's constants* lacks thermodynamic significance. Whilst *f*† values[34] can be calculated to take π_H into account, a number of other anomalies remain.[32] Although multi-factorial expressions such as equation 13 provide good correlation with experimental data, a proper solution to the main problem does not always result.

* Hammett explains[31] that $\Delta G_r = -2.303\ RT \log K$, where K is the equilibrium constant for a reaction, and under special conditions, $\Delta G^\ddagger = -2.303 \log k(h/\varkappa T)$, where h is Planck's constant, and $\varkappa$, Boltzmann's constant. Whence $\Delta G^\ddagger - \Delta G_r = (2.303)\ \rho\sigma$, where ΔG_r and $\Delta G_r^\ddagger$ are respectively standard free energy differences of reactants and products in an equilibrium process, and the free energy of activation of the reaction. Thus, Hammett's ρ and σ constants are thermodynamically significant.

† Where *f* represents the hydrophobic fragmental *constant*, introduced by Rekker[34] to replace π, which is the hydrophobic fragmental substituent.

3 Selective Toxicity

The simple graphical method, which was employed in the preceding section, might be extended to display the relationship between biological activity log $(1/ED_{50})$ and mammalian toxicity $(1/LD_{50})$, and this would facilitate the separation of compounds of high selectivity, *i.e.* those with high biocidal or drug activity and low toxicity, from those of low selectivity. (As far as the author is aware, this approach has never been used before.) Where both biological activities are

[32] A. Albert, 'Selective Toxicity,' 6th edn., Chapman and Hall, London, 1979, pp. 73—75.
[33] S. S. Davis, *J. Pharm. Pharmacol.*, 1973, **25**, 293.
[34] G. G. Nys and R. F. Rekker, *Chim. Ther.*, 1973, **8**, 521.

quadratic in form [*i.e.* log $(1/ED_{50})$ against M and log $(1/LD_{50})$ against M], the new relationship would be expected to be quadratic in form, and this is borne out in practice.

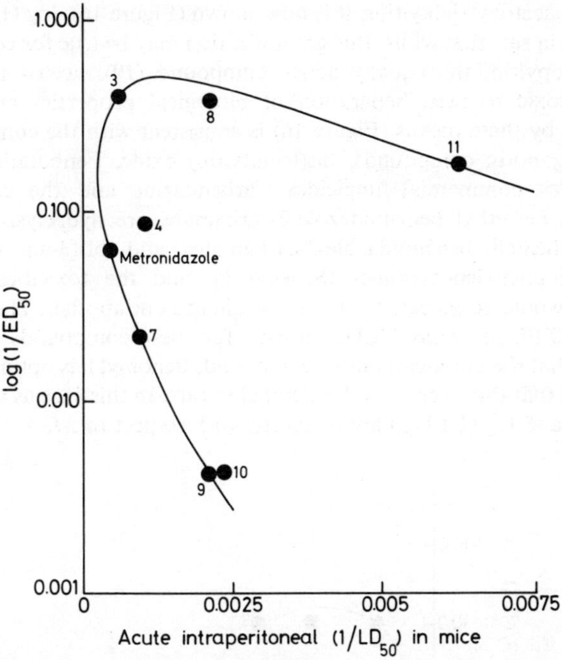

Figure 15 *Log-linear relationship between the anti-parasitic activity* $(1/ED_{50})$ *against the* Trichomonas foetus *infection* in vivo *of some* 1-(*3-chloro-2-hydroxypropyl*) *substituted nitroimidazoles and the acute intraperitoneal toxicity* $(1/LD_{50})$ *in mice.*

Anti-parasitic Drugs.—The new log-linear plot of reciprocal biological action against *Trichomonas foetus versus* intraperitoneal $(1/LD_{50})$ in mice for some 1-(3-chloro-2-hydroxypropyl)-substituted nitroimidazoles has been constructed from the data for various protozoal infections[35] (Figure 15). Both log $(1/ED_{50})$ and $(1/LD_{50})$ are quadratic with respect to M. 1-(3-Chloro-2-hydroxypropyl)-2-methyl-5-nitroimidazole [compound (3), Figure 15] showed much the same spectrum of activities against infections as metromidazole did,[35] and whilst it possesses considerably higher activity than metromidazole towards *T. foetus*, it is equally well tolerated by the mouse (Figure 15). In comparison, compounds (4) [1-(2,3-dichloropropyl)-2-methyl-5-nitroimidazole], (8) [1-(3-chloro-2-hydroxypropyl)-2-isopropyl-5-nitroimidazole], and (11) [1-(3-chloro-2-hydroxy-propyl)-2-nitroimidazole] showed much the same activity towards *T. foetus* as metromidazole, but they were more toxic to mice, and compound (11) was twelve times as toxic as metromidazole. Amongst these structurally related drugs, toxicity to protozoa is separable from that to mammals.

[35] M. Hoffer and E. Grunberg, *J. Med. Chem.*, 1974, **17**, 1019.

Fungicides.—High fungicidal activity has for long been considered to be closely associated with high mammalian toxicity in the case of organotin compounds, and this is reflected *prima facie* by Figures 4 and 6 taken collectively. However, amongst the acetoxytrialkyltins, it is now shown (Figure 16), log (1/MIC) *versus* log ($1/LD_{50}$) in rats that whilst this generalization may be true for compound (9), acetoxytripropyltin, the equally active compound (19), acetoxytrihexyltin, is much less toxic to rats. Separation of biological properties amongst these homologues by these means (Figure 16) is consistent with the continuing small usage of organotin compounds, bis(tributyltin) oxide, Fenbutatin oxide, and Cyhexatin, as commercial fungicides. Carbendazine and the corresponding 'ethyl ester', *i.e.* ethyl benzimidazole-2-carbamate, are hydrolysis products of more complicated benzimidazole-2-carbamates and bis(3-alkoxycarbamoyl-thioureido)-*o*-phenylenediamines (Scheme 1), and the toxicities of all five compounds would be expected to be very similar to one another. The new log–log plot of ($1/10^5ED_{50}$) *versus* $1/LD_{50}$ in rats, for these compounds (Figure 17)[36] now shows that the butyl-carbamoyl compound, Benomyl has optimal fungitoxic activity, and that this agent is well tolerated in rats. In this case as well, both log ($1/10^5ED_{50}$) and log ($1/LD_{50}$) are quadratic with respect to M.

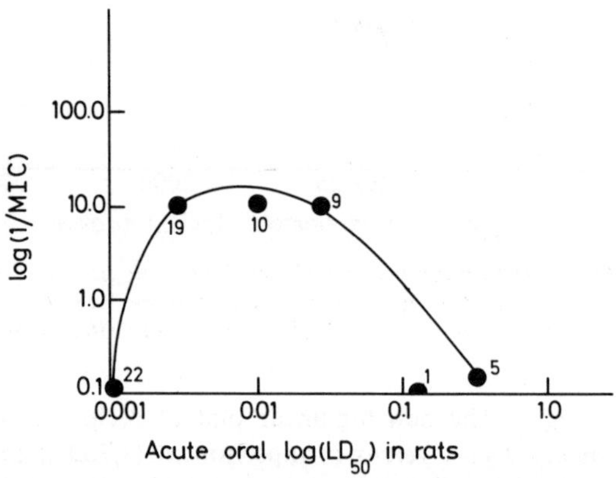

Figure 16 *Log–log relationship between the fungicidal activity* (1/MIC) *against* Penicillium italicum *of acetoxytrialkyltins and the acute oral toxicity* ($1/LD_{50}$) *in rats.*

The retrieval of structure–activity data for drugs and pesticides presents real difficulty, as much is unpublished and consequently the examples (Figures 15—17) considered here, from amongst several alternatives, suffer from inaccuracy through incorporating too few points. Nevertheless, the three new curves exemplified represent trends in relationship between biological activity and mammalian toxicity for the biocides, and they facilitate identification of compounds of high selectivity.

Apparent comparison[37] of Benomyl (methyl 3-butylcarbamoylbenzimidazole-2-carbamate) with thiabendazole, 2-(thiazin-2-yl)benzimidazole and furidazole,

[36] D. R. Clifford and E. C. Hislop, *Proc. 6th Br. Insecticide Fungicide Conf.*, 1971, **1**, 438.
[37] L. V. Edgington, K. L. Khew, and G. L. Barron, *Phytopathology*, 1971, **61**, 42.

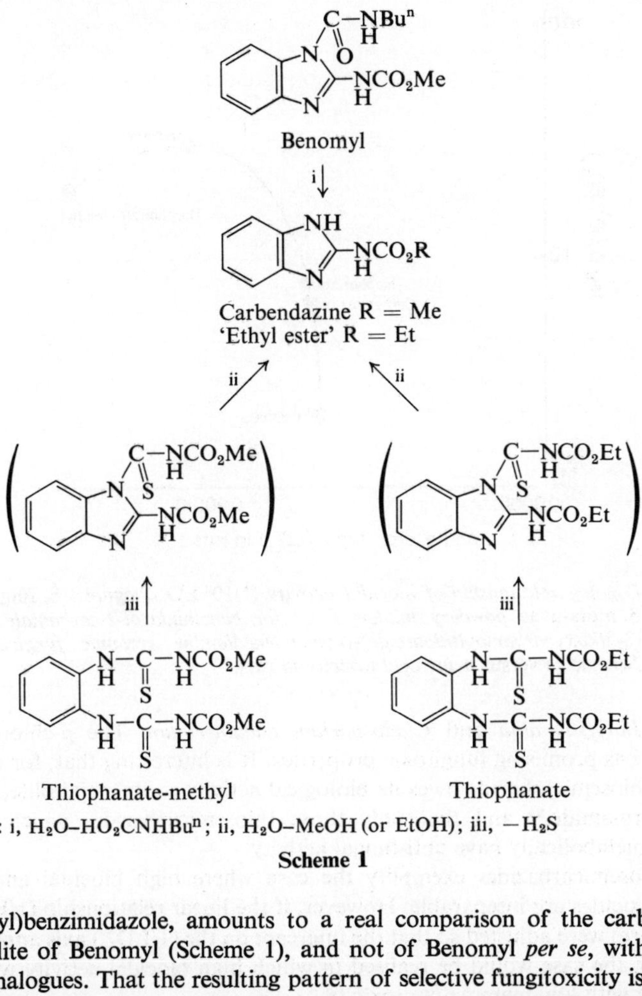

Reagents: i, H_2O–HO_2CNHBu^n; ii, H_2O–MeOH (or EtOH); iii, $-H_2S$

Scheme 1

2-(2-furyl)benzimidazole, amounts to a real comparison of the carbendazine metabolite of Benomyl (Scheme 1), and not of Benomyl *per se*, with the two other analogues. That the resulting pattern of selective fungitoxicity is identical is rather surprising, as biological activity of all three compounds would appear to relate to the benzimidazol-2-yl residue, which is common to all three substances. Because the fungitoxicity of these compounds for various micro-organisms is qualitatively and quantitatively similar, it is possible to construct the linear relationship log $(1/10^5\text{ED}) = 1.25$. High selectivity of Benomyl on this linear relationship stems from its low mammalian toxicity.

At one time, the fungitoxic properties of arylthiosemicarbazine were thoroughly investigated,[38] but these homologues were never used widely, because of adverse mammalian toxicity. Thus, the oral LDL_0 in rats of phenyl-*p*-tolyl- and *p*-chlorophenyl-thiosemicarbazines is *ca.* 50 mg kg^{-1} and the oral LD_{50} is very low, *ca.* 5 mg kg^{-1}. The linear relationship $(1/LD_{50}) = 0.2$ holds for the activities

[38] C. W. Pluijgers and A. Kaars Sijpesteijn, *Ann. Appl. Biol.*, 1966, **57**, 465.

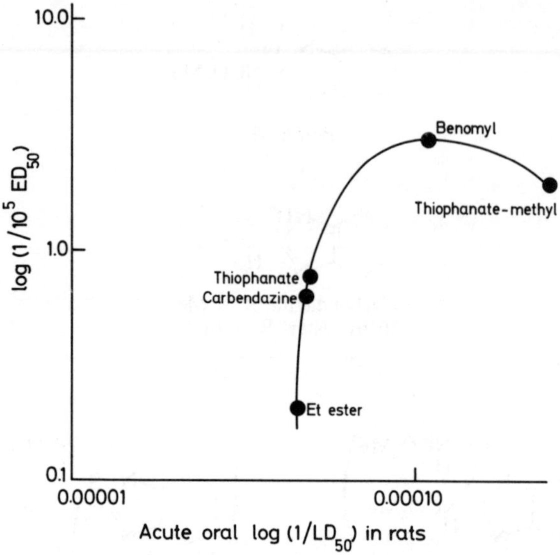

Figure 17 *Log–log relationship of biocidal activity* ($1/10^5$ ED_{50}) *against* S. fulginea *and* S. mors-uvae *powdery mildew fungi for benzimidazol-2-carbamate and bis* (*3-alkoxycarbamoylthioureido*)-o-*phenylenediamine systemic fungicides* (*see Scheme 1*) versus *acute oral toxicity in rats.*

towards *Botyritis albii* and *Cladosporium cucumerinum.* The *p*-chlorophenyl analogue has promising fungitoxic properties. It is interesting that, for example 1-phenylthiosemicarbazide owes its biological activity to its metabolite, phenylazothioformamide,[39] and that only those thiosemicarbazides which can be oxidized metabolically have anti-fungal activity.

Arylthiosemicarbazides exemplify the case where high biocidal and mammalian toxicities are inseparable. However, if the linear relationship ($1/LD_{50}$) = 0.2 (*v. supra*) were adjusted so that the intercept on the ($1/LD_{50}$) axis approached the origin, the case would be realised in which high biocidal activity would be associated with low mammalian toxicity.

The 2-alkylamino-4-hydroxy-5-alkyl-6-methylpyrimidine fungicides developed by ICI workers[40–45] exemplify the principle that high fungicidal activity[46,47] is associated with low mammalian toxicity (oral LD_{50}, > 4 g kg^{-1}) in rats.

[39] A. Kaars Sijpesteijn, C. W. Pluijgers, A. Verloop, and A. Tempel, *Ann. Appl. Biol.*, 1968, **61**, 473.
[40] K. J. Bent, *Ann. Appl. Biol.*, 1970, **66**, 103.
[41] K. J. Bent, A. M. Cole, J. A. W. Turner, and M. Woolner, *Proc. 6th Br. Insecticide Fungicide Conf.*, 1971, **1**, 274.
[42] D. H. Brooks, *Ann. Appl. Biol.*, 1972, **70**, 149.
[43] J. R. Finney and D. W. Hall, *Plant Pathol.*, 1972, **21**, 73.
[44] J. R. Finney, G. M. Farrell, and K. J. Bent, *Proc. 8th Br. Insecticide Fungicide Conf.*, 1975, 667.
[45] M. C. Shephard, K. J. Bent, M. Woolner, and A. M. Cole, *Proc. 8th Br. Insecticide Fungicide Conf.*, 1975, 59.

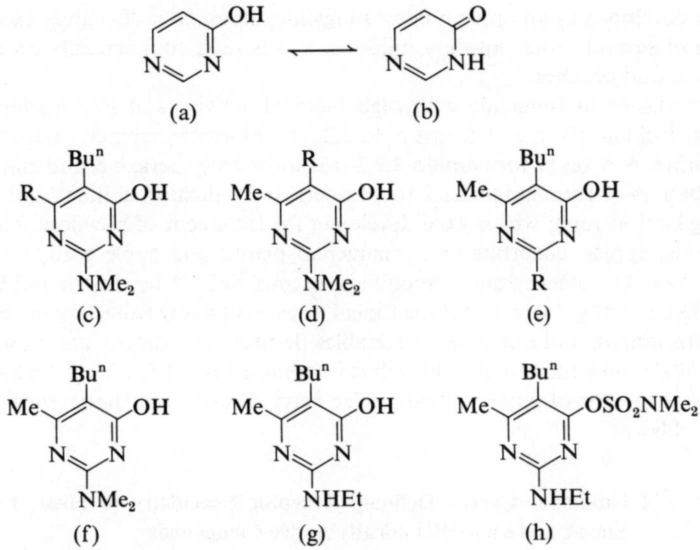

Scheme 2

Actually, the 4-hydroxypyrimidines (a) (Scheme 2) exist as the 4-oxo tautomers (b) both in solution and in the solid state. The O-atom in the 4-position makes for high biological activity, and replacement of the O-function by other substituent groups results either in loss of biocidal activity or in enhanced mammalian toxicity. The preferred substituents [R in formula (c)] in the 6-position were methyl and ethyl. Fungicidal activity is greatest where the 5-alkyl group [R in formula (d)] has from two to five C-atoms, and n-alkyl groups were somewhat more effective than branched chain ones. The alkylamino function in the 2-position [R in formula (e)] proved essential for optimal fungitoxicity. The influence of various 2-substituted amino groups on systemic activity against cucumber and barley mildew was investigated. Of six analogues listed by Woodcock,[46] five gave 90—100% control of the former pathogen, and of these, the 2-dimethylamino analogue, dimethirimil (f), was developed against cucurbit mildew (with only slightly less effective properties against cereal powdery mildews) and the 2-ethylaminoanalogue, ethirimil (g), was developed for its more effective control of cereal mildews. In general, acylation of 4-hydroxypyrimidines does not occur or gives unstable *N*-acyl derivatives, but acylation, for example of dimethirimol in which the bulky 2-dimethylamino group hinders ring substitution, occurred at the O-atom.[48] Several of the resulting *O*-acyl derivatives possessed fungicidal activity (B. P. 1 185 039), and Bupirimate

[46] D. Woodcock, in 'Systemic Fungicides,' ed. R. W. Marsh, Longman Group, London, 1972, pp. 34—85.

[47] K. J. Bent, D. H. Brooks, R. S. Elias, J. R. Finney, C. Shephard, and B. K. Snell, 'Pyrimidine fungicides,' in 'Jealott's Hill: Fifty Years of Agricultural Research,' ed. F. C. Peacock, Imperial Chemical Industries, Plant Protection Division, Bracknell, Berkshire, 1978, pp. 87—97.

[48] B. K. Snell, *J. Chem. Soc.*, 1968, 2358.

(h) was developed as an apple mildew fungicide, although it also gives excellent control of several other powdery mildews, and is used commercially on roses, cucurbits, and peaches.

Other classes of fungicide with high biocidal activity and low mammalian toxicity include (i) the 1-formamido-2,2,2-trichloroethylamines, exemplified by triforine, *N,N'*bis (1-formamido-2,2,2-trichloroethyl)piperazine, and chloraniformethan, *N*-(1-formamido-2,2,2-trichloroethyl)-3,4-dichloroaniline (oral LD_{50} > 2.5 g kg^{-1} in rats), which were developed for treatment of powdery midlews on cereals, apples, cucurbits and ornamental plants, and apple scab;[49–51] and (ii) the *N*-trichloromethylthio compounds, exemplified[52,53] by captan and folpet (oral LD_{50} > 9 g kg^{-1} in rats) for the fungal diseases of many fruits (apples, citrus, cucurbits, grapes, and tomatoes), vegetables (lettuce and onions), and flowering ornamentals, and the structurally related captafol (oral LD_{50} > 2.5 g kg^{-1} in rats), used to control potato blight, coffee berry disease, and the tapping-panel disease of hevea.

4 Unimodal Curves Defining Receptor Specificity to Heat, Light, Sound, and some Biologically Active Compounds

Maximum sensitivity at particular wavelengths characterizes mechano-, photo-, and thermal reception of the sensory organs of higher animals, and on either side of the maximum, the response diminishes in proportion to the divergence of the wavelength from that of optimal sensitivity. The resulting parabolic relationship between sensitivity and wavelength describes the specificity of these receptors. It is well-known that animals show a duplex response to light, as the photo-receptive retina of the vertebrate eye contains both rod and cone receptors, each with its own spectral sensitivity. Photopic vision operates in bright light, as mediated by the cones, and is concerned with colour vision, whereas scotopic vision is effective in dim light, is mediated by the rods, and is unrelated to sensations of colour.[54] The overlapping spectral sensitivities of the two mechanisms are demonstrated by measuring the energy required at each wavelength to produce a response of constant magnitude, sensitivity being the reciprocal of the energy needed to produce the standard response. If the parabolic plot of sensitivity against wavelength is recorded at high light intensity (cone vision), the maximum falls at 0.555 μm, and for low intensity (rod vision), at 0.510 μm (Figure 18). These tenets are supported by the fact that: (i) red glasses were worn during the day by night fighter-pilots to prevent light adaption and rod mechanism insensitivity to dim lights; (ii) where the eyes are subjected to very bright light, there is an inability to see properly in dim light; (iii) night vision can be restored with a

49 W. Ost, V. von Burchhausen, and Ch. A. Drandarevski, *Pestic. Sci.*, 1971, **2**, 219.
50 P. Schicke and K. H. Veen, *Proc. 5th Brit. Insecticide Fungicide Conf.*, 1969, **2**, 569.
51 P. Schicke, K. G. Adlung, and Ch. A. Drandarevski, *Proc. 6th Brit. Insecticide Fungicide Conf.*, 1971, **1**, 82.
52 R. J. Lukens and J. G. Horsfall, *Phytopathology*, 1967, **57**, 876.
53 R. J. Lukens, S. Rich, and J. G. Horsfall, *Phytopathology*, 1965, **55**, 658.
54 G. H. Bell, J. N. Davidson, and H. Scarborough, 'Textbook of Physiology and Biochemistry,' 7th edn., E. and S. Livingstone, Edinburgh, 1968, pp. 808—811.

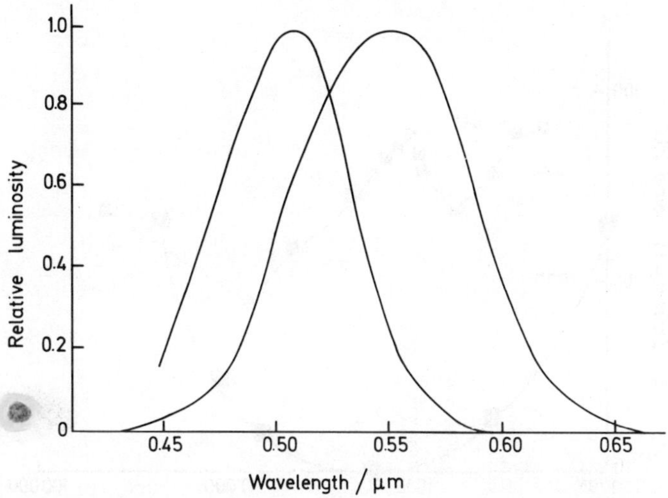

Figure 18 *Overlapping spectral sensitivities of cone vision with* $\lambda_{max.}$ 0.555μm *and rod vision with* $\lambda_{max.}$ 0.510 μm.

small dose of vitamin A, which makes up the rhodopsin concentration of the rod cells; (iv) nocturnal animals have more rods than cones and a reflective surface or tapetum to reflect back light into the eye, after it has passed through the retina; and (v) the eyes of some diurnal animals may contain more cones than rods, for example owls have no rod cells. In response to sound, the human ear is more sensitive to auditory stimulation between 800—8 500 Hz, with an upper limit of *ca.* 16 000 Hz and, in general, the complexity and flexibility of hearing increases with phylo-genetic ascent.[55] Cartilaginous fish respond to sound frequencies of up to 750 Hz, whilst bony ones respond up to 13 000 Hz. In reptiles, the frequency range is 5—10 000 Hz, and in birds, it extends to 25 000 Hz. The bat is one of the most specialized mammals, and its auditory system is sensitive to frequencies of up to 100 kHz.[55] This animal uses a form of echo-location to navigate its flight path and to hunt prey. Unlike the hearing apparatus of vertebrates, that of insects is in general rather limited in function, but locusts are more receptive (Figure 19). The parabolic relationship for the specificity of vertebrate sensory receptors to light and sound, which holds also for those of the mouth and skin towards heat, suggests that some unimodal relationships for biologically active compounds may reflect receptor specificity. The feasibility of this supposition is now tentatively explored.

Thus, in our application of kinetics to structure–activity problems (*q.v.*), expressions (equations 3 and 4) were evolved for receptor response to drugs. It followed that a receptor-binding phenomenon might be implicated (i) in the case of certain sulphonamides,[25] where rate constants were evaluated, and where high tissue concentrations proved disadvantageous to anti-bacterial activity, and

[55] P. N. R. Usherwood, 'Nervous Systems,' The Institute of Biology's Studies in Biology, No. 36, Edward Arnold, London, 1973, pp. 65—79.

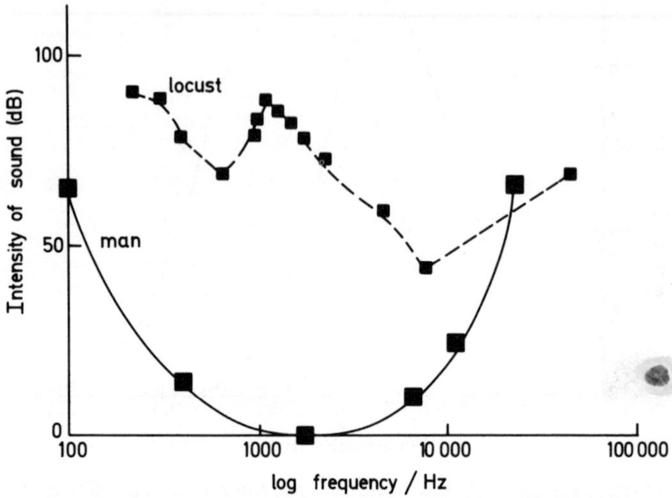

Figure 19 *Comparison of threshold intensity of tympanal organ of man and of the locust for pure tone sounds.*

[Reprinted with permission from P. N. R. Usherwood, '*Nervous Systems*,' 1973, 74. Copyright (1973) Edward Arnold (Publishers) Limited. The figure was modified after B. Uvarov in 'Grasshoppers and Locusts'.[64] Copyright (1966) Cambridge University Press, from which permission was also obtained.]

(ii) in that of ascorbic acid, where a narrow spike (in contrast to a quadratic curve) would represent physiological activity. The response of oats coleoptiles to plant-growth hormones[27] involves a receptor interaction, that was most apparent for the physiological indol-3-ylacetic acid but less evident for synthetic 1-naphthylacetic acid which mimics the natural hormone. Whilst the particularly fine curves[28] for the various acaricidal activities of a series of n-alkyl thiocyanate homologues might be interpreted in terms of receptor specificity, there is no solid evidence for this supposition, and the molluscicidal properties of Boyce and Milborrow's[23] *N*-n-alkyltritylamine homologues are explicable in terms of their lipophilicity, and thus of their penetration to the site of action. Relatively small differences in the nature of the leaving groups that were removed by receptor enzyme to yield the same toxicant made a negligible contribution to the observed activity in this case.[23]

It is further considered that the concept of high activity homologues forming tight-fitting receptor complexes and blocking a vital process in intermediary metabolism, leading to the death of animals, would be consistent with unimodal structure–activity relationships. In this case, departure of the curves from a parabolic shape may reflect, for example, the death of animals from the functional failure of several organs through the expression of a common biochemical lesion in the several biological situations.

Strong evidence[56–58] was presented that the action of Telodrin (1,3,4,5,6,7,8,8-octachloro-1,3,3a,4,7,7a-hexahydro-4,7-methanoisobenzofuran), one of the polychlorinated cyclodiene insecticides,[59] leads to liberation of ammonia in the brain before the onset of convulsions and throughout their course. The α-oxoglutarate, glutamate, and glutamine were utilized in a major ammonia-binding mechanism, and α-oxoglutarate, glutamate, pyruvate, and alanine were utilized in a subsidiary mechanism for ammonia disposal. Calculation[58] showed that glutamine synthesis represented a significant proportion of the total cerebral metabolism during Telodrin intoxication and that, at the maximum rate, it was incommensurate with normal functioning of the tricarboxylic acid cycle in brain cells. (This does not happen in the case of dieldrin,[58] another polychlorinated cyclodiene insecticide, which is not an homologue of Telodrin.) The figures are consistent with eventual deceleration of glutamine synthesis, but it was not certain whether the α-oxoglutarate supply was rate-limiting. Later, in the seizure pattern, the mechanism for ammonia disposal was inadequate, and free ammonia accumulated in cerebral tissues, resulting in the death of animals.

In another example,[60] a ten thousand-fold difference in acute oral toxicity, shown by dogs and rats towards chlorfenvinphos, is commensurate with the concerted interaction of the relatively small differences found in rates of absorption and metabolism, of the availability in circulating blood, of the rate of brain uptake and, above all, of the sensitivity of brain-receptor acetylcholinesterase towards the insecticide, which kills the rats, but not the dogs.

This evidence shows that Telodrin, a well-fitting cyclodiene substrate, caused mitochondrial dysfunction in cerebral tissues, and that chlorfenvinphos fitted rat-brain receptor acetylcholinesterase better than dog-brain enzyme. These examples illustrate that in fact high biological activity may be associated with specific inhibition of intermediary metabolism. Thus, where specific inhibition of intermediary metabolism accounts for the biological activity of an homologous series, receptor specificity would be expected to be a contributing factor.

5 Concluding Remarks

The present chapter discusses the theoretical and experimental basis for currently held views on structure–activity relationships.

It suggests the following: (i) that the joint effect of ionisation and lipophilicity acting as inversely related parameters explains many unimodal structure–activity curves: strong contributions from both give a symmetrical type of curve, which is typical of the sulphonamides, biguanide anti-malarials, and the 4-(1-cyclopropylalkyl)-2,6-dinitrophenol fungicides. On the other hand, the predominance of one factor and near invariability of the other displaces the maximum in the direction of the predominating factor. For example, ionisation of acetoxytrialkyltins is definitive, the low order lipophilicity accounting for the

56 D. E. Hathway, *Arch. Environ. Health*, 1965, **11**, 380.
57 D. E. Hathway and A. Mallinson, *Biochem. J.*, 1964, **90**, 51.
58 D. E. Hathway, A. Mallinson, and D. A. A. Akintonwa, *Biochem. J.*, 1965, **94**, 676.
59 S. B. Soloway, *Adv. Pest. Control Res.*, 1965, **6**, 85.
60 D. H. Hutson and D. E. Hathway, *Biochem. Pharmacol.*, 1967, **16**, 949.

transport characteristics, and the new parabolic curve for the alkyl quaternary ammonium plant-growth substances closely resembles that for the activity of the organotins.

(ii) Parabolic dependence (a) of sulphonamide bacteriostasis on pK_a, such that the optimal pK_a lies between 6 and 8, implies that un-ionised drug penetrates the bacteria, and (b) of barbiturate hypnosis upon octan-1-ol and water distribution emphasizes that the homologues with a favoured balance between lipophilic and hydrophilic factors rapidly reach the receptors and stimulate biological action. 2-Methyl-5-nitroimidazole anti-protozoals and *N*-n-alkyltritylamine molluscicides support the dependence of a parabolic relationship upon lipophilicity.

(iii) Kinetic methods, relating to drug dissociation, elimination, metabolism, penetration into tissues, and receptor-binding, are used to test parameter interaction and to provide a method to check the basis of activities. The plant-growth hormones undoubtedly exemplify receptor binding, but, on balance, the acaricidal activity of n-alkyl thiocynates might be explicable in terms of their lipophilicity.

(iv) The multi-factorial equation (13) takes aromatic substitution into consideration and involves Hammett's ρ and σ constants.

The plot of biocidal activity log $(1/ED_{50})$ against mammalian toxicity $(1/LD_{50})$ for some anti-protozoal 1-(3-chloro-2-hydroxypropyl) substituted nitroimidazole drugs, anti-fungal acetoxytrialkyltins, and benzimidazole-2-carbamates plus metabolically related systemic fungicides give quadratic relationships which facilitate the separation of compounds with high selectivity. Linear relationships result for (i) various benzimidazol-2-yl analogues, where the fungitoxicity is qualitatively and quantitatively similar; (ii) arylthiosemicarbazides, where mammalian toxicity $(1/LD_{50})$ is uniformly high; and (iii) the 2-alkylamino-4-hydroxy-5-butyl-6-methylpyrimidines and their esters, the 1-formamido-2,2,2-trichloroethylamines, and *N*-trichloromethylthio compounds such as captan and folpet, for all of which $(1/LD_{50})$ is consistently low.

The widespread occurrence of parabolic relationships that is shown by the specificity of vertebrate sensory receptors to heat, light, and sound suggests that receptor specificity may contribute to some unimodal structure–activity curves, which mirror chemical stimuli. This possibility is tentatively explored in the last section of the chapter from the standpont of (i) compounds with a physiological role, and (ii) high activity homologues, which might be expected to form well-fitting receptor complexes and to interfere with intermediary metabolism.

Four more points are worth mentioning. The first concerns the reliability of the biological data, presented in this article. These are subject to the error normally associated with such tests, and they have been collected non-selectively from reputable sources, to which reference is made. Accordingly, the assumption has been made that the experimental format on which these data were generated is such as would establish a very satisfactory degree of precision, for example 95% fiducial limits are given for the molluscicidal activities on the perfect parabola which is cited,[23] and 99.5% of fiducial limits apply to the LD_{50} data. Because of the variety of sources, there must be implicit variability of quality and, therefore, it is not possible to provide a meaningful statistical analysis. However, the relationships or trends which have been described are such that they would appear to be entirely inconsistent with a random occurrence. Thus, it is highly improbable that, for example, the biological activity relationships of the acetoxy-trialkyltins, taken singly (Figures 4 and 6) and in combination (Figure 16) as well as the shape of the scatter diagram (Figure 5) representing the toxicity to animals of the twenty six trialkyltins (not homologues) on which measurement has been made, are all quadratic functions, unless these trends are real.

Secondly, the application of different tests to the biological activity of each series of homologues is important to the recognition of the contributing parameters.

Thirdly, this chapter is not intended to be comprehensive. Thus, illustration of structure–activity was sought originally amongst fungicides and anti-bacterials, which differ significantly in their toxicities for unicellular organisms and mammals, partly on account of differences in transport characteristics between unicellular and mammalian membranes. For example, carcinogenicity correlates well with mutagenicity measured in mammalian cells, but not with that in Ames' bacteria, unless a molecular size or lipophilicity parameter is included in the relationship.[61] Insecticides, which would have provided relevant structure–activity data, were excluded because of extensive treatment[26,62,63] particularly from the standpoint of lipophilicity. Selective toxicities were unavailable for drugs concerned with disease states, and whilst some reference is made to herbicides in the narrative, they represent a very special case, as the mode of action of many of them involves mechanisms absent from animals.

Finally, interaction of two inversely related parameters, in the way that has been discussed, seems to be commensurate with the present evidence relating to structure–activity.

[61] N. K. Scribner, B. Woodworth, G. P. Ford, and J. F. Scribner, *Carcinogenesis*, 1980, **1**, 715.
[62] T. R. Fukuto, *Bull. Org. Mond. Sante*, 1971, **44**, 31.
[63] R. L. Metcalf, *Bull. Org. Mond. Sante*, 1971, **44**, 43.

Chapter 3 Measurement of a Carcinogenic Exposure

1 Introduction and Relevance

Druckrey and Küpfmüller[1,2] first applied pharmacological methods to the experimental induction of tumours in rodents and thereby imposed measurement upon cancer science. They found[1,2] the relation:

$$dt^n = k \tag{1}$$

where d is the daily dose, expressed in mg day^{-1}, t is the period of induction or latency of tumours, expressed usually in days or months, k is a proportionality constant, and n is a small positive integer, which is evaluated from the slope of the linear plot of log d against log t for the carcinogens in question (*v. infra*).

For chronically administered small doses of 3 mg day^{-1} of 4-dimethylamino-azobenzene (Butter Yellow) in rats, t amounted to 350 days, but for larger doses of 30 mg day^{-1}, t was 34 days. The total dose dt proved to be almost constant, except for very small dose levels, $\leqslant$1 mg day^{-1}, where the product of the factors gave a smaller value, thereby suggesting that chronic administration of very small amounts of chemical carcinogen may be more effective in producing tumours, hepatomas in the case of Butter Yellow, than larger doses administered over a shorter period of time. Entirely independently of Druckrey and Küpfmüller (*loc. cit.*), Bryan and Shimkin[3] demonstrated a dose-response relationship for the yields of murine skin sarcomas, after single injections of either 20-methyl-cholanthrene or 3,4-benzopyrene.

The validity of equation 1 was tested further[4] by a series of 'stop experiments', which employed interrupted administrations of Butter Yellow, and which afforded the results that would be expected. 'Stop experiments' were made subsequently[5] with 4-dimethylaminostilbene, which elicits ear-duct tumours, and this work amply confirmed Druckrey's propositions.[1,2,4] The value of n (equation 1) for Butter Yellow, 4-dimethylaminostilbene, and 3,4-benzopyrene was found to be respectively 1, 3, and 4.

These feeding experiments stressed above all the importance of the induction

[1] H. Druckrey and K. Küpfmüller, 'Dosis und Wirkung,' Editio Cantor, Aulendorf-im-Württemberg, 1949.
[2] H. Druckrey and K. Küpfmüller, *Z. Naturforsch., Teil B*, 1948, **3**, 254.
[3] W. R. Bryan and M. B. Schimkin, *J. Nat. Cancer Inst.*, 1943, **3**, 503.
[4] H. Druckrey, in 'Chemical Carcinogenesis: Mechanisms of Action,' Ciba Foundation Colloquium, 1959, pp. 110–130.
[5] D. Schmähl, C. Thomas, and K. König, *Z. Krebsforsch.*, 1963, **65**, 342.

period, which is known to be long, often > 20 years, for human beings, who may have been exposed inadvertently to relatively large amounts of a particular carcinogen or carcinogens. Druckrey's experiments and the contemporaneously developing theory of genetics led him to realize[4] that his evidence relates to cellular inheritance through the modification of cellular genetic material in a very significant way.

It would now appear[6] that it ought to be possible to make 'marker experiments' in which estimations of biologically significant nucleoside analogues formed in target-organ (for example liver tissue in the case of vinyl chloride) DNA, after periods of exposure to small—very small amounts of the carcinogen, would provide some measure of the heritable genetic injury incurred for the dose levels used. An essential corollary of the method would be the retention of the animals, which had been exposed, until their death, in order to determine whether they succumbed to the tumours in question. It might be feasible that some animals, exposed above a certain dose-level, would contain measurable amounts of the significant nucleoside analogue(s) in their target cells, commensurate with cancer induction. In others, the levels of significant nucleoside analogue(s) would fall near or below the limits of detection and they might die later of natural causes, as the induction period corresponding to the very small amounts of carcinogen that they had received would be considerably longer than the normal life-span of the animals.

In general, there might be considerable difficulty in the implementation of such a procedure for a specific compound because, although many interactions of ultimate carcinogens with DNA have been elucidated *in vivo* resulting in several products (nucleoside analogues), there is little knowledge as to which of these would account for mutagenicity/carcinogenicity. The absence of such information might introduce error into estimates which may have been made of the 'carcinogenic exposure' of animals. In any case, for the assessment of the human situation, it is implicit that a very awkward extension would have to be made from the experiments in animals and, at best, this would involve several approximations.

Such an experiment was planned in 1975 for the exposure of animals to vinyl chloride by inhalation,[6] but only very preliminary data were obtained. It must be said that such a method is not now entirely novel, although it would have been at that time, and work might be mentioned on the methylation of DNA guanine residue by dimethylnitrosamine[7] and on the lack of methylation of guanine residues by dichlorvos.[8] In the former case, dimethylnitrosamine alkylated kidney nucleic acids to about the extent of one-ninth of those of the liver at 100 $\mu g\ kg^{-1}$, but at $< 14\ \mu g\ kg^{-1}$ no alkylation of kidney nucleic acids was detected.

It was considered[6] that it would be impossible to derive dose-response data at very low dose levels by conventional carcinogenicity testing 'because at the anticipated dose-levels, too many animals to be practicable would be necessary

[6] D. E. Hathway, in 'Foreign Compound Metabolism in Mammals,' ed. D. E. Hathway, The Chemical Society, London, 1979, vol. **5**, pp. 190—243.
[7] M. I. Diaz Gomez, P. F. Swann, and P. N. Magee, *Biochem. J.*, 1977, **164**, 497
[8] M. F. Wooder, A. S. Wright, and L. J. King, *Chem.-Biol. Interact.*, 1977, **19**, 25.

to give a satisfactory degree of significance' even on the assumption of no spontaneous tumours occurring in the control groups. A proper risk analysis therefore involves the implementation of other sorts of experiment.

2 Chemical Carcinogenesis and Mutagenicity

Present doctrine on chemical carcinogenesis relates to a multi-stage process, which includes an initial, apparently irreversible initiation that involves direct interaction of the carcinogen or a reactive metabolite with target-cell nucleic acids. One feature common to chemical mutagens and carcinogens is therefore their reaction with nucleic acids in biological systems through the formation of electrophiles.[9] Support for a formal relationship between carcinogenesis and mutagenesis rests: (i) on the strong correlation between the carcinogenic potential of chemical substances and mutagenicity;[10,11,35] (ii) on the well-known photodimerization of some dT residues of DNA in the induction of cancer by radiation;[12] and (iii) on the correlation, amongst the simple alkylating agents,[13] of the alkylation of a larger proportion of O^6-position sites of dG in comparison with those at *N*-7 with powerful carcinogenicity and of a much smaller proportion of *O*-6 sites in comparison with those at *N*-7 with weak carcinogenicity.

It would appear therefore that the established mutation of micro-organisms by a given chemical compound ought to provide a clear warning as to the risk of its possible carcinogenic action in mammals, especially if there are corresponding dose-response data available for the mutagenicity concerned. In any case, it is easier and much more economical to make measurements in micro-organisms than in mammals, and reduction to an ideal system or a more ideal system is integral to advances in science. Furthermore, the Ames test of mutagenicity (see section 3) is capable of facile extension to include mediation by the drug-metabolizing enzymes of mammalian tissue. However, the possibility of false positives must be borne in mind. For example, methylene dichloride does not appear to be carcinogenic in animals and in man,[14] but it behaves as a mutagen in the Ames test[14] through its metabolic transformation by the bacteria into a sufficient quantity of reactive metabolite to give a response.[14a]

It is worthwhile mentioning at this stage in the discussion that Druckrey[4] defined cell multiplication in an organ by the expression:

$$N = N_{\text{fin}}\,(1 - e^{t/T}) \qquad (2)$$

[9] H. Bartsch and P. L. Grover, in 'Scientific Foundations of Oncology,' ed. T. Symington and R. L. Carter, Heinemann Medical, London, 1976, pp. 334—342.

[10] B. N. Ames, J. McCann, and E. Yamasaki, *Mutat. Res.*, 1975, **31**, 347; B. N. Ames, *Science*, 1976, **191**, 241; B. N. Ames, 'European Environ. Mutagen Soc. Mtg.,' Edinburgh, 1977.

[11] R. Montesano and H. Bartsch, *Mutat. Res.*, 1976, **32**, 179.

[12] R. B. Setlow and R. W. Hart, in 'Proc. 5th Internat. Congr. Radiation Res. (Seattle), 1974,' eds. O. F. Nygaard, H. I. Adler, and W. K. Sinclair, Academic Press, New York, 1975, p. 879.

[13] D. E. Hathway and G. F. Kolar, *Chem. Soc. Rev.*, 1980, **9**, 241.

[14] I.A.R.C. Monographs, 'Evaluation of Carcinogenic Risk of Chemicals to Man, Volume 20 (Some halogenated hydrocarbons),' Agency for Research on Cancer, Lyon, France, 1979, pp. 449—465.

[14a] T. Green, *Mutat. Res.*, 1983 in the press.

where N_t is the number of cells at time t, N_{fin} gives the final value, and T is a time constant.

He explains that 'the cells no longer behave as parts of an organ, but as individuals within a population. Normal cells are therefore capable of multiplying exponentially, similarly to cancer cells'. Later in that article,[4] reference is made to the normal cells as constituents of an organ-limited growth, and maintenance of an homeostatic cell number, *viz.*

$$N_t = N_{max}\,(1 - e^{-t/T})$$

and to cancer cells as individuals in a population with exponential cell multiplication, *viz.* equation 3:

$$N_t = N_0 e^{t/T} \tag{3}$$

This concept[4] is taken up by Zimmer[15] with regard to a mutation process, comprising m mutational events in each of n cells, which was rate-limiting with regard to tumour induction.

The fraction of individual animals with tumours N^*/N_0 might be represented theoretically by the expression:

$$N^*/N_0 = (1 - e^{-kD})^{mn} \tag{4}$$

where D is the dose and k is a proportionality constant.

A schematic representation on a linear logarithmic plot of the fraction of animals without tumours, *viz.* log $(1 - N^*/N_0)$ as a function of dose D, would reduce to log N/N_0 as a function of D, and this approaches a straight line with the intercept log mn at $D = 0$, thereby enabling an estimate of the number of targets mn to be made. Studies of simple alkylating agents of the two types recognized by Hathway and Kolar[13] give straight lines,[15] which extrapolate to log 1, *i.e.* $mn = 1$.

Any variations in the sensitivity of the cells to the agents in this way lead to a decrease in the extrapolation number.[15] The conclusion that can be drawn in this event is that 'tumour induction depends on a single mutation in a single cell, and that the dose-response curve is linear from zero dose'.

Ehrenberg, an acknowledged expert in the measurement of a carcinogenic exposure and in the meaningful interpretation of cognate information, found[16] that, if the dose-response curve (*v. supra*) contains terms of an higher order of the dose than that taken into account, considerable attention ought to be paid to whether the experimental evidence implies a linear relationship at low doses and to the slope. It ought to be clearly stated that the involvement of a single cell in the mathematical argument agrees with the monoclonal origin of many tumours.[17]

Even at this early stage in the discussion, the force of the latter arguments suggests that ways may be found for avoiding the extension of data from experiments made in animals to the human situation. Such methodology would make

[15] K. G. Zimmer, 'Studies in Quantitative Radiation Biology,' Oliver and Boyd, Edinburgh, 1961.
[16] L. Ehrenberg, *Int. J. Rad. Biol.*, 1977, **31**, 503.
[17] P. J. Fialkow, *N. Eng. J. Med.*, 1974, **219**, 26.

use: (i) of extensive mutagenic investigations in diverse organisms, including the estimation of risk from mutation in relation to that from ionising radiation, *i.e.* the rad-equivalence (*v. infra*); and (ii) of an innate (inborn) biological monitoring system, which is capable of functioning both internally in the body with respect to estimates of exposure and externally with respect to determinations of dose *vs.* mutagenic response. Furthermore, the dose-response relationships for bacteria, yeasts, higher plants, and small test animals to mutagens would be expected to apply also to man. The same proposition seems to be valid also for cancer induction[18] (section 6).

3 Quantitative Mutagenicity Data

In accord with previous discussion (see section 2), great attention has been given, notably by Bartsch *et al.* at the International Agency for Cancer Research at Lyon, by the Ehrenberg School in Stockholm, by Loprieno *et al.* dell' Universitá Pisa, by Purchase *et al.* at ICI's Central Toxicology Laboratory, and above all by Ames' School at Berkeley, California, to the generation of quantitative mutagenicity data for industrial chemicals and pesticides. The work has involved the use of several interesting, and in some ways novel, biological systems, including the higher plants,[19-21] yeasts,[22-25] bacteria,[26-37] *Drosophila*,[38,39] and mammalian cell lines including Chinese hamster V-79 cells.[40-42] In particular, the

[18] C. J. Calleman, L. Ehrenberg, B. Jansson, S. Osterman-Golkar, D. Segerbäck, K. Svensson, and C. A. Wachtmeister, *J. Environ. Path. Toxicol.*, 1978, **2(2)**, 427.
[19] S. Osterman-Golkar, L. Ehrenberg, and C. A. Wachtmeister, *Radiat. Bot.*, 1970, **10**, 303.
[20] L. Ehrenberg, S. Osterman-Golkar, D. Singh, and U. Lundquist, *Radiat. Bot.*, 1974, **15**, 185.
[21] J. Velemínský, S. Osterman-Golkar, and L. Ehrenberg, *Mutat. Res.*, 1970, **10**, 169.
[22] H. Marquardt, F. K. Zimmermann, and R. Schwaier, *Z. Vererburgsl*, 1964, **95**, 82.
[23] N. Loprieno, R. Barale, C. Bauer, S. Baroncelli, G. Bronzetti, A. Cammellini, A. Cinci, C. Corsi, C. Leporini, R. Nieri, M. Nozzolini, and C. Serra, *Mutat. Res.*, 1974, **25**, 197.
[24] D. J. Brusich and H. Andrews, *Mutat. Res.*, 1974, **26**, 491.
[25] N. Loprieno, R. Bardle, S. Baroncelli, H. Bartsch, G. Bronzetti, A. Cammellini, C. Corsi, D. Frezza, R. Nieri, C. Leporini, D. Rosellini, and A. M. Rossi, *Cancer Res.*, 1977, **36**, 253.
[26] I. Turtóczky and L. Ehrenberg, *Mutat. Res.*, 1969, **8**, 229.
[27] S. Neale, *Mutat. Res.*, 1972, **14**, 155.
[28] U. Rannug, R. Göthe, and C. A. Wachtmeister, *Chem.-Biol. Interact.*, 1976, **12**, 251.
[29] A. Camus, B. Bertram, F. W. Kruger, C. Malaveille, and H. Bartsch, *Z. Krebsforsch.*, 1976, **86**, 293.
[30] C. Malaveille, H. Bartsch, A. Barbin, A. M. Camus, R. Montesano, A. Croisy, and P. Jacquignon, *Biochem. Biophys. Res. Commun.*, 1975, **63**, 363.
[31] A. Kolman and L. Ehrenberg, *Mutat. Res.*, 1978, **49**, 297.
[32] B. N. Ames, F. D. Lee, and W. E. Durston, *Proc. Natl. Acad. Sci., USA*, 1973, **70**, 782.
[33] J. McCann, V. Simmon, D. Streitwieser, and B. N. Ames, *Proc. Natl. Acad. Sci., USA*, 1975, **72**, 3190.
[34] J. McCann, N. E. Spingarn, J. Kobori, and B. N. Ames, *Proc. Natl. Acad. Sci., USA.*, 1975, **72**, 979.
[35] I. F. H. Purchase, E. Longstaff, J. Ashby, J. A. Styles, D. Anderson, P. A. Lefêvre, and F. R. Westwood, *Nature*, 1976, **264**, 624.
[36] J. Ashby and J. A. Styles, *Nature*, 1978, **271**, 452
[37] P. D. Lawley, *Mutat. Res.*, 1974, **23**, 283.
[38] O. G. Fahmy, M. J. Fahmy, J. Massasso, and M. Ondrej, *Mutat. Res.*, 1966, **3**, 201.
[39] L. Pasternak, *Arzneim.-Forsch.*, 1964, **14**, 802.
[40] E. Huberman, H. Bartsch, and L. Sachs, *Int. J. Cancer*, 1975, **16**, 639.
[41] E. Huberman, L. Aspiras, C. Heidelberger, P. L. Grover, and P. Sims, *Proc. Natl. Acad. Sci., USA*, 1971, **68**, 3195.
[42] E. Huberman and L. Sachs, *Int. J. Cancer*, 1974, **13**, 326.

Ames test[32] has been developed as a very important and reproducible screen for chemical mutagens.[10,11,28–30,32–36] This test employs genetically manipulated *Salmonella typhimurium* strains, which are capable of detecting the sort of specific mutagenicity that may be involved, for example, either base-pair-substitution by special strains or frame-shift mutations by other special strains. As has been mentioned already (see section 2), the incorporation of tissue drug-metabolizing enzymes into the Ames test affords a very versatile system, which has the capacity to simulate the various biological situations that occur in mammals.

Consideration of the shape of the dose-response curves for the initiation of mutagenicity by chemicals is important to an understanding of the dose-response for cancer induction. Thus, for example, in the chlorophyll mutation system for measuring forward mutation in barley,[43,44] many alkylating agents showed an exponential dose-response with a linear component at low dose levels.[45] The presence of this linear component of the dose-response relationship was confirmed later in *E. coli*[26,27,46] and other bacteria,[10,11,28–37] and also in plant seeds[19,20,47]and growing plants.[21,48] Ionising radiation causes dose-dependent mutagenesis in bacteria, plants, and small rodents, such as mice.[49] The linear relationship produced is paralleled by an increased incidence of tumours with increasing radiation both in the experimental induction of tumours in animals and in the case of human populations which had been exposed to low doses of radiation.[50,51] Thus, there is a strong supposition that a dose-response relationship for chemically induced cancer will also have a linear dose component. This is due to: (i) the linear dose-response of tumours induced by radiation in mammals (*v. supra*); (ii) the strong correlation between the carcinogenicity and mutagenicity of chemical compounds;[10,11,52] and (iii) the linear dose-response of mutation, initiated both by radiation and by chemical substances (*v. supra*).

It ought to be clearly stated that much of the carcinogenicity testing of chemical substances has been made, especially in the past, to give purely qualitative risk assessments, and that some dose-response investigations[53] have been most concerned with the duration of the period of induction. Paucity of quantitative data stresses the need for dose monitoring (see section 5). Despite this limitation, the importance of quantitative mutagenicity data to the cancer situation cannot be over-emphasized. In this connotation, the usefulness of

[43] A. Gustafsson, 'Proc. 2nd Radiobiol. Symp., Liege,' 1954, pp. 282—284.
[44] L. Ehrenberg, in 'Chemical Mutagens,' ed. A. Hollaender, Plenum Press, New York, 1971, pp. 365—386.
[45] L. Ehrenberg, U. Lundquist, S. Osterman, and B. Sparrman, *Hereditas*, 1966, **56**, 277,
[46] L. Ehrenberg, K. D. Hiesche, S. Osterman-Golkar, and I. Wennberg, *Mutat. Res.*, 1974, **24**, 83.
[47] L. Ehrenberg and A. Gustafsson, *Hereditas*, 1957, **43**, 595.
[48] K. Lindgren, 'The mutagenic effect of ethylene oxide in air,' Thesis, University of Stockholm, 1971.
[49] W. L. Russel, L. B. Russel, and E. M. Kelly, *Science*, 1958, **128**, 1546.
[50] A. Stewart and G. W. Kneale, *Lancet*, 1970, **i**, 1185.
[51] UNSCEAR, A report of the United Nations Scientific Committee on the Effects of Atomic Radiation, Vol. 11 (A8725), 27th Session, Supplement no. 25, United Nations, New York, 1972.
[52] E. C. Miller and J. A. Miller, in 'Chemical Mutagens,' ed. A. Hollaender, Plenum Press, New York, 1971, pp. 83—120.
[53] H. Druckrey, R. Preussmann, S. Ivankovic, and D. Schmähl, *Z. Krebsforsch.*, 1967, **69**, 103.

measurement, for example, in terms of rad-equivalence, is important, particularly with regard to a standard dose.

The concept of rad-equivalence stems from the linear dose-response mutation, initiated both by radiation and chemical substances [see (iii) above]. Clearly, this concept is meaningful, and measurement of significant equivalence is possible, if the following conditions are satisfied.

(i) Radiation and chemicals must be interchangeable in the test-system concerned.

(ii) The doses, defined as the product, *viz.* of the flux of radiation and the period of exposure and of the concentration of the chemical compound and the period of exposure, are realistic only where, keeping the product constant and varying the two factors in opposite ways, the biological effect remains the same over a wide range of concentration and time.

(iii) The two dose-response curves ought to be strictly similar and, in this case, the principle of Searle's[54] 'doubling doses' for the estimation of genetic risks is relevant.

(iv) The activities both of radiation and of the test compound depend on the experimental conditions and the effect that is measured, and the possibility that they may not vary in parallel must be continually taken into consideration.[55]

It ought to be said that the substances, for which quantitative mutagenicity data have been obtained in the several papers which have been mentioned (*v. supra*), are, for the most part, direct alkylating agents or they belong to the nitrosamides and nitrosamines or they are vinyl chloride-related compounds. The way in which these chemical mutagens or their ultimate reactive metabolites react with nucleic acid has been analysed in a discussion paper[13] both in terms of S_N1 and S_N2 mechanisms and in those of soft and hard acids and bases. Great attention has been paid by Ehrenberg *et al.* (*loc. cit.*) to the relevant physicochemical properties of the substances which they investigated, particularly to Swain and Scott[56] *n* and *s* values. Such considerations have an important bearing on the sort of chemical substances which act as mutagens, and possibly as carcinogens, in mammals.

4 'Extrapolation' of Carcinogenicity Data from Animals to Man

Quantitative extension of toxicity data, derived in animals, to the human situation depends on the assumption that physiological parameters in animals and man are strictly comparable and, for example, a comparison of the toxicity of cancer chemotherapeutic agents in dogs, hamsters, mice, monkeys, and rats and in human subjects might be cited.[57] Ehrenberg *et al.*[46] draw attention to

[54] A. G. Searle, 'Use of doubling doses for the estimation of genetic risks,' in 'Radiological Protection, First European Symp. on Rad-Equivalence,' ed. R. Chanet, 1977, pp. 133—145.

[55] R. Latarjet, 'Quantitative mutagenesis by chemicals and radiation: Prerequisites for the establishment of rad-equivalences, in Radiobiological Protection, First European Symp. on Rad-Equivalence,' ed. R. Chanet, 1977, pp. 154—168.

[56] C. G. Swain and C. B. Scott, *J. Am. Chem. Soc.*, 1953, **75**, 141.

[57] E. J. Freireich, E. A. Gehan, D. P. Rall, L. H. Schmidt, and H. E. Skipper, *Cancer Chemother. Rep.*, 1966, **50(4)**, 219.

three problem areas. The first concerns the rate of pulmonary absorption. For resting or nearly resting animals, the mouse value is valid. In man at rest, the relative pulmonary ventilation is approximately one-tenth of the mouse value, *i.e.* 0.1 and 1 ml min^{-1} g^{-1} respectively, whereas for man in moderate exercise, the value may be set at one-half of that for the resting mouse. Secondly, in the absence of other data, the mouse λ-value may be used to estimate λ, the rate of elimination, in man. Thirdly, there is the matter of the steady-state of a foreign compound in an organ, which is distal to the site of entry in a mammal as large as man. There is no information to decide whether the concentration concerned approximates to the average body content of the compound. However, for a rapidly diffusing compound, it is felt that there would be a linear relationship between exposure and tissue doses within a few minutes of administration, because of the efficiency of mammalian transport systems, and irrespective of the size of the mammal exposed. On this assumption, Ehrneberg *et al.*[46] calculated the testis dose, *i.e.* the germinal dose as opposed to the somatic one, in a resting man to be 0.06 μmol kg^{-1} h/p.p.m. h and, in a man at moderate exercise, to be 0.28 μmol kg^{-1} h/p.p.m. h. Such a study[57] as the one mentioned previously might involve the use of safety factors. Further difficulty may arise, as few comparisons of 'late effects' have been made.[58] Mechanisms of tumour induction in different mammals are essentially the same, but species sensitivity, for example, between a particular species of animal and man to a chemical carcinogen, arises from differences in the differential between uptake and elimination, in the distribution amongst the organs of the body, in metabolism, and in the immune response of the various tissues.

It is a paradox that whilst mammals are prone to cancer, experiments in animals afford a rather crude way of identifying carcinogenic action. Thus, for example,[59] an experiment involving groups with 59 animals/group does not detect a carcinogenic risk of $< 5\%$, and such a risk would be unacceptable where human beings are concerned. Low risk would require animal experiments involving thousands or hundreds of thousands of animals, and such data would be valid only if the huge group(s) of unexposed, control animals did not display spontaneous tumours. Any incidence of spontaneous tumours would greatly diminish the sensitivity of the animal test system. In fact, the possibility that spontaneous tumours may occur provides a very good reason against attempting to extend the data, found in conventional carcinogenicity testing, to man.

The rate at which the total dose of a chemical carcinogen is administered to animals presents another problem. Thus, in the case of a polycyclic aromatic hydrocarbon, which causes cancer through a single administration, it has been found[60] that the same dose, administered chronically over a long period of time, elicits an increased tumour yield. In the general case, this finding would mean that exposure to lower doses of carcinogen over a long period of time is likely to be more effective in inducing tumours than brief exposure to an higher dose-

[58] D. G. Hoel, D. W. Gaylor, R. L. Kirschstein, U. Saffiotti, and M. A. Schneiderman, *J. Toxicol. Environ. Health*, 1975, **1**, 133.
[59] G. Zbinden, in 'Progress in Toxicology: Special Topics,' Springer-Verlag, Berlin, 1973, vol. **1**, p. 18.
[60] W. W. Payne and W. C. Hueper, *Am. Ind. Hyg. Assoc. J.*, 1960, **21**, 350.

level. This supposition is confirmed by the induction of hepatomas through the administration of very small dose-levels of Butter Yellow over a prolonged period of time,[1,2] and the same was true also for the induction of ear-duct carcinoma through administration of very small dose-levels of 4-dimethylamino-stilbene.[5] It might be argued *ab initio* that for a toxic chemical carcinogen, the administration of large doses might kill the animals, which would not have died from acute toxicity had they been submitted to long-term exposure at lower dose-levels, although they would succumb eventually to tumours. Moreover, under rate-limiting conditions of target-tissue concentration, such reaction as would have occurred would be sufficient to initiate the sequence of events leading to cancer after a very considerable induction period. However, mitigating circumstances might arise through the presence of cellular nucleo-philes, like glutathione, protecting the nucleic acids from attack, for example, by electrophilic epoxide. Such a situation might afford an instance of competitive reaction kinetics, in which, theoretically, exposure to high dose-levels of carcino-gen would present a much greater risk than lower ones over a longer period.

An inverse relationship has been found between dose and a power of the latency period.[1,2,4,5] From Druckrey and Küpfmüller's law (equation 1), it follows that:

$$t = t_0\, (d_0/d)^{1/n} \tag{5}$$

in which a usual value for n, say $n = 3$, might be substituted. Whence (equation 5), it follows that the long period for the appearance of tumours in mice of 15 months following a dose of 1 $\mu g\ g^{-1}$ body-weight of 20-methylcholanthrene is reduced for a dose of 1 mg g^{-1} to 1.5 months. This has been taken to indicate that, at least theoretically, it should be possible to find a dose so low that the mean period of induction of tumours would exceed the normal life-span of the species of animal under investigation. Indeed, Batten and Hathway[61] have applied such a calculation to the interesting oxidative *N*-dephenylation that yielded infinitesimal quantities of 2-naphthylamine *in vivo*. No *N*-hydroxylation and no other metabolites of 2-naphthylamine were ever found in the bladder of the dogs so exposed. Predictably, no bladder cancer resulted from the corresponding carcinogenicity testing with *N*-phenyl-2-naphthylamine, and epidemiological investigations[62,63] have not revealed any incidence of bladder cancer, above the normal, national level for spontaneous tumours, in operators who have been exposed in their working place.

It is feasible, however, that as the variation in latency increases with diminish-ing dose, a small dose may give individual latency times within the usual life-span, although the mean latency for the group of exposed animals as an whole exceeds the life-span, and such a calculation as the foregoing one does not take account of this limitation.

Another problem arises from the discrepancy in genetic make-up between animals and a human population. Thus, experimental animals are genetically

[61] P. L. Batten and D. E. Hathway, *Br. J. Cancer*, 1977, **35**, 342.
[62] C. A. Veys, M. D. Thesis, University of Liverpool, 1973.
[63] A. J. Fox, D. C. Lindars, and R. Owen, *Br. J. Ind. Med.*, 1974, **31**, 140.

well-characterized and, in an inbred colony, animals of the same age are similar in size. They are exposed to a single chemical carcinogen in their lifetime. At the start of an experiment, all the animals are strictly comparable, and the environment is rigorously controlled for them throughout the test. None of these conditions apply to human populations. In addition, there is a wide variation in the sensitivity of individual subjects towards any particular carcinogen, and this factor mitigates as well against the quantitative extension of carcinogenicity data found in animals.

Nevertheless, despite all the limitations, which have been raised, dose-response investigations would appear to be very worthwhile. The fact that mathematical models can be applied to epidemiological data emphasizes the importance of such dose-response investigations in experimental animals to the control of human exposure in the working environment. Interesting dose-response investigations have been reported, for example, for radiation carcinogenesis by Brown,[64] for urethane carcinogenesis by Schmähl, Port and Wahrendorf,[65] and for vinyl chloride carcinogenesis by Maltoni and Lefemine:[66–69] the last-named investigations involved exposure by inhalation. A dose-dependence for tumours in urethane carcinogenesis was demonstrated[65] both in the rat and mouse experiments. Maltoni and Lefemine[68] draw attention to a dose-response relationship in rats for vinyl chloride-induced liver angiosarcomas and nephroblastomas, at the lower dose ranges.

In respect of 'the extrapolation' of carcinogenicity data from animals to man, it ought to be clearly stated that, whilst human beings are exposed generally in their lifetime to several carcinogens, the introduction of any particular chemical carcinogen into this complicated biological situation exerts an incremental effect with regard to the total incidence of tumours, from zero dose of the carcinogen concerned. The foregoing supposition is entirely independent of whatever mathematical model is used[70] (see also ref. 71). This conclusion is valid for tumours of monoclonal origin.[17]

5 Dose Monitors

Whilst the energy absorbed by unit mass of tissue provides a definition of the tissue dose of ionizing radiation in an organ of the body, it is more difficult to define a dose for a chemical carcinogen or mutagen. Thus, if D_e is the exposure dose, then:

$$D_e = \int_{t_1}^{t_2} C_e \mathrm{d}t \qquad (6)$$

[64] J. M. Brown, *Health Phys.*, 1976, **31**, 231.
[65] D. Schmähl, R. Port, and J. Wahrendorf, *Int. J. Cancer*, 1977, **19**, 77.
[66] C. Maltoni and G. Lefemine, *Atti Accad. Naz. Lincei, Cl. Sci. Fis. Mat. Nat. Rend.*, 1974, **[8]56**, 1.
[67] C. Maltoni and G. Lefemine, *Environ. Res.*, 1974, **7**, 387.
[68] C. Maltoni and G. Lefemine, *Ann. N. Y. Acad. Sci.*, 1975, **246**, 195.
[69] C. Maltoni, *Environ. Health Perspectives*, 1977, **21**, 1.
[70] K. S. Crump, D. G. Hoel, C. H. Langley, and R. Peto, *Cancer Res.*, 1976, **36**, 2973.
[71] J. Ashby and J. A. Styles, *Br. Med. Bull.*, 1980, **36[1]**, 63.

where C_e is the time-dependent concentration of the foreign compound concerned, for example, in the atmosphere, and the times t_1 and t_2 denote the start and end of exposure.

Thus, the exposure dose may be defined as the integral of the concentration function with respect to time, over the limits of the experiment.

Similarly, the amount of foreign compound kg^{-1} of body weight is used to express the dose, administered enterally or parenterally. Clearly, this value is directly proportional to D_e, provided that the rate of absorption remains constant. Moreover, as the rates of distribution, metabolism, and elimination vary with the different chemical substances in question, the tissue dose is not proportional to the integral of the concentration in the whole animal nor to the quantity absorbed.

If D_t be the tissue dose, then:

$$D_t = \int_{t_1}^{t_2} C_t \mathrm{d}t \qquad (7)$$

where C_t is the concentration of ultimate carcinogen integrated over the limits t_1, t_2 or after 0.00.

Again, D_t might be defined as the number of potential genotoxic events/cell,[72] and this might approach closest to the radiological dose.

Other considerations, in this context, relate to the sites in DNA with which reactive chemical carcinogens or their ultimate metabolites react, and the *O*-6 position of dG residues is important, particularly to simple alkylating agents.[13]

D_t is probably the most suitable basis for estimates of risk, and in this respect, there has been some change of ground (*cf.* section 1) in the arguments, which have developed in this discussion. At the outset (section 1), it was tacitly assumed that actual estimations might be made.

The tissue dose, D_t (equation 7) of an alkylating agent RX will be directly proportional to the product, RY, of reaction with a nucleophile Y in the tissue concerned.

$$\mathrm{RX} + \mathrm{Y} \xrightarrow{k} \mathrm{RY} + \mathrm{X} \qquad (8)$$

$$[\mathrm{RY}]/[\mathrm{Y}] = k[\mathrm{RX}]t = kD\mathrm{t} \qquad (9)$$

The proportionality constant, k, is the 2nd order rate constant for the reaction in equation 8. This means that the reaction product, RY, must be stable chemically throughout the period of experimental exposure, and that Y and RY should not be subject to turnover, repair, *etc.*

It was these concepts which provided the reason for employing proteins as the nucleophiles, Y (equations 8 and 9) for dose monitoring (*v. infra*). Ehrenberg *et al.*[46] have utilized this idea to monitor the doses of alkylating agent, resulting from the exposure of living mice to an atmosphere containing ethylene oxide. It ought to be stated clearly that the mutagenic activity of ethylene oxide had

[72] C. Ramel, 'Ambio Special Report,' 1973, no. 3, 15.

been demonstrated previously in *Drosophila*[73] and barley,[47,74,75] and was known to be an effective initiator of chromosomal aberrations.[76] In this work,[46] the degree of alkylation of tissue proteins was used in the determination of D_t (*v. supra*) in resting mice, which were exposed for 1—2 h to air containing 1—35 p.p.m. of ethylene oxide.

The values for D_e were thus *ca.* 0.03—0.2% of the LD_{50} for ethylene oxide.

The results obtained,[46] D_e and D_t for various tissues, agreed with the absorption of all the ethylene oxide by alveolar ventilation, with rapid distribution throughout all of the body organs, and with a rapid detoxication of the ethylene oxide, followed by the rapid excretion of ethylene oxide metabolites from the body. When the average slope of the curves for the alkylation of spleen and testis protein of 0.23 nmol hydroxyethyl/g protein/p.p.m. h (equation 10) was used:[46]

$$[RY]/[Y] = 0.23 \times 10^{-9} = kD_t \qquad (10)$$

Whence, if $k = 4 \times 10^{-4}$ l g^{-1} h^{-1}:

$$D_t = 0.58 \ \mu\text{mol h/p.p.m. h} \qquad (11)$$

(Such values would seem to be representative of the dose with respect to somatic and germinal tissues.)

These results[46] infer that an exposure dose of 1 p.p.m. h gives an absorption of 2.5 μmol kg^{-1} $\simeq$ 2.5 μmol l^{-1}.

If an exponential time dependence for absorbed ethylene oxide be assumed,[46] then the mean life ($1/\lambda$) of ethylene oxide would be 0.23 h, which corresponds to a value for $t_{0.5}$ ($t_{0.5} = \ln 2/\lambda$) of 9 min for inspired ethylene oxide.[46]

However, when an animal is exposed chronically to a compound which is present in the atmosphere at a concentration of C_e mol/l of air, the amount, which is absorbed in time t, is given by the expression:

$$x = KC_et \text{ mol kg}^{-1}$$

where K is a proportionality constant.

If the average rate of consumption, *i.e.* the sum of metabolism, elimination, and displacement from the tissue concerned, be assumed to be:

$$dy/dt = \lambda(x - y)$$

where y is the amount consumed in time t, then the concentration will be:

$$C_t = (x - y) = K.C_e(1 - e^{-\lambda t})/\lambda$$

i.e. the concentration reaches a steady-state value $C_{ss} = KC_e/\lambda$.

90 and 95% of the steady-state concentration will be reached after 3.3 and 4.3 biological lives respectively. For ethylene oxide, with a $t_{0.5}$ value of 9 min, this corresponds to 30—40 min from the beginning of the exposure. The value $t_{0.5} =$ 9 min was confirmed[46] by i.p. injection of ethylene oxide.

[73] I. A. Rapoport, *Dokl. Akad. Nauk SSSR*, 1948, **60**, 469.
[74] L. Ehrenberg, A. Gustafsson, and U. Lundquist, *Acta Chem. Scand.*, 1956, **10**, 492.
[75] L. Ehrenberg, A. Gustafsson, and U. Lundquist, *Hereditas*, 1959, **45**, 351.
[76] J. Moutschen, M. Moutschen-Dahmen, and L. Ehrenberg, *Hereditas*, 1968, **60**, 267.

From an analysis of the various experiments, it appeared[46] that this value of $t_{0.5}$ may be an under-estimate by a factor of >1.5.

Finally, the degree of alkylation of tissue DNA agreed approximately[46] with what would be predicted on the basis of the values found for D_t (*v. supra*). It must be said, however, that in some cases the amounts of tissue DNA were very small indeed and that, with hindsight, not necessarily the best methods were used in fact for measuring 7-(2-hydroxyethyl)guanine.

In further considerations, which emphasized the importance of abundance, accessibility, and stability, erythrocyte haemoglobin and spermatozoa DNA appeared theoretically to be most suitable macromolecules for this sort of dosimetry (see equations 8 and 9).

Circulating haemoglobin was accordingly employed in three studies.[77–79] In man, haemoglobin has a biological lifetime of approximately 4 months. On the assumption that this time estimate holds also for the alkylated macromolecule, then haemoglobin might be used not only for monitoring acute exposures but also for doses arising from chronic exposures. Accordingly haemoglobin has been used to monitor mice, exposed to ethylene oxide by inhalation; the animals were killed and exsanguinated at different times after treatment.[77] On account of the random alkylation of erythrocytes of different age and of the stability of alkylated haemoglobin, the amounts of alkylated amino acids in the protein decreased linearly with time, and reached zero value after approximately 40 days, *i.e.* the life-span of erythrocytes in mice.[77] Metabolic incorporation of ethylene oxide into the haemoglobin macromolecule is brought about mainly through the alkylation of cysteinyl residues to give *S*-(2-hydroxyethyl)cysteinyl ones and of histidinyl residues to give *N*-3-(2-hydroxyethyl)-histidinyl ones.[78]

In work with the two dose monitors for following the fate of ethylene oxide,[46,77,78] the liver tissue proteins contained approximately the same amount of *S*-(2-hydroxyethyl)cysteinyl residues as the erythrocyte haemoglobin, although incorporation into liver protein was an order of magnitude higher than that into haemoglobin. These results[77,78] agree with the rapid distribution of ethylene oxide throughout the mammalian body to yield the same dose (D_t) in all of the organs.[46]

6 Validity of the Dose–Response Approach to Chemical Cancer in Man

Contingent upon the problem of the human subject exposed to chemical carcinogens in his occupation or (as pollutants) in his environment is the matter (i) of monitoring the target-organ dose (D_t) and (ii) of using the mutagenic activity of ionising radiation as a standard for the measurement of risk associated with unit target dose. Reference might be made here to the comparison of the linear

[77] S. Osterman-Golkar, L. Ehrenberg, D. Segerbäck, and I. Hällström, *Mutat. Res.*, 1976, **34**, 1.

[78] L. Ehrenberg, S. Osterman-Golkar, D. Segerbäck, K. Svensson, and C. J. Calleman, *Mutat. Res.*, 1977, **45**, 175.

[79] D. Segerbäck, C. J. Calleman, L. Ehrenberg, G. Löfroth, and S. Osterman-Golkar, *Mutat. Res.*, 1978, **49**, 71.

low-dose portion of the dose–response curves for alkylating agents and their rad-equivalence, which was proportional to the rate of reaction of nucleophiles of relatively low reactivity.[13] Furthermore, it has been established that the rad-equivalence of several alkylating agents was approximately the same in bacteria, plants, and mammals (see ref. 46 and section 3). Hence, the assumption might be made that the scope of the rad-equivalence, which has been established, includes the human subject. This eventuality permits of an estimate of the risk of heritable damage to be made, using the value of D_t, which would be determined in man. Despite the lack of experiments, which would provide a comparison of dose–response curves with respect to chemicals and radiation in the same strains of experimental animal, it has been suggested (Ehrenberg *et al.*, many ref. including 46, 80, and 81) that the rad-equivalence of mutation, which has been established, might be applied to the context of cancer (*v. supra*). This would avoid the inherent difficulty of attempting to extend the carcinogenicity data found in small laboratory animals to human populations (see section 4).

In their paper,[18] Calleman *et al.* make use of the continuous monitoring of atmospheric ethylene oxide of a sterilization plant and of the availability of the blood of operatives, exposed to relatively well-defined doses (D_e) of ethylene oxide. Interestingly, a preliminary risk estimate made in 1974,[46] from D_t values in mice, was found to be largely confirmed.

In the exposed persons, erythrocyte haemoglobin was used as the dose monitor, and the degree of alkylation was measured as *N*-3-(2-hydroxyethyl)-histidinyl residues by mass fragmentometry.[18] The resulting data are consistent with fast elimination from tissues ($\lambda = 4.6\ h^{-1}$, *i.e.* a biological $t_{0.5}$ of *ca.* 9 min) found in mice. At the rate of respiration for light work, an exposure of 1 p.p.m./h which resulted in a D_t value of 1×10^1 mrad-equiv.,[18] was consistent with a low degree of risk.[18] Epidemiologically, ethylene oxide, in common with radiation, would appear to be associated with leukaemias rather than with solid tumours. Calleman *et al.*[18] report that in the industrial establishments, with which they were concerned in 1964, an average exposure level of 5—10 p.p.m. of ethylene oxide obtained, and accordingly their estimate of 10 mrad-equiv. (p.p.m. h)$^{-1}$ would correspond to 3 rad-equiv. week^{-1}. In 100 workers, exposed for 10 years, the collective dose would be 1.2×10^5 mrad-equiv., and the most likely value of the risk to middle-aged persons of radiation-induced leukaemia might be *ca.* 30×10^{-6} rad^{-1}. Hence, on this basis, during the working period of 10 years, $30 \times 10^{-6} \times 1.2 \times 10^5 = 3.6$ cases of leukaemia would be predicted, of which one might appear before the end of the 10-year period. It might be necessary to include an uncertainty factor of 2 to give a more realistic assessment.

At the German sterilization plant studied by Calleman *et al.*,[18] the weekly exposure dose was 9×10^2 p.p.m. h, corresponding to a weekly risk of 6 rad-equiv., so that *ca.* 3 cases of leukaemia would be expected to occur under such

80 L. Ehrenberg, in 'Mutagenesis in Sub-Mammalian Systems,' ed. G. E. Paget, M. P. T. Press, New York, 1979, pp. 73—88.

81 S. Hussain and L. Ehrenberg, *Abh. Dtsch. Akad. Wiss. Berlin, Kl. Math.-Naturwiss.-Tech.*, 1977, **9**, 95.

working conditions during 10 years involving 100 operatives. Such a prediction seems to have been realized, as 3 cases of leukaemia were found, and at least two of them were of the type, which is known to be induced by ionising radiation.

The scope of this exercise is too slight for ethylene oxide to be classified as a frank (human) carcinogen. Thus, for example, World producers of ethylene and manufacturers of ethylene oxide as a chemical intermediate would be seen to observe more stringent precautions with regard to the possible occupational hazard and safety of their operatives than are commonly taken for sterilisation purposes. Epidemiological data are unavailable for ethylene oxide.[82] Nevertheless, the Ehrenberg School has sounded a clear warning regarding the risk attributable to this substance, and the correlation[18] between the incidence of overt leukaemia in man and their dosimetry and calculation is very impressive.

It cannot be denied that, in the general case, target-organ DNA is a much better model of heritable genetic injury (see section 1) than erythrocyte haemoglobin, but measurement in haemoglobin may have special relevance for leukaemia. However, the preferred model may be inaccessible: (i) because the measurements which were discussed in section 1 are very difficult to make despite conspicuous advances in very sensitive mass fragmentometry, spectrophotofluorimetry, *etc.*; (ii) because both the range-finding and the numbers of measurements to confer statistical significance are uncertain; and (iii) because this method would require awkward extension of data found in animals to man. When the foregoing limitations are taken into account, the dose monitoring of the Ehrenberg School and their risk analysis would seem to be realistic, under the prevailing circumstances.

[82] IARC Monographs, 'Evaluation of Carcinogenic Risk of Chemicals to Man,' vol. 11 (Cadmium, nickel, some epoxides, miscellaneous industrial chemicals and general considerations on volatile anaesthetics), Agency for Research on Cancer, Lyon, France, 1976, pp. 157—167.

Part II

Relation between Dose and Effect and Time

Chapter 4 Biological Action

1 Application of the Law of Mass Action to Drug–Receptor Interactions

If a drug X (where the word drug is being used in the widest sense, as meaning any compound that is capable of exerting a biological action in mammals) combines with a receptor R to afford a complex RX, which produces a response, then:

$$\mathrm{R} + \mathrm{X} \underset{k_2}{\overset{k_1}{\rightleftarrows}} \mathrm{RX}$$

$$\frac{[\mathrm{R}][\mathrm{X}]}{[\mathrm{RX}]} = \frac{k_2}{k_1} = K_{\mathrm{x}}$$

where K_{x} is the dissociation constant of the complex. Then, if $[\mathrm{R_T}]$ is the total concentration of receptors, since $[\mathrm{R_T}] = [\mathrm{R}] + [\mathrm{RX}]$:

$$\frac{[\mathrm{RX}]}{[\mathrm{R_T}]} = \frac{[\mathrm{X}]}{K_{\mathrm{x}} + [\mathrm{X}]}$$

If the response (Δ) is proportional to the concentration of RX, then $\Delta = k_3$ [RX] and the maximum response ($\Delta_{\mathrm{max.}}$), obtained when all of the receptors are occupied, is $\Delta_{\mathrm{max.}} = k_3[\mathrm{R_T}]$. Whence:

$$\Delta = \Delta_{\mathrm{max.}} \frac{[\mathrm{RX}]}{[\mathrm{R_T}]}$$

or

$$\Delta = \frac{\Delta_{max.}[X]}{K_x + [X]} \tag{1}$$

For this hyperbolic function, $\Delta = 0$ when $[X] = 0$, and $\Delta \rightarrow \Delta_{max.}$ when $[X] \rightarrow \infty$. When $\Delta = \frac{1}{2}\Delta_{max.}$, $K_x = [X]$, which means that K_x may be expressed in terms of mol^{-1}.

The derivation of equation 1 is identical with that of the Michaelis–Menten equation:

$$v = \frac{V_{max.}[S]}{K_m + [S]}$$

which defines the quantitative relationship between the enzyme reaction rate v and the substrate concentration [S], if either the maximum velocity $V_{max.}$ or the lumped K_m is known, but in this case, $v = k_3$ [ES] refers to the dissociation of a steady-state intermediate. No such assumption relates to the analogous proportionality $\Delta = k_3[RX]$.

The equations derived here (*v. supra*) are generally applicable, and they include as a class enzyme–substrate and enzyme–inhibitor interactions.

At this stage in the treatment, it would be expedient to ask what assumptions were made in the derivation of equation 1. Firstly, there is the so-called 'assumption of occupancy', *viz.* that the response is proportional to the receptors occupied. This assumption is satisfactory where enzyme–substrate and enzyme–inhibitor phenomena are concerned, *i.e.* where the receptor is an enzyme, as the concentration either of enzyme-bound substrate or of inhibitor is a measure of the response. But, with regard to drug effects in general, there is no way of knowing whether such occupancy is valid. A second assumption, that one molecule of drug combines with one receptor, is the simplest possible reaction mechanism, which is implicit both in the derivation of equation 1 and of the Michaelis–Menten equation. Thirdly, a negligible fraction of total drug is combined in this way, so that in equation 1, the term which refers to uncombined drug [X] might be replaced by the total drug concentration $[X_T]$. This assumption is true, for example, for zone A in the zone behaviour of enzymes.[1] Thus, equation 1 holds for drug-binding experiments in which uncombined drug is measured. However, in those cases where the criterion of effect is provided by the biological action, and only the total drug that was added to the system is known, it is conventional to assume zone A behaviour (*v. supra*).

One of the most widely used transformations of equation 1 is the double reciprocal equation:

$$\frac{1}{\Delta} = \frac{K_x}{\Delta_{max.}[X]} + \frac{1}{\Delta_{max.}} \tag{2}$$

which is analogous to the Lineweaver–Burk equation,[2] and which represents

[1] O. H. Straus and A. Goldstein, *J. Gen. Physiol.*, 1943, **26**, 559.
[2] J. L. Webb, 'Enzyme and Metabolic Inhibitors,' Academic Press, New York, 1963, vol. 1.

a straight line of slope $K_x/\Delta_{max.}$ and an intercept $1/\Delta_{max.}$ on the ordinate. The advantage of this transformation is that $\Delta_{max.}$ may be deduced more accurately than from the corresponding (hyperbolic) plot of Δ against [X], where $\Delta_{max.}$ is measured asymptotically. The intercept on the abscissa of the double reciprocal plot is $-1/K_x$. Equation 2 is used widely for the analysis of antagonisms, particularly of enzyme inhibitions. (*cf.* ref. 3*a*).

An antagonist Z, which causes inactivation of the receptor so as to prevent effective combination with the drug, irrespective of concentration [X], is said to be non-competitive.* Thus, (i) Z might combine irreversibly with R at the same site as X would have done in the absence of Z; (ii) Z might combine at a different site and so prevent a conformational change in R, essential for combination with X and the production of a characteristic response; or (iii) Z might produce a conformational change in R, which would destroy the reactivity of the site where X would interact. Essentially, the degree of antagonism and its feasible reversibility are unrelated to [X]. The total number of available receptor sites for a drug, under specific experimental conditions, would be diminished by a fixed concentration of antagonist, but the remaining receptors retain unchanged affinity towards X, *i.e.* provided that there are spare receptors, when the concentration of antagonist is small this type of antagonism appears to be reversible. (But, for higher concentrations of antagonist, the block will not be reversed by more agonist, and this condition has been described as unsurmountable by Gaddum, Khan Hameed, Hathway, and Stephens.[3b]) In a double reciprocal plot, $\Delta_{max.}$ would be lowered in direct proportion to the decrease in free receptors and the intercept on the ordinate would increase, but that ($-1/K_x$) on the abscissa remains unchanged.

On the other hand, an antagonist is said to be competitive* if it combines reversibly with the same receptor sites as the drug. In competitive antagonism, $\Delta_{max.}$ remains unaltered, as a high enough ratio of X: Z brings about complete occupation of the receptors by X, irrespective of the presence of Z. In the double reciprocal plot, the intercept on the ordinate remains unchanged, but the affinity, *i.e.* the intercept on the abscissa ($-1/K_x$), would be lowered. Conversely, the generation of such results by experiment is held to establish competitive antagonism.

Equations involving double reciprocal plots for competitive and non-competitive (drug) antagonisms have been derived.[2] Good examples of the use of the double reciprocal plot for determining the nature of antagonisms are provided by: (i) the inhibition of the oxidative *N*-demethylation of a morphine analogue by chlorpromazine, which is a competitive inhibitor;[5] and (ii) the antagonism of exogenous histamine in animals, where the nature of the receptors was ignored, and where effects on the blood pressure were used to monitor biological action.

* The terms competitive and non-competitive were used in the present context by D. W. Woolley in a book[4] which the author read thirty years ago.

3 (*a*) J. E. Dowd and D. S. Riggs, *J. Biol. Chem.*, 1965, **240**, 863; (*b*) J. H. Gaddum, Khan A. Hameed, D. E. Hathway, and F. F. Stephens, *Q. J. Exp. Physiol.*, 1955, **40**, 49.

4 D. W. Woolley, 'A Study of Antimetabolites,' John Wiley and Sons, New York, 1952, pp. 64, 68 *et. seq.*

5 A. Rubin, T. R. Tephly, and G. J. Mannering, *Biochem. Pharmacol.*, 1964, **13**, 1007.

In the latter experiment, diphenhydramine acted as a competitive antagonist,[6] and ergotamine acted uncompetitively.[6]

2 Chemical Nature of Receptors

At this stage in the narrative, it might be suitable to discuss briefly the nature of some different receptors.

The Receptor as an Enzyme.—One of the first connections between the discovery and the action of drugs was made by Stedman,[7,8] who showed that physiostigmine blocked the acetylcholinesterase *in vitro*, which is normally responsible for the destruction of acetylcholine immediately after it has completed transferring a nerve impulse across the nerve–muscle junction. (At the time when Stedman carried out these experiments, the neurotransmitter function of acetylcholine had just been discovered.[9,10]) Stedman went on to show that physiostigmine contracts the pupil of the eye because it is a strong inhibitor of acetylcholinesterase in the nerve–muscle synapse, thus allowing the muscle to be contracted by the acetylcholine, which leaks from the nerve ending between impulses.[11] It was this work[7,8,11] and the specification of enzyme requirements,[12] which established the fact that a receptor can be an enzyme. Since then, despite the enormous difficulty of extracting this enzyme intact from various cell-wall fractions to which it is bound, acetylcholinesterase has been isolated from several tissues.[13–16] The isolation of the insulin-receptor protein from fat-cell envelopes presented a more formidable problem.[17–19]

The Receptor as a Nucleic Acid.—Accumulation of aminoacridines in the nuclei of cells was known from their use in vital staining,[20] and the reason for the coplanarity of these molecules became clear twenty years later when Lerman showed[21] the intercalation of aminoacridines between folds of DNA, where they are held by van der Waals forces and ionic bonds to the phosphate anions. Consequential increase in the melting temperature correlated with the interference caused to the unwinding of the strands and to the normal functioning of DNA. It was shown afterwards[22] that the antibacterial property of the amino-

6 G. Chen and D. Russell, *J. Pharmacol.*, 1950, **99**, 401.
7 E. Stedman, *Biochem. J.*, 1926, **20**, 719.
8 E. Stedman, *Nature*, 1926, **159**, 194.
9 O. Loewi, *Pflüg. Arch. ges. Physiol.*, 1921, **189**, 239.
10 O. Loewi and E. Navratil, *Pflüg. Arch. ges. Physiol.*, 1926, **214**, 678.
11 E. Stedman, *Am. J. Physiol.*, 1929, **90**, 528.
12 E. Stedman and E. Stedman, *Biochem. J.*, 1931, **25**, 1147.
13 R. Miledi, P. Molinoff, and L. T. Potter, *Nature*, 1971, **229**, 554.
14 S. Ehrenpreis, J. H. Fleisch, and T. W. Mittag, *Pharmacol. Rev.*, 1969, **21**, 131.
15 J. P. Changeaux, J. C. Meunier, and M. Huchet, *Mol. Pharmacol.*, 1971, **7**, 538.
16 J. P. Changeaux, T. R. Podleski, and L. Wofsy, *Proc. Natl. Acad. Sci., USA*, 1967, **58**, 2063.
17 P. Cuatrecasas, *Proc. Natl. Acad. Sci., USA*, 1969, **63**, 450.
18 P. Cuatrecasas, *J. Biol. Chem.*, 1971, **246**, 7265.
19 P. Cuatrecasas, *Proc. Natl. Acad. Sci., USA*, 1972, **69**, 1277.
20 S. Strugger, *Jen. Z. Naturwiss.*, 1940, **73**, 97.
21 L. S. Lerman, *J. Mol. Biol.*, 1961, **3**, 18.
22 J. Hurwitz, J. J. Furth, M. H. Malamy, and M. Alexander, *Proc. Natl. Acad. Sci., USA*, 1962, **48**, 1222.

acridines results from the blocking of the DNA-template requirement of DNA and RNA polymerases. Thus, the study of the structure–activity relationships of aminoacridines and their physically related analogues firmly established the role of nucleic acids as receptors.

That DNA is the eventual receptor for steroid hormones may be investigated by using the antagonist role of actinomycin D, which is a specific inhibitor of DNA function. However, in the case of steroids, sequential receptors are involved and the first of these are proteins. Pioneering binding studies involving [^{3}H]-17β-oestradiol of high specific activity had shown[23] that a receptor protein, specific to oestrogens, was present in the uterus, vagina, and anterior pituitary gland. This work was extended to the successful isolation of receptor from these tissues by ultracentrifugal methods.[24] Similarly, progesterone was shown to have high specificity for the oviduct.[25] The resulting steroid–receptor complexes diffuse into the nucleus of the same cell, where they bind to native chromatin, and in this way DNA codon is derepressed and produces the requisite m-RNA, which in turn uses cytoplasmic ribosomes to synthesize characteristic protein. The physiological response to the hormone in question takes place when the foregoing steps have been completed, and occurs approximately 1 h after administration.[26] Amongst further examples are the following: (i) the androgen, dihydrotestosterone, bound specifically to an acidic protein in androgen-dependent tissue such as the prostate gland.[27] (ii) Corticosteroids bind specifically to a protein in the hepatic cytosol and some cells, and the resulting complex enters the nucleus where it is bound to DNA. This leads to the formation of a specific m-RNA, which is suppressed by actinomycin D (*v. supra*), and which in turn produces enzymes characteristic of the corticosteroid.[28] By means of affinity chromatography, corticosteroid-binding globulin has now been isolated.[29] (iii) A rather similar sequence regulates the diuretic effect of aldosterone.[30]

Vitamin D_3 exerts its effect on Ca^{2+} absorption through its inductive action on DNA in the cells lining the intestine.[31] Through m-RNA, the insect steroid hormone, ecdysone, induces DNA to form key enzymes concerned with the synthesis of the phenol, *N*-acetyl-3,4-dihydroxyphenethylamine that subsequently reacts with cuticular protein to stimulate moulting.[32] Amongst the plants hormones: (i) the gibberellins induce DNA to synthesize α-amylase in barley endosperm;[33] and (ii) both the cytokinins and the auxins stimulate DNA to synthesize specific RNA.[34]

23 E. V. Jensen and H. I. Jacobson, *Recent Prog. Horm. Res.*, 1962, **18**, 387.
24 D. Toft and J. Gorski, *Proc. Natl. Acad. Sci., USA*, 1966, **55**, 1574.
25 B. W. O'Malley and A. R. Means, *Science*, 1974, **183**, 610.
26 N. R. Cohen, *Biol. Rev., Cambridge Philos. Soc.*, 1966, **41**, 503.
27 K. M. Anderson and S. Liao, *Nature*, 1968, **219**, 277.
28 C. E. Sekeris, *Biochem. J.*, 1971, **124**, 43.
29 W. Rosner and H. L. Bradlow, *J. Clin. Endocrinol.*, 1971, **33**, 193.
30 I. S. Edelman, R. Bogoroch, and G. A. Porter, *Proc. Natl. Acad. Sci., USA*, 1963, **50**, 1169.
31 M. R. Haussler and A. W. Norman, *Proc. Natl. Acad. Sci., USA*, 1969, **62**, 155.
32 P. Karlson and C. E. Sekeris, *Biochim. Biophys. Acta*, 1962, **63**, 489.
33 J. E. Varner and G. R. Chandra, *Proc. Natl. Acad. Sci., USA*, 1964, **52**, 100.
34 A. G. Matthysse and M. Abrams, *Biochim. Biophys. Acta*, 1970, **199**, 511.

The Receptor as a Co-enzyme.—A great deal of work on the antibacterial action of Fe^{2+} complexes of 8-hydroxyquinoline or dimethyldithiocarbamic acid and on its prevention by a small concentration of Co^{2+} suggested that the metal complexes oxidatively destroy lipoic acid, which is the co-enzyme essential to the oxidative decarboxylation of pyruvate.[35,36] Furthermore, pyruvate was found to accumulate in the medium.[35] Thus, lipoic acid is implicated as the receptor for the antibacterial metal complexes.

Concluding Remarks.—Isolation of some receptors and direct evidence for the presence of others provide a sound basis for the concept of 'receptors', which was put forward tentatively by Langley[37] in 1878, and which was developed (*v. supra*) to explain biological action, notably by A. J. Clark, John Gaddum, and E. J. Ariens during the following century. The present author remembers that the late Professor D. K. de Jongh in his preface to Ariens' book[38] used as a simile for the receptor a beautiful but elusive woman, to whom the experimental pharmacologist had addressed many messages, and who sometimes sent back her responses. Although the pharmacologist had assembled for himself an image of what this beautiful woman was like, he could not have claimed at that time (1964) to have seen her, although one day he may do so. That then unforeseeable day has dawned, and we now know very much more about receptors and biological action than hitherto.

3 The Log Dose–Response Curve

It is more often convenient in experimental pharmacology to show the relationship between dose and response directly, rather than by a double reciprocal plot.

In this connection, log dose–response plots are greatly preferred to dose–response ones for the following reasons: (i) linear plots are easier to treat statistically than the corresponding hyperbolae; (ii) drugs which produce the same effect by the same mechanism, but which differ in potency, afford parallel linear plots; and (iii) a wide range of doses can be represented by a single graph.

Let us determine to what extent log dose–response curves can be described by equations based on the law of mass action.

If f is the fraction of a maximum response registered by a particular dose, then:

$$f = \frac{\Delta}{\Delta_{max.}} = \frac{[RX]}{[R_T]}$$

Whence, by equation 1:

$$f = \frac{[X]}{K_x + [X]}$$

[35] A. K. Sijpesteijn and M. J. Janssen, *Antonie van Leeuvenhoek*, 1959, **25**, 422.
[36] A. Albert, M. Gibson, and S. Rubbo, *Br. J. Exp. Pathol.*, 1953, **34**, 119.
[37] J. Langley, *J. Physiol.*, 1878, **1**, 339.
[38] E. J. Ariens, 'Molecular Pharmacology,' Academic Press, New York, 1964.

or

$$[X] = K_x\left(\frac{f}{1-f}\right)$$

But, if $[X_T] - [RX]$ be substituted for $[X]$ and $f[R_T]$ for $[RX]$, then:

$$[X_T] = K_x\left(\frac{f}{1-f}\right) + f[R_T] \quad (3)$$

This expression provides a measure of total drug in terms of free and bound forms. It will be seen that equation 3 holds for drug–response relationships, where the 'assumption of occupancy' applies, where the combining ratio of drug to receptor is unity, and where no assumption is made about the particular fraction of the total drug that is bound to receptors (*v. supra*).

If in equation 3 the $f[R_T]$ term, representing bound drug, is very much smaller than $K_x[f/(1-f)]$, representing free drug, it might be omitted. For any moderate values of f, this simplification can be made if $[R_T]$ is small compared with K_x, for example, if $[R_T]/K_x < 1/10$. This amounts to zone A approximation, where nearly all of the drug molecules are free, even at receptor saturation. Thus:

$$[X_T] = K_x\left(\frac{f}{1-f}\right) \quad (3a)$$

However, if $[R_T]$ is very large compared with K_x, the expression $K_x[f/(1-f)]$, representing free drug, becomes negligible for any moderate values of f and may be omitted.

This amounts to zone C approximation, in which almost no drug molecules are free, and in this case:

$$[X_T] = f[R_T] \quad (3c)$$

Binding is stoicheiometric, either because the drug–receptor dissociation constant is very small or because the receptor concentration is very large.

It will be seen that the same equation and log dose–response curve would be given by an irreversible drug–receptor combination.

Between the behaviour described by equations 3a and 3c is that of zone B, which is described by the full equation 3.

Simplification of equation 3 is brought about by means of the ratio $[R_T]/K_x$, *i.e.* the concentration of receptors expressed in terms of the drug–receptor dissociation constant. Equation 3 becomes:

$$\frac{[X_T]}{K_x} = \frac{f}{1-f} + f\left(\frac{[R_T]}{K_x}\right)$$

The three forms of this equation can be plotted as log dose–response curves, so that the abscissa represents dose, expressed in terms of the drug–receptor dissociation constant.

Thus, essentially, f is plotted against $\log([X_T]/K_x)$.

The curve for zone A is the symmetrical sigmoid, with an inflexion at $f = 0.5$, and is identical with the graphical representation of the Henderson–Hasselbalch[39,40] equation. Equation 3a may be re-written:

$$\log [X] = \log K_x + \log\left(\frac{f}{1-f}\right)$$

This is equivalent to:

$$\log [H^+] = \log K_a' + \log\left(\frac{HA}{A^-}\right)$$

$$= \log K_a' + \log\left(\frac{\beta}{1-\beta}\right)$$

where β is the undissociated fraction.

Inversion describes the plot of ionised fraction as a function of pH, *viz.* $pH = pK_a + \log$ [proton acceptor]/[proton donor].

Zone A log dose–response curves for a series of generically related drugs, like those ionisation-pH curves for a set of acids, are parallel sigmoids with invariant slopes at their mid-points. The mid-point is found by differentiation. Thus:

$$d \ln [X] = d \ln\left(\frac{f}{1-f}\right) = \left(\frac{df}{f(1-f)}\right)$$

$$df/d \log [X] = 2.303 f(1-f)$$

At the mid-point, $f = 0.5$, and $df/d \log [X] = 0.576$.

For zone C, the theoretical curve is described by the logarithm form of equation 3c:

$$\log f = \log ([X_T]/[R_T])$$

in which the molar ratio of drug to receptor determines the fractional response. This log dose–response curve is not sigmoid, and differentiation gives a mid-point of 1.15, which is double that of the zone A curve.

Log dose–response curves for zone B assume shapes between the ones for zone A and zone C.

Finally, in sections 1—3 of this chapter, the assumption was made that one molecule of drug combines with one receptor site, and this concept appears to be a rational one. There is a strong supposition that an interpretation based on the law of mass action and the 'assumption of occupancy' is correct in most cases, because of the high incidence amongst experimental results of values which approximate to 0.575 for the mid-point slope of log dose–response curves. However, other combining ratios are feasible and, for example, a cross-linking

[39] P. Henderson, *J. Am. Chem. Soc.*, 1908, **30**, 954.
[40] K. A. Hasselbalch, *Biochem. Z.*, 1917, **78**, 112.

agent would yield a drug–receptor combining ratio of 1: 2, and Ariens has considered the possibility of a drug acting at more than one receptor site.[41]

4 Alternative Concepts to the 'Assumption of Occupancy'

Fractional Occupancy Threshold.—If the receptors do not have a rate-limiting role in the reactions leading to biological action, no drug effect will arise unless a particular 'fractional occupancy threshold' is exceeded. This alternative concept to the one put forward in section 1 (*v. supra*) merits consideration, as a similar concept applies to some examples of enzyme inhibition. If the drug–receptor molecular combining ratio is 1: 1, f_0 is the fractional occupancy threshold (of receptors) below which no drug effect is obtained, and the maximum drug effect ($f = 1.0$) occurs at receptor saturation, then in zone A:

$$[X_T] = K_x \left\{ \frac{f + [f_0/(1 - f_0)]}{1 - f} \right\} \qquad (4a)$$

and in zone C:

$$[X_T] = [R_T]\{f + f_0(1 - f)\} \qquad (4c)$$

In these cases, the curve representing fractional occupancy $\left(\frac{[RX]}{[R_T]}\right)$ is no longer identical with that representing the fractional response f. The latter curve is shifted farther away from the ordinate, *i.e.* to the right, and its gradient increases the greater the value of f_0. For zone A, the mid-point slope cannot exceed 1.15, which is twice the slope for the conventional zone A curve (*v. supra*).

For zone C, the mid-point slope can increase without limit as the value of f_0. increases. For example, for an f_0 value of 0.5: in zone A, when $f = 0.5$ the log dose–response slope is 0.863, and in zone C, when $f = 0.5$ the log dose–response slope is 3.45. For a very large excess of receptors, for example when $f_0 = 0.9$, the log-response slope might be so steep that it would mimic an 'all-or-none' type of response.

A result of the displacement of curves for biological action to the right of receptor occupancy ones is that the experimentally determined log dose–response will underestimate the real affinity of the drug for the receptor; *i.e.* $ED_{50} > K_x$.

The properties of carbonic anhydrase inhibitors illustrate the influence of excess of receptors. Carbonic anhydrase catalyses CO_2 hydration, $CO_2 + H_2O \rightleftharpoons H^+ + HCO_3^-$, and therefore the presence of a sufficient $[H^+]$ to acidify the tubular urine necessitates the operation of this enzyme. Predictably, if enzymic activity is inhibited,[42,43] the urine becomes alkaline, and assay of HCO_3^- is a measure of carbonic anhydrase inhibition.

Spare Receptors.—An important corollary of the concept of a 'fractional occupancy threshold' (*v. supra*) is the implication of a reservoir of receptors. It

[41] E. J. Ariens, ref. 38, p. 341.
[42] T. H. Maren, *J. Pharmacol.*, 1963, **139**, 140.
[43] J. T. Edsall, *Harvey Lectures*, 1966—1967, **62**, 191.

might be argued that: (i) the 'all-or-none' discussion (section 4) might have been used to treat the transition from weak drug effects to weak competitive antagonisms, which is found in practice, and (ii) phenomena such as non-competitive antagonism, competitive antagonism, auto-inhibition, *etc.* have their origin in the simple type of biological action described in section 1, in which case, the concepts of a threshold phenomenon and spare receptors seem to have evolved naturally from first principles.

A. J. Clark's[44] 'atropine anomaly' provides a good illustration of the spare receptors hypothesis. If a heart in a tissue bath is treated with a small dose of atropine and then re-tested with acetylcholine, the log dose–response curve will be shifted farther way from the ordinate, *i.e.* to the right, and increasing doses of atropine will shift the curve progressively further to the right. Clark (*loc. cit.*) found that these curves were essentially parallel, and that each ten-fold increase (for example) in atropine concentration resulted in a ten-fold increase in acetylcholine to afford the same response. At successive atropine concentrations, the same maximum response was obtained in each case, provided that the acetylcholine concentration was high enough to bring it about. If the mass-action law and the 'occupancy assumption' hold, when maximum response was obtained in presence of atropine, the receptors ought to have been occupied entirely by acetylcholine molecules (and the atropine ones to have been displaced). In this case, if the contents of the tissue bath were replaced successively by some high acetylcholine concentrations, and finally replaced by a fresh solution, devoid of acetylcholine and atropine, the heart ought to have regained its initial sensitivity to acetylcholine. However, it was found[44] that the diminished sensitivity, caused by the atropine, persisted. The atropine effect disappeared eventually with sequential washing, but the rate of removal in the washings is the same irrespective of whether acetylcholine is present in the wash liquor. Thus, this antagonism, which is apparently competitive, is practically irreversible, and is unaffected by the presence of the agonist.

If the affinity of acetylcholine for the receptors is assumed to be low, and maximum muscle response was obtained when only a small fraction of the receptors was occupied, the antagonism by atropine becomes explicable. Thus, if the total number of receptors is n, and if 0.01 n in combination with acetylcholine is sufficient to bring about maximum response, then 99% of the receptors are 'spare receptors'. If atropine blocks irreversibly 90% of the receptors, then 0.10 n are left for interaction with acetylcholine. Clearly, it will now require 10% occupancy to produce the 0.01 n necessary for maximum response. Since the law of mass action predicts that fractional occupancy is determined only by the concentration of free ligand, a much higher acetylcholine concentration will now be required. Hence, the shifts to the right of the log dose–response curves are accounted for, and this gives the appearance of competitive antagonism. There is however a limit to this process, as when the antagonist occupies such a large proportion of receptor sites that insufficient free receptors are available for normal, maximum response by a physiological concentration of agonist.

[44] A. J. Clark, *J. Physiol.*, 1926, **61**, 547; R. B. Barlow, 'Introduction to Chemical Pharmacology', Methuen, London, 2nd edn. 1964, pp. 214—220.

It ought to be explained that although potent agonists such as acetylcholine behave in the presence of antagonists in the way which has been described (*v. supra*), for just so long as spare receptors are available weak agonists do not. By definition, a weak agonist requires a high fractional occupancy to produce a response and, even then, it is unable to effect the maximum response which this tissue is capable of giving. This means that no spare receptors are present, and antagonists would lower immediately such response as has been produced.

The spare receptors hypothesis helps to explain a response such as neurotransmission, which is extremely rapid in onset and termination, and which is very sensitive to exceedingly low and transient changes in agonist concentration. A reservoir of spare receptors, a rapid rate constant for the dissociation of the drug–receptor complex, and a correspondingly low affinity value contribute to a mechanism for responses to very low concentrations of agonist.

5 Unspecific Compounds

A category of drugs, which are not mediated directly by receptors, and which produce unspecific effects, include the osmotic diuretics, mannitol and urea, osmotic cathartics such as magnesium sulphate, the antacids, and compounds such as ammonium chloride, which acidify the urine. Absorption of an osmotic diuretic is followed by its glomerular filtration and the increased osmolarity of tubular urine, with the result that water reabsorbed against a high osmotic gradient produces diuresis. As both Mg^{2+} and SO_4^{2-} cross the wall of the gut slowly, the lumen retains an osmotic equivalent of water. Inorganic and organic bases and ion-exchange resins, taken orally, neutralize gastric acidity. As NH_4^+ is metabolized into urea, ammonium chloride contributes to the $[H^+]$ of the body fluids:

$$2\,NH_4Cl + CO_2 \longrightarrow CO(NH_2)_2 + H_2O + 2\,HCl$$

Volatile general anaesthetics, such as chloroform, diethyl ether, halothane, nitrous oxide, and 1,1,2-trichloroethylene, constitute another category of drug for which the drug–receptor concept is not directly applicable, and it was found[45–47] that the oil–water partition coefficients of this apparently heterogeneous category of compound paralleled their anaesthetic potency. This finding suggested that the physiological functioning of the lipid membranes surrounding neuronal tissues might have been modified through preferential partitioning of the anaesthetics *per se*. On the other hand, the representation of the living cell by such a simple model is not entirely satisfactory, and Ferguson[48] was able to show without recourse to any model system that anaesthetic action was explicable in terms of the thermodynamic activity of the compound (*v. infra*). Essentially, Ferguson[48] realised that in Meyer's experiments[47] with volatile compounds, the conditions approximated to equilibrium, as the test animals were maintained at a steady state of depression for a considerable period of time. Whilst

[45] H. H. Meyer, *Arch. Exp. Pathol. Pharmakol.*, 1899, **42**, 109.
[46] E. Overton, 'Studien über die Narkosen,' Gustav Fischer, Jena, 1901.
[47] K. H. Meyer, *Trans. Faraday Soc.*, 1937, **33**, 1062.
[48] J. Ferguson, *Proc. R. Soc.*, 1939, **B 127**, 387.

the concentration of anaesthetic gas in the biophase was not measured, the chemical potential in all phases at equilibrium would be the same, and consequently the concentration in the biophase would be identical with that in the inhalation mixture, which was determined.

Now the chemical potential is given by:

$$\mu = \frac{\delta G}{\delta N}$$

where G is the Gibbs Free Energy and N the number of molecules, T and P being constant.

If μ_0 is the chemical potential in a standard state, and μ that of the anaesthetic gas, with a partial pressure p_t in the inhalation mixture, then:

$$\mu = \mu_0 + RT \ln (p_t)$$

The value RT in (p_t/p_s), where p_s is the saturation vapour pressure of the compound at the temperature of the experiment, would represent the difference in Gibbs Free Energy between the molecule in a steady state and that in the biophase.

Ferguson[48] used p_t/p_s as an indication of the 'thermodynamic activity' of the compound in question, and he employed Meyer's[47] values to obtain p_t and tables of physical constants for p_s.

Although the range of compounds differed widely in the concentrations (>200-fold) that would be necessary to produce depression, the fraction p_t/p_s was roughly constant. The only assumption that is implied to obtain Ferguson's results is that the experiments be made under equilibrium conditions.

The implication is that, for these unspecific compounds, biological action depends on the thermodynamic activity, *i.e.* that ΔG, the difference in Gibbs Free Energy between standard and biologically active states, is approximately the same for most of the compounds, irrespective of the absolute values of G. In the search for an entirely new anaesthetic from amongst a very wide range of halogenofluoroalkanes, Suckling[49] made use of the constant value of p_t/p_s. Thus, he was able to predict the corresponding values for p_t from those of p_s for the individual compounds, and hence to deduce the concentrations which would produce deep anaesthesia. The discovery of halothane,[49] which is the best volatile general anaesthetic known, provided further evidence for the thermodynamic approach.

Thus, the biological action of unspecific drugs, which is not mediated by receptors, can be explained in physico-chemical terms.

The category of unspecific compounds also includes the possibility of a drug reacting with a small molecular species *in vivo*, and such a phenomenon may be illustrated by the case of penicillamine. In Wilson's disease, defective synthesis of caeruloplasmin causes Cu^{2+} to accumulate in the liver and brain, where the resulting injury may be prevented and/or to some extent restored by administration of penicillamine which complexes with Cu^{2+}, the copper complex

[49] C. W. Suckling, *Br. J. Anaesth.*, 1957, **29**, 466.

being eliminated in the urine. But, in rheumatoid arthritis, treatment with penicillamine is followed by increased excretion of copper, lowered concentrations of caeruloplasmin in body fluids, and other effects which do not match changes in the disease state. In this case, penicillamine seems to behave as an immuno-stimulant.

6 Conclusion

Many findings in experimental pharmacology, and in toxicology (see chapter 5), are explained by the simple concepts of biological action, which have been described in sections 1 and 3—5, and it is hard to justify a more refined analysis[38,50] because of practical difficulties in making measurements to support the theory.

[50] H. Druckrey and K. Küpfmüller, 'Dosis und Wirkung,' Editio Cantor KG, Aulendorf im Württemberg, 1949.

Chapter 5 Extension of Simple Theory to Toxicology

1 Introduction

Mathematical treatment of biological action (see chapter 4) applies unconditionally to the ideal state, such as the tissue-bath situation, but *in vivo*, for example, the distribution, metabolism, and elimination of the pharmacologically active principle or principles (as active metabolites may be formed, which would contribute to drug action) as well as the action of natural, physiological agonists would have to be taken into account. Unlike both the naturally occuring and the synthetic drugs, which possess a high degree of molecular conformation and hence of specificity, pesticides are made to react in general with the more ill-defined receptors of several different species, whether they be insects in the case of insecticides or dicotyledonous and grass weeds in that of herbicides, and this produces further complication. Thus, clearly, whilst the mammalian toxicities both of pesticides and of industrial chemicals arise adventitiously, 'these are the stuff that toxicology is made of'. The present chapter attempts to interpret some examples of these toxicities from the point of view of pharmacology (*v. supra*), in which considerable progress has been made.

2 Drugs as Agonists

The idea that drugs behave as agonists seemed to be worthwhile exploring because, as has been mentioned (chapter 4), several important ones, for example insulin, aldosterone, the androgens, corticosteroids, oestrogens, and progestins, act in that way at special receptor sites. Whilst these substances are undoubtedly powerful drugs that are used widely in medicine, it might be argued that they are also naturally occurring, physiological agonists. On the other hand, morphine for which there is no endogenous counterpart acts as an agonist at an authenticated opoid receptor or receptors in the brain,[1–3] and other morphine narcotics, such as levorphanol, also act there; naloxone behaves as a specific antagonist. Again, the benzodiazepine anxiolytic drugs act at an anxiolytic receptor,[4,5] which is entirely different from the opoid receptor. In a similar vein, it is well known that acetylcholine and congeners act both at a muscarine receptor, for which

1 A. Goldstein, L. Lowney, and B. Pal, *Proc. Nat. Acad. Sci., USA*, 1971, **68**, 1742.
2 C. Pert and S. Snyder, *Science*, 1973, **179**, 1011.
3 C. Pert and S. Snyder, *Mol. Pharmacol.*, 1974, **10**, 868
4 C. Braestrup, R. Albrechtsen, and R. Squires, *Nature*, 1977, **269**, 702.
5 A. Young, S. Zukin, and S. Snyder, *Proc. Nat. Acad. Sci., USA*, 1974, **71**, 2246.

atropine is the most studied antagonist, and at a nicotinic receptor, for which tubocurarine and decamethonium (and suxamethonium) constitute two classes of antagonist. However, despite the structural relationship to the naturally occurring purines, there is no known barbiturate receptor, and the initial premise seems to be an over-simplification, as it is not true for all of the drugs where there is a clear receptor involvement. Thus, whilst isoprenaline simulates adrenaline in its behaviour as an agonist at the catecholamine β-receptor,[6–8] pinadolol and propranolol are antagonists, *viz.* 'β-blockers', and other drugs in this series behave in part as agonists and in part as antagonists with regard to the β-receptor. In another situation, in studies with heart slices,[9] therapeutic dose-levels of digitoxin have been shown not to inhibit the Na^+ pump, but to stimulate K^+-uptake, and there is a clear agonist action with regard to the Na/K ATP-ase receptor. With isolated guinea-pig atria, low concentrations of ouabain stimulate K^+-uptake, but higher ones inhibit it.[10] Further work[11] showed that extracellular K^+ competes for the binding and inhibitory effect of doses of ouabain, and that the binding of ouabain to both high- and low-affinity sites is to the Na pump. Thus, the cardiac glycosides play an agonist role, and the different affinity sites may be considered to reflect different states of the same population of receptors.

Whilst there is a clear trend running through these arguments, the boundaries between the agonist/antagonist role for drugs is blurred. What seems to emerge, not perhaps surprisingly, is that drugs (in the strictly medicinal sense) act at special receptor sites in the body, and whilst many drugs behave as agonists (*v. supra*), other ones function as antagonists. It will be seen (sections 3—6) that toxicants do not give the same sort of picture.

3 Toxicants as Antagonists, in Cases where there is Clear Receptor Involvement

Many toxicants, for example pesticides, appear to function as antagonists of various description (see chapter 4) in cases where there is clear receptor involvement, for example where the receptor is an identifiable enzyme system. It follows that many such toxicants behave as metabolic inhibitors.

(a) Agents, such as the unspecific weed-killer DNOC, uncouple oxidative phosphorylations (equation 1) associated with the respiratory chain by which

$$\text{NADH} + \text{H}^+ + 3\,\text{ADP} + 3\,\text{P}_i + \tfrac{1}{2}\,\text{O}_2 \longrightarrow \text{NAD}^+ + 4\,\text{H}_2\text{O} + 3\,\text{ATP} \quad (1)$$

approximately 40% of the energy released during electron transport would be recovered. They therefore permit the oxidation of NADH by O_2 (equation 2)

$$\text{NADH} + \text{H}^+ + \tfrac{1}{2}\,\text{O}_2 \longrightarrow \text{NAD}^+ + \text{H}_2\text{O} \qquad \Delta G_0 = -52.7\ \text{kcal} \quad (2)$$

[6] E. Brown, G. Aurbach, D. Hauser, and F. Troxler, *J. Biol. Chem.*, 1976, **251**, 1232.
[7] M. Maguire, R. Wiklund, H. Anderson, and A. Gilman, *J. Biol. Chem.*, 1976, **251**, 1221.
[8] L. Williams, L. Jarett, and R. Lefkowitz, *J. Biol. Chem.*, 1976, **251**, 3096.
[9] T. Godfraind, *Arch. Int. Pharmacodyn.*, 1973, **206**, 384.
[10] T. Godfraind and M. Lesne, *Br. J. Pharmacol.*, 1972, **46**, 488.
[11] T. Godfraind and J. Ghysel-Barton, *Nature*, 1977, **265**, 165.

without the coupled phosphorylation of three molecules of ADP (equation 3).

$$3\ ADP + 3\ P_i \longrightarrow 3\ ATP + 3\ H_2O \qquad \Delta G_0 = 21.9\ \text{kcal} \tag{3}$$

These uncouplers: (i) will stimulate the respiration of isolated mitochondria suspended in a medium deficient in phosphate or phosphate acceptor, and sometimes even in a medium containing phosphate plus acceptor; (ii) will abolish ATP; (iii) will enhance the normally very low ATP-ase activity of mitochondria and will hydrolyse additions of ATP; and (iv) will inhibit the isotopic exchange reaction in which inorganic phosphate, labelled with ^{32}P, exchanges rapidly with the terminal phosphate group of ATP in the absence of electron transport, *i.e.* the P_i-ATP exchange reaction, as well as the ADP–ATP exchange reaction and the exchange of O atoms of the water of the medium and those of P_i.

A chemical coupling hypothesis for the mechanism of oxidative phosphorylation, which implicates high-energy intermediates, has been proposed and is based in part on the characteristics of polynitrophenol inhibitors such as DNOC, and of oligomycin on the separate reaction steps. Specific proteins, known as coupling factors, have been isolated, which are capable of restoring phosphorylation in sub-mitochondrial particles, but the high-energy intermediates (*v. supra*) have never been found. Present evidence suggests that the intact membrane structure is essential to oxidative phosphorylation.[12–14]

Alternatively, the 'chemiosmotic hypothesis' suggests that electron transport provides the energy for creating a pH or electrical potential gradient across the inner mitochondrial membrane, which would serve as the immediate source of energy for oxidative phosphorylation.[15,16] The properties of the uncoupling agent are consistent with its being absorbed into the relevant membrane of the chemiosmotic model, where it would act as a proton carrier. By these means, the $[H^+]$ concentration on both sides of the membrane would equalize and the pH gradient, vital for ATP formation, would be discharged.

Finally, it ought to be made clear that in mammals liberation of heat energy by uncoupling agents, which antagonize the synthesis of energy-rich ATP, produces fever.

(b) Another example is presented by the toxicity of fluoroacetate, which has been used as a rodenticide, and which is known to cause convulsions in pigeons. Investigation[17] showed (i) that in contrast to F^-, fluoroacetate did not affect guinea-pig, rat, or pigeon brain respiration, and (ii) that when guinea-pig kidney particles were exposed to fluoroacetate, the resulting decrease in O_2-uptake (fumarate substrate) was followed by accumulation of citrate, but not of acetate. These results and the fact[18] that the injection of guinea-pigs and rats with fluoroacetate produced increased concentrations of citrate in several

12 A. L. Lehninger, 'The Mitochondrion,' W. A. Benjamin, New York, 1964.
13 E. C. Slater, 'Flavins and Flavoproteins,' Elsevier, Amsterdam, 1966.
14 H. A. Lardy and S. M. Ferguson, *Ann. Rev. Biochem.*, 1969, **38**, 991.
15 P. Mitchell, *Biol. Rev.*, 1965, **41**, 445.
16 P. Mitchell and J. Moyle, *Eur. J. Biochem.*, 1969, **7**, 471; P. Mitchell, *Theoret. Exp. Biophys.*, 1969, **2**, 159.
17 C. Liebecq and R. A. Peters, *Biochim. Biophys. Acta*, 1949, **3**, 215.
18 P. Buffa and R. A. Peters, *J. Physiol.*, 1949, **110**, 488.

tissues implicated the tricarboxylic acid cycle. It was Ogston's[19] renewed interest in Emil Fischer's three-point attachment of substrate to enzyme that suggested that the introduction of an asymmetrical centre into citric acid itself might lead to enzyme-complex formation with fluorocitrate, which would be commensurate with the metabolic inhibition that had been found. This supposition was confirmed: (i) by the isolation of crystalline fluorocitrate from a kidney preparation, reinforced with ATP and Mg^{2+}, and treated with fluoroacetate;[20] (ii) by the fact that intracisternally administered fluorocitrate was more toxic than fluoroacetate in anaesthetized animals;[21] and (iii) by the inhibition of aconitase,[22–24] but not of isocitrate dehydrogenase,[25] by fluorocitrate.

Whilst the fluorocitrate antagonism of aconitase accounts adequately for the deadly toxicity of fluoroacetate in rodents (which led to the banning of the use of fluoroacetate for environmental puposes), there seems to have been some debate about whether the same explanation applies to the cerebral effects (*v. supra*), but any objection would now appear to be unjustified, provided that the cerebral utilization of NH_4^+ be taken into consideration (see chapter 9)

(c) In all probability, more is known about the toxicity of organophosphates and carbamates than about that of any other agents. Such substrates are powerful antagonists of acetylcholinesterase (AChE) receptor protein. Not only has the role of acetylcholinesterase *vis-à-vis* the agonist, acetylcholine (chapter 4, section 2) been described, but the muscarinic and nicotinic receptor sites (chapter 5, section 2) have been investigated. In addition, in the case of the substrates, the well-known 'nerve gases' provided a range of highly toxic organophosphates, with lethal doses in the range 0.1—10 mg kg^{-1}, from which the organophosphate insecticides were developed. Some organophosphates and carbamates show marked selectivity towards particular esterases. The true cholinesterase, AChE, is present mainly in erythrocytes, the brain and nervous tissue. It is vital to nerve transmission, and is the acetylcholine-hydrolysing enzyme which is inhibited by excess of substrate. (It hydrolyses acetyl-β-methylcholine.) By contrast, serum pseudo-cholinesterase, which also hydrolyses acetylcholine, is not inhibited by excess of substrate and hydrolyses acetyl-β-methylcholine poorly. Unlike AChE, it has no physiological function, and its activity can be obliterated without harming the mammal concerned.

It would be inappropriate to consider the mechanism of antagonism/inhibition of organophosphates at this stage, as this subject is described under kinetics (section 4).

The kinetics of carbamate inhibition by cholinesterase has been investigated, and Goldstein[26] has shown that their form depends on the so-called zone of behaviour (chapter 4). Where the inhibitor is in great excess (zone A), Michaelis–Menten treatment is adequate, but where the enzyme is in excess (zone C),

19 A. G. Ogston, *Nature*, 1948, **162**, 963.
20 P. Buffa, R. A. Peters, and R. W. Wakelin, *Biochem. J.*, 1951, **48**, 467.
21 A. B. Hastings, R. A. Peters, and R. W. Wakelin, *J. Physiol.*, 1953, **120**, 51P.
22 J. F. Morrison and R. A. Peters, *Biochem. J.*, 1954, **56**, xxxvi.
23 J. F. Morrison and R. A. Peters, *Biochem. J.*, 1954, **58**, 473.
24 R. A. Peters, *Biochem. J.*, 1961, **79**, 261.
25 W. D. Lotspeich, R. A. Peters, and T. H. Wilson, *Biochem. J.*, 1952, **51**, 20.
26 A. Goldstein, *J. Gen. Physiol.*, 1944, **27**, 529.

different equations are necessary. Myers[27] has corrected Goldstein's results[28] to conform with steady-state kinetics. Carbamates afford competitive antagonism with regard to cholinesterase, and inhibition may be lowered by washing, dialysis, or dilution, or by addition of substrate. The dissociation time for the enzyme (inhibition) complex is also slow, but this is independent of the carbamate concentration employed.[29] In many cases, equilibrium is never attained, as the inhibition increases and then decreases because of carbamate metabolism. Thus, carbamates behave more as alternative substrates, with very low turnover values, than as 'true' inhibitors.[30] But, even if carbamates are regarded in this way, (i) the inhibited enzyme might be expected to complex with the whole carbamate molecule, in which case hydrolysis might involve transient carbamoylation of the esteratic site, or (ii) the inhibited enzyme might be carbamoylated at the esteratic site, when competition with the inhibition would involve hydrolysis of the carbamoylated enzyme. (The latter possibility is analogous to that of the organophosphates, which give relatively stable phosphorylated enzymes.) Other work[31] supports the second supposition, as reactivation rates of inhibited enzymes were found to depend only on the nature of the *N*-substituents; thus, dimethylcarbamoylcholine and dimethylcarbamoyl fluoride gave the same inhibited enzyme, presumably the dimethylcarbamoylated ChE.

Whilst eserine-type carbamates are bound initially both to esteratic and to anionic sites of ChE (in contrast to most organophosphates, which attack only the esteratic site, and Methylene Blue, atropine, *etc.* which combine with the anionic site), carbaryl-type carbamates bind to the anionic site, and very precise structure–activity relationships apply to this group of insecticides.

(d) The anti-coagulative properties of 4-hydroxycoumarins such as dicoumarol, and rodenticides such as warfarin, present a far more complicated picture than the antagonisms discussed under items (a)—(c) (*v. supra*). Quick and Collentine's (1950) hypothesis[32] that warfarin and vitamin K combined with a single enzyme, which was concerned with prothrombin synthesis, now seems to be an over-simplification. On the other hand, it is well-established that the undoubted antagonism of vitamin K and warfarin, both in living animals and in a perfused liver preparation, is non-competitive. Warfarin sensitivity decreases the more that an *in vitro* system is simplified. This and other evidence suggests that the carboxylase system, which contributes γ-carboxylated amino acids to prothrombin protein, is influenced indirectly by warfarin, and not by direct antagonism.

Various propositions have been made: (i) Bell and Matschiner[33] suggested that the control point for warfarin is vitamin K epoxide reductase, and that warfarin blocks the regeneration of vitamin K, which is essential to the carboxylase system; (ii) Goodman *et al.*[34] indicated that the warfarin receptor might be

[27] D. K. Myers, *Biochem. J.*, 1952, **52**, 46.
[28] A. Goldstein, *Arch. Biochem.*, 1951, **34**, 169.
[29] I. B. Wilson, *Arch. Int. Pharmacodyn.*, 1955, **104**, 204.
[30] D. K. Myers, *Biochem. J.*, 1956, **62**, 556.
[31] I. B. Wilson, M. A. Hatch, and S. Ginsburg, *J. Biol. Chem.*, 1960, **235**, 2312.
[32] A. J. Quick and G. Collentine, *J. Lab. Clin. Med.*, 1950, **36**, 976.
[33] R. G. Bell and J. T. Matschiner, *Nature*, 1972, **237**, 32.
[34] S. R. Goodman, R. M. Houser, and R. E. Olson, *Biochem. Biophys. Res. Commun.*, 1974, **61**, 250.

an allosteric modifier of the carboxylase system, and in that way it would be sensitive both to concentrations of warfarin and to those of vitamin K. Meanwhile, the isolation of a warfarin-receptor protein,[35] which reacts with warfarin and phylloquinone, focuses attention on the influence of this receptor on the vitamin K-dependent carboxylation system.[36,37] It is feasible that the two systems might integrate in some way with different members in an electron-transport chain.

(e) The extreme toxicity of cyanide and hydrogen sulphide results from the terminal inhibition, which they effect with the mitochondrial respiratory chain (equation 4).[38]

$$\text{NAD} \rightarrow \text{FP} \rightarrow \text{CoQ} \rightarrow \text{cyt b} \rightarrow \text{cyt c}_1 \rightarrow \text{cyt c} \rightarrow \text{cyt a} + \text{a}_3 \rightarrow \text{O}_2 \qquad (4)$$

The Fe^{III} form of cytochrome a + a_3 can accept electrons from reduced cytochrome c to assume the Fe^{II} state, which is oxidized in turn by molecular oxygen to regenerate the Fe^{III} form. Evidence[39,40] shows that the cytochrome a + a_3 system is a complex (*M* 240 000) that consists of six possibly identical subunits, each of which contains a single haem A group and a Cu atom. When these are associated into a hexameric complex, two of the subunits show a different absorption spectrum from the others; these are known as cytochrome a, and the four remaining subunits, which correspond to cytochrome a_3, react directly with O_2, whereas cytochrome a does not. The assumption is made that electrons received by cytochrome a subunits are transferred to cytochrome a_3 subunits, which deliver them to oxygen (equation 5).

$$\begin{aligned} &2\text{cyt c(II)} + 2\text{ cyt a(III)} \rightleftharpoons 2\text{ cyt c(III)} + 2\text{ cyt a(II)} \\ &2\text{ cyt a(II)} + 2\text{ cyt a}_3\text{(III)} \rightleftharpoons 2\text{ cyt a(III)} + 2\text{ cyt a}_3\text{(II)} \\ &2\text{ cyt a}_3\text{(II)} + \tfrac{1}{2}\text{ O}_2 + 2\text{ H}^+ \rightleftharpoons 2\text{ cyt a}_3\text{(III)} + \text{H}_2\text{O} \end{aligned} \qquad (5)$$

[The Cu atoms of the cytochrome a_3 subunits give characteristic e.s.r. signals and undergo Cu^{II} to Cu^{I} transitions during electron transfer to O_2 (equation 5).]

Cyanide, at a concentration of 10^{-8}M, and also hydrogen sulphide completely inhibit the cytochrome a + a_3 complex by binding strongly to cytochrome a_3(III), thereby blocking electron transfer from cytochromes c and a.[41] By these means, cellular respiration is stopped, and the effect on the poisoned mammal is so profound that, whilst CN^- and HS^- may inhibit other enzymes, those effects are not expressed. The concept of one toxic mechanism dominating several subsidiary ones in a terminal situation will be mentioned again in chapter 9.

35 M. T. Searcey, C. B. Graves, and R. E. Olson, *J. Biol. Chem.*, 1977, **252**, 6260.
36 J. A. Sadowski and J. W. Suttie, *Fed. Proc.*, 1976, **35**, 662.
37 R. M. Houser, J. P. Jones, A. Fausto, E. J. Gardner, F. C. Lee, and R. E. Olson, *Fed. Proc.*, 1976, **35**, 1353.
38 W. S. Caughley, W. J. Wallace, J. A. Volpe, and S. Yoshikawa, 'The Enzymes,' ed. P. D. Boyer, Academic Press, New York, 3rd edn., 1976, vol. 13, p. 300.
39 B. G. Malmström, *Quart. Rev. Biophys.*, 1974, **6**, 389.
40 R. Lemberg and J. Barrett, 'Cytochromes,' Academic Press, New York, 1973, p. 4 *et seq.*
41 Q. H. Gibson, C. Greenwood, D. C. Wharton, and G. Palmer, 'Oxidases and Related Redox Systems,' ed. T. E. King, H. S. Mason, and M. Morrison, John Wiley and Sons, New York, 1965, vol. 2, pp. 595, 596.

(f) Inhibitors of gas transport differ from metabolic inhibitors in that they make the physical separation of the lungs and tissues into an effective barrier, and they have ideally no direct effect on intermediary metabolism. Thus, their action must be described in terms of physiological, and not biochemical, systems.

Carbon monoxide reacts with haemoglobin and myoglobin. The affinity of haemoglobin for CO is much greater than for O_2, and under those conditions where sufficient amounts of these gases are present so that little uncombined haemoglobin remains the distribution of haemoglobin between the ligands is given by equation 6.

$$K = \frac{[\mathrm{HbCO}]\,\mathrm{pO_2},}{[\mathrm{HbO_2}]\,\mathrm{pCO}} \tag{6}$$

where K is the partition coefficient; it has a value of 210 for man[42] which means that the affinity of human haemoglobin for CO is two hundred and ten times greater than that for O_2.

When all of the haemoglobin is converted into carboxyhaemoglobin or oxyhaemoglobin, the fractions which are transformed in this way are derived from equations 7 and 8.

$$\frac{[\mathrm{HbCO}]}{[\mathrm{HbCO}] + [\mathrm{HbO_2}]} = K.\frac{\mathrm{pCO}}{\mathrm{pO_2} + K.\mathrm{pCO}} \tag{7}$$

$$\frac{[\mathrm{HbO_2}]}{[\mathrm{HbCO}] + [\mathrm{HbO_2}]} = \frac{\mathrm{pO_2}}{\mathrm{pO_2} + K.\mathrm{pCO}} \tag{8}$$

Experimental findings show that when very little CO is present in the air, a relatively large proportion of the haemoglobin is converted into carboxyhaemoglobin, and this explains the very poisonous nature of the gas when such gas mixtures are inhaled. The results indicate also that in a person, who is poisoned with CO, and who is administered pure O_2 instead of air, there will be a favourable rate of conversion of carboxyhaemoglobin into oxyhaemoglobin (see section 5). The high blood concentration of O_2 in such a case will tend to displace CO from carboxyhaemoglobin by mass action (equation 9).

$$\mathrm{HbCO} + \mathrm{O_2} \rightleftarrows \mathrm{HbO_2} + \mathrm{CO} \tag{9}$$

CO will be eliminated by the pulmonary route.

Haldane[43] pointed out that anoxic symptoms caused by CO poisoning greatly surpass in severity those of anaemia, where the blood O_2 content is the same in the two conditions. The main reasons for the difference between the CO poisoning and anaemia seem to be the alteration of the dissociation curve produced by partial conversion of haemoglobin into carboxyhaemoglobin,

[42] J. Sendroy, S. H. Lui, and D. D. Van Slyke, *Am. J. Physiol.*, 1929, **90**, 511.
[43] J. B. S. Haldane, *J. Physiol.*, 1912, **45**, xxii.

and the lack of cardio-respiratory adjustment to CO poisoning.[44,45] In order to account for all of the data,[44,45] it is necessary to consider the blood supply to the brain, which is the organ that is most susceptible to injury through lack of O_2. When the O_2-tension in blood from the brain was estimated as the rate of O_2 used, and the blood-flow, the arterial O_2-content, and the O_2 dissociation were all specified, the results indicated that no important symptoms ought to be found below 30% saturation of the blood with CO, but above 40% saturation, a rapidly progressive toxicity would occur. It follows that it is possible to account for the toxicity of CO in mammals solely in terms of its reaction with haemoglobin (Scheme 1).

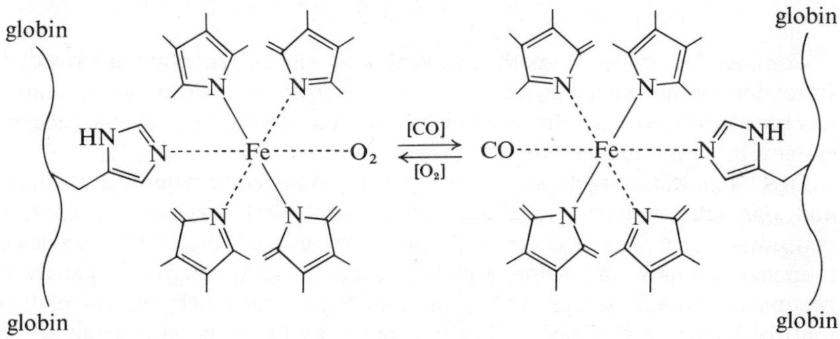

Scheme 1

(g) Another type of toxic action has to do either (i) with the reaction of toxic metals, such as lead and mercury and their derivatives (*e.g.* the organo mercurials) with biologically functional groups, or (ii) with the reaction of toxic substances, *e.g.* the dithiocarbamates, as well as of CN^- and HS^-, with the biologically functional metals belonging to prosthetic groups.

Mercurials, such as *p*-chloromercurio benzoate (PCMB) and *p*-chloromercuriophenyl sulphonate (PCMPS), exemplify the first class of agent, and like the parent metal and its inorganic compounds, they owe their toxicity to mercaptide formation. Whilst the detailed mode of action has not been elucidated, definitive studies have been made on the generation of mercaptides with sulphydryl enzymes.

Thus, reaction of PCMPS with rabbit-muscle glyceraldehyde-3-phosphate dehydrogenase[46] caused enzyme inactivation when 3 moles of inhibitor had been bound and the 2 moles of bound DNP had been released. Both effects were instantaneously reversed by addition of cellular nucleophiles such as cysteine. Although the *prima facie* evidence suggests involvement of SH groups in the binding of nucleotide, in fact conformational changes are involved[47,48] (Scheme 2).

[44] F. J. W. Roughton and R. C. Darling, *Am. J. Physiol.*, 1944, **141**, 17.
[45] N. Joels and L. G. C. E. Pugh, *J. Physiol.*, 1958, **142**, 63.
[46] S. F. Velick, *J. Biol. Chem.*, 1953, **203**, 563.
[47] S. F. Velick, *J. Biol. Chem.*, 1958, **233**, 1455.
[48] P. D. Boyer and A. R. Schültz, in 'Sulphur in Proteins,' ed. R. Benesch *et al.*, Academic Press, New York, 1959, p. 199.

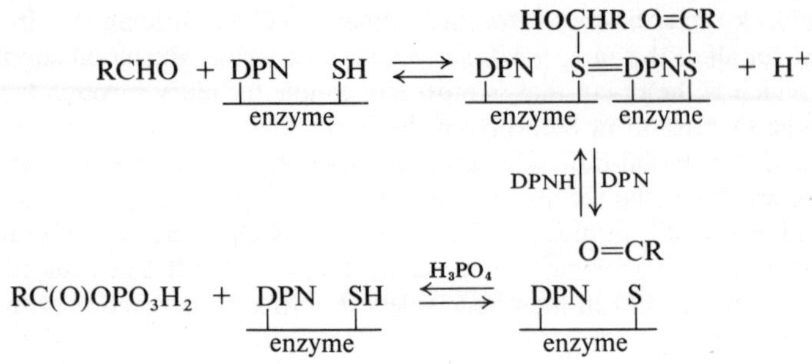

Scheme 2

Considerable evidence, both chemical and kinetic, supports intermediate formation of an acyl enzyme.[49–51] The chemistry of mercaptide formation has been discussed from the viewpoint of specificity in respect of other enzyme systems including muscle phosphorylase.[52–54]

DDC fungicides, such as sodium dimethyldithiocarbamate and its ferric and zinc salts, ferbam and ziram, inhibit sulphydryl enzymes and enzymes dependent upon iron and copper. Chefurka[55] showed that DDC fungicides inhibited strongly the sulphydryl-dependent house-fly enzymes, glucose-6-phosphate dehydrogenase and 6-phosphonogluconate dehydrogenase, and that the antagonism might be alleviated partly by the addition of cysteine. He concluded that DDC fungicides act on sulphydryl-dependent enzymes of the aerobic hexose monophosphate oxidation pathway. Goksøyer[56] found that DDC compounds do not inhibit respiration by blocking ATP, but by inhibition of succinic dehydrogenase. Kaars Sijpesteijn and Janssen[57] concluded from their own work and that of others that DDC fungicides inhibit enzymes with an essential dithiol grouping, and they suggested that enzymes thus inhibited are dependent on dihydrolipoic acid as co-enzyme. Owens' work[58] indicated that ferbam and thiram inhibit at least one enzyme in the synthesis of citrate from acetate. As the toxicity of ferbam and thiram depends on their capacity to produce free radicals, and as ziram cannot form them, Owens[58] suggested that the inactivation of aconitase by ziram would involve the abstraction of Fe from the enzyme and its replacement by Zn to afford the more stable Fe–DDC chelate.

Twenty years' research was summarized by Ludwig and Thorn,[59] who proposed that the DDC type of dithiocarbamate cannot be separated properly

[49] O. J. Koeppe, P. D. Boyer, and M. P. Stulberg, *J. Biol. Chem.*, 1956, **219**, 569.
[50] I. Krimsky and E. Racker, *Science*, 1955, **122**, 319.
[51] E. Racker and I. Krimsky, *J. Biol. Chem.*, 1952, **198**, 731.
[52] N. B. Madsen and C. F. Cori, *J. Biol. Chem.*, 1956, **233**, 1055.
[53] N. B. Madsen and F. R. N. Gurd, *J. Biol. Chem.*, 1956, **223**, 1075.
[54] N. B. Madsen, *J. Biol. Chem.*, 1956, **223**, 1067.
[55] W. Chefurka, *Enzymologia*, 1956, **18**, 209.
[56] J. Goksøyr, *Univ. Bergen Årbok. Naturvitensk. Rekke*, 1958, 1.
[57] A. Kaars Sijpesteijn and M. J. Janssen, *Antonie van Leeuwenhoek J. Microbiol. Serol.*, 1959, **25**, 422.
[58] R. G. Owens, in 'Developments in Industrial Microbiology,' ed. B. Miller, Plenum Press, New York, 1960, vol. 1, p. 187.
[59] R. A. Ludwig and G. D. Thorn, *Adv. Pest Control Res.*, 1960, **3**, 219.

from the ethylenebisdithiocarbamate type, which includes nabam and zineb. The nabam-type fungicides share all of the reactions of the DDC type *in vivo*, and they have some additional ones. This greater reactivity is associated most probably with the mobile H on the N atom, which is present in the nabam molecule but absent from DDC ones.

Complication arises when operatives, who have been exposed occupationally to dithiocarbamates, take alcoholic drinks. These compounds, by inhibiting the liver NAD-dependent acetaldehyde dehydrogenase, cause toxic acetaldehyde to accumulate and thereby block detoxication of the ethanol. This information led to the development of the disulphuram treatment for alcoholism.

(h) The possibility that O_2-toxicity involved the antagonism of essential cellular reactions goes back to the time of Bert,[60] and, by the time of the World War II studies by Bean, Dickens, and Stadie *et al.* (*v. infra*), some investigations of the mechanism of O_2-toxicity had been made. Thus, it had been established (i) that O_2 was capable of inactivating a number of enzymes,[61,62] and (ii) that the respiration of brain homogenates and slices was depressed significantly under hyperbaric oxygenation.[63–65] These early observations were extended greatly by the work of Dickens[66,67] and of Stadie *et al.*[68–75] (*v. supra*), who found that, although some enzymes were resistant to O_2-toxicity, many others were easily inhibited by O_2 at high pressures and even at the concentration present in air. Sulphydryl enzymes were especially susceptible to O_2-toxicity.[67,68] Experimental conditions were very important, as some enzymes that were readily inactivated *in vitro* were resistant to O_2-toxicity *in vivo*, and, as normal, physiological metabolites, coenzymes, and metal ions influenced enzyme inhibition by O_2 *in vitro*.[64,66,67,69,75]

Despite the conclusive demonstration of enzyme inhibition by O_2,[76] there has been some reluctance to conclude that the inhibitory effects of O_2 on metabolism are the direct cause of the symptoms of O_2-toxicity in the intact animal.[77–79]

[60] P. Bert, 'La Pression Barométrique,' Masson and Cie, Paris, 1878.
[61] J. W. Bean, *Physiol. Rev.*, 1945, **25**, 1.
[62] W. C. Stadie, B. C. Riggs, and N. Haugaard, *Am. J. Med. Sci.*, 1944, **207**, 84.
[63] K. A. C. Elliott and B. Libet, *J. Biol. Chem.*, 1942, **143**, 227.
[64] P. J. G. Mann and J. H. Quastel, *Biochem. J.*, 1946, **40**, 139.
[65] H. van Goor and J. Jongblood, *Arch. Neerl. Physiol.*, 1942, **26**, 407.
[66] F. Dickens, *Biochem. J.*, 1946, **40**, 145.
[67] F. Dickens, *Biochem. J.*, 1946, **40**, 170.
[68] N. Haugaard, *J. Biol. Chem.*, 1946, **164**, 265.
[69] W. C. Stadie and N. Haugaard, *J. Biol. Chem.*, 1945, **161**, 153.
[70] W. C. Stadie and N. Haugaard, *J. Biol. Chem.*, 1945, **161**, 181.
[71] W. C. Stadie and N. Haugaard, *J. Biol. Chem.*, 1946, **164**, 257.
[72] W. C. Stadie, B. C. Riggs, and N. Haugaard, *J. Biol. Chem.*, 1945, **160**, 191.
[73] W. C. Stadie, B. C. Riggs, and N. Haugaard, *J. Biol. Chem.*, 1945, **160**, 209.
[74] W. C. Stadie, B. C. Riggs, and N. Haugaard, *J. Biol. Chem.*, 1945, **161**, 175.
[75] W. C. Stadie, B. C. Riggs, and N. Haugaard, *J. Biol. Chem.*, 1945, **161**, 189.
[76] N. Haugaard, *Physiol. Rev.*, 1968, **48(2)**, 311.
[77] H. C. Davies and R. E. Davies, in 'Handbook of Physiology, Respiration,' ed. W. O. Fenn and H. Rahn, *Am. Physiol. Soc.*, Washington D.C., 1965, section 3, vol. 11, pp. 1047—1058.
[78] F. Dickens, in 'Neurochemistry,' ed. K. A. C. Elliott, I. H. Page, and J. H. Quastel, Thomas, Springfield, Illinois, 2nd edn., 1962, pp. 851—869.
[79] N. Haugaard, in 'Oxygen in the Animal Organism,' ed. F. Dickens and E. Neil, Macmillan, New York, 1964, pp. 495—505.

Haugaard[76] gives two reasons for this. 'First, inactivation of enzymes *in vitro* appeared to be too slow in onset to account for the symptoms that occurred so rapidly in the intact animal. Second, no conclusive demonstration had been made that any enzyme, in any organ of the intact animal, was inhibited during exposure of the animal to O_2 at an elevated pressure.'

There are now several examples of the inactivation *in vivo* of enzymes which are essential to intermediary metabolism, some of which are given in Table 1.

Table 1

Biochemical description	*Enzyme*	*Organism*	*Ref.*
Pyruvate oxidation[a]		*S.aureus, E.coli, Azotobacter, etc.*	80–84
α-Oxoglutarate oxidation[a]		*Azotobacter*	84
Acetate dissimilation[a]	Phosphate transacetylase	*Azotobacter*	85
Citric acid cycle[a]	Aconitase	Pea seed	86
Citric acid cycle[a]		Potato tuber	87

[a]All of these examples (*v. supra*) were described by N. Haugaard,[76] and some further examples are appended (*v. infra*).

NAD+ biosynthesis	Quinolinate synthetase	*E. coli*	88, 89
Aromatic amino-acid biosynthesis		*E. coli*	90, 91
Branched chain amino-acid biosynthesis	Dihydroxyacid dehydratase	*E. coli*	92, 93
Purine biosynthesis	Aminophosphoribosyl transferase	Human placenta	94
Purine biosynthesis	Aminophosphoribosyl transferase	*B. subtilis*	95

A continuing search for other enzymes that are altered by O_2-toxicity and the thorough investigation of those chemical reactions which bring about

[80] J. Caldwell, *Nature*, 1964, **201**, 514.
[81] E. S. Guzman Barron, *J. Biol. Chem.*, 1936, **113**, 695.
[82] M. J. Wolin, J. B. Evans, and C. J. Niven, *Arch. Biochem. Biophys.*, 1956, **58**, 356.
[83] M. J. Dilworth and C. A. Parker, *Nature*, 1961, **19**, 520.
[84] M. J. Dilworth, *Biochim. Biophys. Acta*, 1962, **56**, 127.
[85] M. J. Dilworth and I. R. Kennedy, *Biochim. Biophys. Acta*, 1963, **67**, 240.
[86] G. G. Pritchard, *J. Expl. Botany*, 1961, **12**, 353.
[87] J. Barker and L. W. Mapson, *Proc. Roy. Soc.*, 1955, **143**, 523.
[88] R. L. Brunker and O. R. Brown, *Microbios*, 1971, **4**, 193.
[89] O. R. Brown in 'Biochemical and Clinical Aspects of Oxygen,' ed. W. S. Caughey, Academic Press, New York, 1979, pp. 755—766.
[90] D. E. Boehme, K. Vincent, and O. R. Brown, *Nature*, 1976, **262**, 418.
[91] J. A. Fee in 'Oxygen and Oxy-radicals in Chemistry and Biology,' ed. M. A. J. Rodgers and E. L. Powers, Academic Press, New York, 1981, in the press.
[92] O. R. Brown and F. Yein, *Biochem. Biophys. Res. Commun.*, 1978, **85**, 1219.
[93] J. A. Fee, A. C. Lees, P. Z. Bloch, P. L. Gilliland, and O. R. Brown, *Biochem. Int.*, 1981, **1**, 304.
[94] M. Itakura and E. W. Holmes, *J. Biol. Chem.*, 1979, **254**, 333.
[95] R. L. Switzer, M. R. Maurizi, J. Y. Wong, J. S. Brabson, and E. Meyer in 'Limited Proteolysis in Micro-organisms,' ed. G. Cohen and H. Holzer, DHEW Publication No. (NIH) 79-1591, US Government Printing Office, Washington, DC.

enzyme inhibition, would seem to provide a promising approach to a more detailed understanding of O_2-toxicity.[96]

It ought to be made clear at this stage that a rival theory, which made free radicals responsible for O_2-toxicity,[97] has been the subject of investigation for over one-quarter of a century. This proposition was made soon after the time when Waters, one of the protagonists of free-radical chemistry, wrote a famous book,[98] and at the time when free-radical chemistry was beginning to enjoy a wide reputation. In the present context, what became known as 'the superoxide theory' rested on the assumption (i) the O_2^- is formed in biological systems, (ii) that O_2^- is extremely toxic to cellular constituents, and (iii) that superoxide dismutases destroy O_2^-, and are therefore vital to the protection of aerobiasis.[99]

$$2\,O_2^- + 2\,H^+ \longrightarrow H_2O_2 + O_2$$

This theory achieved a measure of immediate credibility, as considerable evidence supported premise (i). Only much later did more intensive research and reasonable chemical supposition[96] begin to undermine the position of the superoxide theory.

With regard to proposition (iii), whilst the occurrence of superoxide dismutases has been found to be widespread, and many observations[99–105] have been brought together in support of this hypothesis, some conflicting results have been exposed, and some of the foregoing observations (*q.v.*) are capable of alternative explanation. Thus, a more extensive survey of micro-organisms showed the presence of superoxide dismutase in varying amounts in a variety of strictly anaerobic organisms.[106–112] Whilst there is no correlation between the amounts of dismutase in the anaerobes and their capacity to withstand O_2, and even the presence of this enzyme in organisms that never encounter O_2 does not agree with present ideas about cellular economy, the significance of these results is uncertain. However, the fact that other aerobic organisms consume O_2 and

96 J. A. Fee in 'Oxygen and Life: Second BOC Priestley Conference,' Special Publication No. 39, The Royal Society of Chemistry, London, 1981, pp. 77—97.
97 R. Gersham, D. L. Gilbert, S. W. Nye, P. Dwyer, and W. O. Fenn, *Science*, 1954, **119**, 623.
98 W. A. Waters, 'The Chemistry of Free Radicals', The Clarendon Press, Oxford, 2nd. edn., 1948.
99 J. M. McCord, B. B. Keele, and I. Fridovich, *Proc. Nat. Acad. Sci. USA*, 1971, **68**, 1024.
100 H. M. Hassan and I. Fridovich in 'Strategies of Microbial Life in Extreme Environments,' ed. M. Shilo, Verlag-Chemie, Weinheim, 1979, pp. 179—193.
101 H. M. Hassan and I. Fridovich, *J. Biol. Chem.*, 1977, **252**, 7667.
102 J. A. Fee, A. C. Lees, P. L. Bloch, and F. C. Neidhardt, in 'Biochemical and Clinical Aspects of Oxygen,' ed. W. S. Caughey, Academic Press, New York, 1979, pp. 635—658.
103 H. M. Hassan and I. Fridovich, *J. Biol. Chem.*, 1979, **254**, 10846.
104 H. M. Hassan and I. Fridovich, *Arch. Biochem. Biophys.*, 1979, **196**, 385.
105 H. M. Hassan and I. Fridovich, *Rev. Inf. Diseases*, 1979, **1**, 357.
106 J. Hewitt and J. G. Morris, *FEBS Lett.*, 1975, **50**, 315.
107 F. P. Tally, B. R. Goldin, N. V. Jacobus, and S. Z. Gorbach, *Infect. Immunity*, 1977, **16**, 20.
108 D. G. Lindmark and M. Müller, *J. Biol. Chem.*, 1974, **249**, 4634.
109 E. C. Hatchikian and Y. A. Henry, *Biochemie*, 1977, **59**, 153.
110 J. Carlsson, J. Wrether, and G. Beckman, *J. Clin. Microbiol.*, 1977, **6**, 280.
111 E. M. Gregory, W. E. C. Moore, and L. V. Holdeman, *Appl. Environ. Microbiol.*, 1978, **35**, 988.
112 S. Kanematsu and K. Asada, *FEBS Lett.*, 1978, **91**, 94.

form O_2^-, but lack dismutase,[113–115] contradicts the concept of the requirement of dismutases for aerobiasis.

In a similar vein, the alleged induction of Mn protein (*i.e.* a dismutase) in *E. coli* strains, and their improved resistance to hyperoxia is misleading,[80,93,116] as neither hyperoxia nor the inducing agent is bacteriocidal. It would now appear from other work[90,102,117,118] that in fact the inducing process brings about some sort of adaptation of the cell contents.

If the second part, (ii), of the superoxide theory is considered, no reaction of O_2^- has proved to be toxic to a cell. In fact, O_2^- rather like F^- is pretty unreactive, and it appears not to be responsible for various degradative reactions attributed to it, where O_2^- is undoubtedly present but where superoxide dismutase serves to protect the substrates in question. In addition, fundamental O_2^- chemistry, and careful studies[119] of the effect of O_2^-, H_2O_2, and metal ions on biological substances, as well as reasonable chemical supposition about the availability of intracellular-ion participation in Fenton chemistry, imply that neither O_2^- nor Fenton-initiated O_2^- reactions are likely to cause toxicity.

On the present evidence, the conclusion is drawn that the production of free radicals does not account for O_2-toxicity, and that future progress with this problem stems from the alternative sensitive enzyme approach (*v. supra*).

The foregoing treatment of toxicants as antagonists is not meant to be exhaustive, but rather to delineate underlying principles. Several cases apart from the ones already mentioned, including the biochemical changes responsible for aldrin/dieldrin and Telodrin convulsive states, CCl_4-induced fatty infiltration of the liver, and paraquat poisoning, will be discussed under the heading of 'mechanisms of toxicity' (chapter 9). Whilst irradiation presents contingent material, it is felt that this is a special subject in its own right, and as it is very difficult to separate the resulting enzyme activations and inhibitions, inhibition due to radiation will be excluded from present considerations. Finally, in example (h), the fact that extensive researches were implemented on the superoxide theory, which was subsequently proved to be largely irrelevant to O_2-toxicity, stresses the need to ensure that the biochemical changes which are being investigated are relevant to the causative mechanism.

4 Kinetics of Inhibition

There is a strong supposition that in those cases where a toxicant functions as an antagonist, and where the receptor is a single enzyme system, the toxic effects might be explained in terms of enzyme inhibition. It would now appear that, inasmuch as the kinetics have been investigated, this concept is reasonably correct.

Thus, if an organophosphorus ester (O.P.) AB combines with receptor cholinesterase (RH) to give a relatively stable (phosphorylated) product (RA), then:

113 P. Norrod and S. A. Morse, *Biochem. Biophys. Res. Commun.*, 1979, **90**, 1287.
114 T. Kirby, J. Blum, I. Kahane, and I. Fridovich, *Arch. Biochem. Biophys.*, 1980, **201**, 551.
115 C. Deeters-Joris, A.-M. Vandevoorde, and P. Baudhuin, *Biochem. J.* 1975, **150**, 31.
116 O. R. Brown, H. F. Howitt, J. L. Stees, and W. S. Platner, *J. Lipid Res.*, 1971, **12**, 692.
117 P. L. Bloch, T. A. Phillips, and F. C. Neidhardt, *J. Bact.*, 1980, **141**, 1409.
118 D. P. Nierlich, *Ann. Rev. Microbiol.*, 1978, **32**, 393.
119 J. A. Fee, in 'Metal Ion Activation of Dioxygen,' ed. T. G. Spiro, John Wiley and Sons, New York, 1980, pp. 209—237.

$$RH + AB \xrightarrow{k_a} RA + BH \qquad (1)$$

where k_a is the rate constant for combination of AB with RH.

As the concentration of inhibitor is at least 10 times that of the enzyme, the bimolecular reaction (equation 1) almost always affords first-order kinetics. AB probably reacts with the prosthetic group (catalytic centre), as the addition of substrate greatly diminishes the rate of reaction of O.P.s with enzyme. In that connexion, this and other evidence[120–123] show that the structural requirements of the substrate (AB) resemble those of effective inhibitors. Accordingly, the inclusion of a Michaelis complex (see equation 2) into equation 1 would appear relevant. Thus:

$$RH + AB \underset{k_{-1}}{\overset{k_{+1}}{\rightleftharpoons}} RHAB \xrightarrow{k_{+2}} RA + BH \qquad (2)$$

Substrate saturation phenomena, for example, would be consistent with such complex formation, *i.e.* the rate of phosphorylation ought to be maximal, if all of the unphosphorylated enzyme were present in complex form.

k_{+2} was fairly rapid, and Main *et al.*[124,125] established the conditions necessary for its measurement (equation 3). Thus:

$$\frac{[AB]}{k} = \frac{[AB]}{k_{+2}} = \frac{K_a}{k_{+2}} \qquad (3)$$

where k is the first-order rate constant for formation of RA with a given [AB], and K_a is a constant analogous to K_m for hydrolysis of AB to BH (it is in fact the [AB] when the rate of enzyme phosphorylation is one-half of the maximum rate).

Thus, K_a may be regarded as a measure of the affinity of AB for RH, and is an expression of the association–dissociation of the complex RHAB (equation 2). Some phosphorylated enzymes may be unstable, and in that case, equation 2 may be extended to the form of equation 4:

$$RH + AB \underset{k_{-1}}{\overset{k_{+1}}{\rightleftharpoons}} RHAB \xrightarrow{k_{+2}} BH + RA \xrightarrow{k_{+3}} RH + AOB \qquad (4)$$

$$\ln\left(\frac{[RH_0]}{[RH_0] - [RA]}\right) = \frac{k_{+2}\ [AB].t}{K_a + [AB]} \qquad (5)$$

[120] W. N. Aldridge, *Biochem. J.*, 1953, **53**, 62.
[121] A. S. V. Burgen and F. Hobbiger, *Br. J. Pharmacol.*, 1951, **6**, 593.
[122] D. F. Heath and M. Vandekar, *Biochem. J.*, 1957, **67**, 187.
[123] T. R. Fukuto, R. L. Metcalf, R. B. March, and M. G. Maxon, *J. Am. Chem. Soc.*, 1955, **77**, 3670.
[124] A. R. Main and F. Iverson, *Biochem. J.*, 1966, **100**, 525.
[125] A. R. Main and W. C. Dauterman, *Nature*, 1963, **198**, 551.

where $[RH_0]$ is the total enzyme concentration, t is the time of reaction, and $K_a = (k_{+2} + k_{-1})/k_{+1}$.

When the concentration of RHAB is negligible, equation 4 reduces to equation 1, in which case:

$$\ln\left(\frac{[RH_0]}{[RH_0] - [RA]}\right) = k_a[AB].t \tag{6}$$

When $[AB] \leqslant K_a$, it follows from equations 5 and 6 that $k_a = k_{2+}/K_a$. If

$$RA + H_2O \xrightarrow{k_{+3}} RH + AOH \qquad (7) \quad [\text{see } (4)]$$

the integrated form corresponding to (7) is $\ln\left(\frac{[RA_0]}{[RA]}\right) = k_{+3}\, t$, where $[RA_0]$ is the initial concentration of the phosphorylated enzyme. Furthermore, Aldridge and Reiner[126] considered: (a) reversible inhibition of AChE by two O.P.s.; (b) the influence of substrate on reversible inhibition; and (c) the influence of substrate on progressive inhibition.

In the case of (a), the rate constant, k, for a given inhibitor concentration is defined by equation 8:

$$k = \frac{(k_{+2}/K_a)\,[AB]}{1 + [AB]/K_a} \tag{8}$$

This rearranges to give equation 3 (*v. supra*).

When $[AB]/k$ is plotted against $[AB]$, the slope is $1/k_{+2}$, and the intercept is K_a/k_{+2}. But an alternative mechanism (equation 9) affords an analogous equation (equation 10) to equation 3.

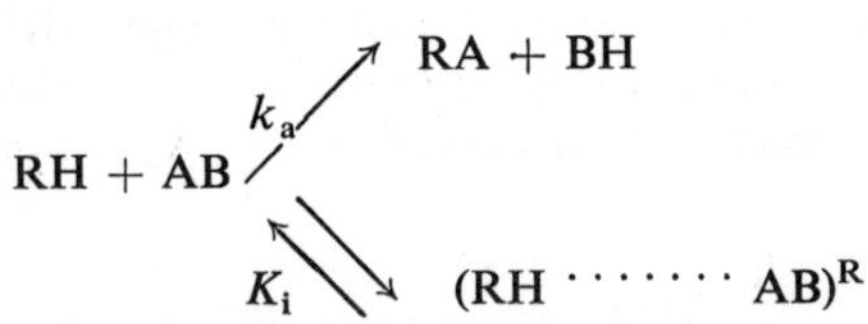

(9)

$$\frac{AB}{k} = \frac{1}{k_a} + \frac{[AB]}{k_a K_i} \tag{10}$$

Thus, according to whether the mechanism is defined by equation 4 or 9, a graph of $[AB]/k$ *vs.* $[AB]$ would give either k_a and K_i (equation 10) or K_a and k_{+2} (equation 3).

[126] W. N. Aldridge and E. Reiner, *Biochem. J.*, 1969, **115**, 147.

In the case of (b), the results have been analysed by the method of Hunter and Downs,[127] using equation 11:

$$\frac{v[\mathrm{AB}]}{v_o - v} = K_i + \frac{K_i[\mathrm{S}]}{K_m} \tag{11}$$

where v_o is the enzymic activity in the absence of inhibition, and v is the enzymic activity in the presence of inhibition.

In the case of (c), the first-order rate constant (k') for progressive inhibition in the presence of substrate for the system described by equation 9 is defined by equation 12:

$$k' = \frac{k_a[\mathrm{AB}]}{1 + \frac{[\mathrm{S}]}{K_m} + \frac{[\mathrm{S}]}{K_{ss}} + \frac{[\mathrm{S}]^2}{K_m K_s} + \frac{[\mathrm{AB}]}{K_i} + \frac{[\mathrm{AB}][\mathrm{S}]}{K_m K_i}} \tag{12}$$

Enough has been said to show that the inhibitory process is identical with substrate reactions. The hydrolysis of substrates is pH-dependent, and the inhibition of AChE by O.P.s has been shown to be a function of pH.[128,129] Finally, the inhibition of AChE by high concentrations of the natural substrate has been shown also to have inhibitor implications.[130–132]

As the P atom of the O.P. can be recovered from the phosphorylated enzyme as a serine derivative after degradation,[133,134] a serine residue(s) in AChE would appear to be involved in the catalytic process, despite the fact that serine is not a reactive molecule *per se*.[135]

The same sort of phenomenon to the foregoing holds as well in the case of AChE inhibition by the carbamates ROC(O)NHR′. Monomethyl- and dimethyl-carbamates react with AChE to give carbamoylated enzymes,[136,137] which are unstable (see equation 4); free enzyme is regenerated from monomethyl- and dimethyl-carbamoylated AChE with $t_{0.5}$ values respectively of 30 and 56 min at pH 8 and 25 °C.[138] Other carbamoylated AChE are much more stable. Some K_{+2} and K_a values have been determined, and Main *et al.* (*loc. cit.*) showed that for eserine, k_{+2} = 10.8 min^{-1} and K_a = 3.3 μM, and for phenylmethylcarbamate, k_{+2} = 7.1 min^{-1} and K_a = 26 μM. Thus, O.P.s and carbamates react with AChE to produce relatively stable acylated enzymes.

127 A. Hunter and C. E. Downs, *J. Biol. Chem.*, 1945, **157**, 427.
128 I. B. Wilson and F. Bergmann, *J. Biol. Chem.*, 1950, **185**, 479.
129 D. Nachmansohn, 'Chemical and Molecular Basis of Nerve Activity,' Academic Press, New York, 1959, pp. 120, 121.
130 K. B. Augustinsson, *Acta Physiol. Scand.*, 1948, **15**, Suppl. 52, 1.
131 D. Nachmansohn, ref. 129, p. 49.
132 I. B. Wilson and F. Bergmann, *J. Biol. Chem.*, 1950, **186**, 683.
133 N. K. Schaffer, S. C. May, and W. H. Summerson, *J. Biol. Chem.*, 1953, **202**, 67.
134 N. K. Schaffer, S. C. May, and W. H. Summerson, *J. Biol. Chem.*, 1954, **206**, 201.
135 R. D. O'Brien, in 'Metabolic Inhibitors,' ed. R. M. Hochster and J. H. Quastel, Academic Press, New York and London, 1963, vol. 2, pp. 205—241.
136 I. B. Wilson, M. A. Hatch, and S. Ginsburg, *J. Biol. Chem.*, 1960, **235**, 2312.
137 I. B. Wilson, M. A. Harrison, and S. Ginsburg, *J. Biol. Chem.*, 1961, **236**, 1498.
138 E. Reiner and W. N. Aldridge, *Biochem. J.*, 1967, **105**, 171.

(Because of their greater lability, carbamoylated enzymes have not been degraded to give amino-acid derivatives.)

The kinetic approach to cyanide poisoning and interaction with the respiratory chain does not seem to have progressed very far, although the interaction itself (section 3) is well-established. However, early work[139] with yeast cells showed that CN^- reacted with at least three sites in the respiratory chain, that CN^- inhibition was non-competitive with respect to O_2-uptake, and that K_i values for the rate-limiting reaction and for the fast terminal oxidase reaction were respectively, 3.7×10^{-5} and 1.4×10^{-5}.

5 Antidotes to Poisoning, with Special Reference to Antagonism

There is a strong supposition that in those cases (i) where antagonism is competitive (*q.v.*), potent antidotes would compete with the action of the toxicants concerned. But, (ii) where antagonism is non-competitive, and where biochemical lesions are formed, the only antidotes that are feasible would react rapidly with the still unchanged toxicant.

(i) Organophosphate insecticides (sections 3 and 4) provide outstanding exemplification of those toxicants that behave as competitive antagonists; in this case, the receptor is acetylcholinesterase AChE. A clue to the possibility that suitable antidotes might be found arose from the storage of phosphorylated enzyme in buffer, by which some 50% of the AChE activity was eventually restored (see also equations 4 and 8—10, section 4), and solutions of stronger nucleophiles such as hydroxylamine were found to be more favourable; but the rate of reaction by such means was too slow to be practical. On the basis of work by Wilson *et al.* (*v. supra*),[140] agents such as pralidoxime iodide (1) were developed

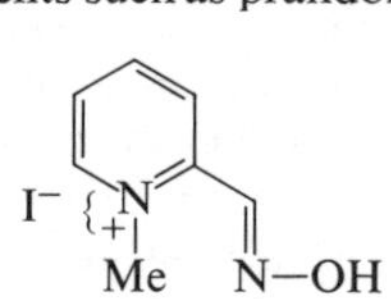

(1)

which, when injected i.v., counteracted the action of organophosphates by reactivating inhibited synaptic AChE. Thus, pralidoxime was found to be effective in human subjects poisoned with parathion.[141] Further work showed that animals treated with pralidoxime had high cerebral concentrations of acetylcholine,[142,143] which would have protected their lives, had they been subjected to organophosphate poisoning. Thus, besides reversing the phosphorylation of receptor protein in poisoned subjects, such antidotes may also act directly on synaptic receptor AChE. Atropine, in combination therapy against organophosphate poisoning, acts in a complementary way to the oxime. It does not

[139] R. J. Winzler, *J. Cellular Comp. Physiol.*, 1943, **11**, 229.
[140] I. B. Wilson and S. Ginsburg, *Biochim. Biophys. Acta*, 1955, **18**, 168.
[141] T. Namba and K. Hiraki, *J. Am. Med. Assoc.*, 1958, **166**, 1834.
[142] M. P. Milosevic, *J. Pharm. Pharmacol.*, 1969, **21**, 469.
[143] M. P. Milosevic, *Br. J. Pharmacol.*, 1970, **39**, 732.

antagonize the action of organophosphates at the neuromuscular junction, but by binding to synaptic receptor replaces acetylcholine, and blocks synaptic transmission.

In methaemoglobinaemia, where circulating erythrocyte haemoglobin has been oxidized to the Fe^{III} form, methaemoglobin, there is a natural tendency towards recovery. Methaemoglobin is reduced in low concentration to haemoglobin by a series of red-cell enzymes. The system, which is active in nitrite-methaemoglobinaemia, depends on DPN-reducing dehydrogenases, and in man this system deals with 5—10% of total pigment h^{-1}, whereas in aniline–phenylhydroxylamine-methaemoglobinaemia, reduction involves TPN-reducing dehydrogenases, including enzymes capable of decarboxylating glucose 6-phosphate. For methaemoglobinaemia treatment, the chemical changes involved in the reduction of methaemoglobin must not be coupled to haemoglobin oxidation, and several redox dyes, such as Methylene Blue (MB), meet these conditions. Thus,

$$\text{MB} + \text{TPN system} + \text{glucose} \longrightarrow \text{leuco MB} + \text{oxidation products} + CO_2$$

$$\text{leuco MB} + O_2 \longrightarrow \text{MB} + H_2O_2$$

$$\text{leuco MB} + \text{methaemoglobin} \rightleftarrows \text{MB} + \text{haemoglobin}$$

In this case, the presence of O_2 keeps the concentration of free haemoglobin very low. Equilibrium favours methaemoglobin reduction, and as the dehydrogenase systems are very active, Methylene Blue acts as an effective redox carrier which allows methaemoglobin to be reduced at the expense of glucose oxidation. Intravenous injection of Methylene Blue affords a fifty-fold acceleration in methaemoglobin reduction.

Experiments on the rate of removal of CO from circulating blood (section 3) have given conflicting results,[144,145] but inhalation of O_2 instead of air affords a six-fold acceleration in CO elimination, and the addition of CO_2 to the O_2 supply is alleged to increase the rate still more. It is about the composition of the O_2–CO_2 mixtures for resuscitation that controversy has been concerned, but the result of CO poisoning depends on the pO_2 in the brain and the duration of hypoxia. Provided that alveolar pO_2 is roused promptly by O_2 administration, the latter stages of recovery are relatively unimportant. On balance, whilst O_2–CO_2 mixtures may be superior to O_2 alone, the improvement may not amount to as much as has been claimed.[146–150] The fact that vitamin K may be used as an effective antidote against warfarin poisoning provides strong evidence for Quick and Collentine's[32] hypothesis that warfarin and vitamin K combine with the flavoprotein, vitamin K reductase.[151] However, as has been discussed (section 3),

144 F. J. W. Roughton and R. W. Root, *Am. J. Physiol.*, 1945, **145**, 239.
145 J. L. Lillienthal, *Pharmacol. Rev.*, 1950, **2**, 324.
146 K. W. McDonald and W. D. M. Paton, *Br. Med. J.*, 1955, **1**, 313.
147 K. W. McDonald and W. D. M. Paton, *Br. Med. J.*, 1955, **1**, 664.
148 Y. E. Henderson and H. W. Haggard, *J. Pharmacol.*, 1920, **16**, 11.
149 M. Nicloux, H. Nerson, J. Stahl, and J. Weill, *C.R. Soc. Biol.*, 1925, **92**, 174.
150 M. Nicloux, H. Nerson, J. Stahl, and J. Weill, *C.R. Soc. Biol.*, 1925, **92**, 178.
151 F. Marki and C. Martius, *Biochem. Z.*, 1960, **333**, 111.

this antagonism at any rate in an *in vitro* preparation does not appear to be competitive, and other evidence (*v. supra*) suggests that the antagonism concerned may be indirect.

(ii) Cyanide is an outstanding case of a toxicant which behaves as a non-competitive antagonist, and which produces a well-authenticated biochemical lesion (see section 3). Accordingly, antidotal procedures for a victim of poisoning deal with the detoxication of ingested CN^-.

Mitochondrial sulphur transferase (rhodanese) accommodates sub-lethal doses of CN^- (equations 13 and 14).[152–154]

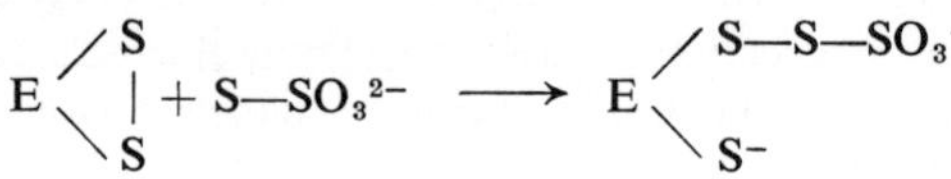
(13)

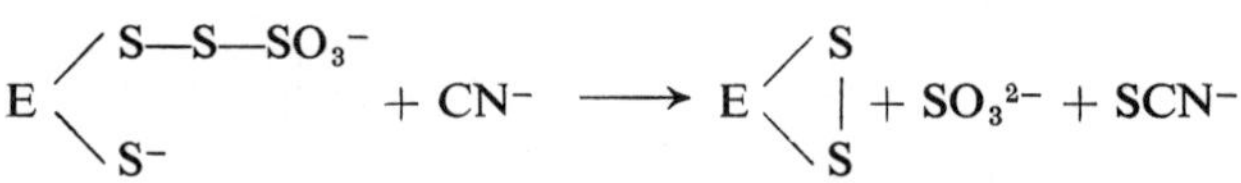
(14)

By these means, CN^- is converted into the non-toxic SCN^-, which is excreted in the urine and saliva.[152,153] Sulphur transferase is distributed widely in the mitochondria of the body, and the activity is greatest in the liver, the decreasing order of activity being frog > rabbit > cow > man > dog.[153] It has been found[155] that a whole dog liver has sufficient sulphur-transferase activity to catalyse the transformation of 4015 mg of cyanide in 15 min, and the whole sketetal muscle of the dog contained enough sulphur transferase activity to metabolize 1763 mg of cyanide. Thus, the mitochondrial sulphur-transferase activity of the body would appear adequate to prevent the inactivation of mitochondrial cytochrome a_3 by ingested CN^-, but the supply of sulphur substrate is limiting. Schmiedeberg[156] discovered the occurrence of thiosulphate *in vivo*, and this has been confirmed[157,158] more recently. Cysteine, cystine, glutathione, and β-mercaptopyruvic acid, which are not sulphur substrates, can act as sulphur donors.[159,160] However, mobilisation of sulphur from all sources is insufficient.

On this account, aqueous solutions of sodium thiosulphate are injected i.v. in cases of CN^- poisoning to enhance its detoxication (equations 13 and 14). This antidotal procedure supplements nitrite treatment, in which aqueous solutions of sodium nitrite are also injected i.v. The NO_2^- oxidizes a proportion of the circulating haemoglobin Fe^{II} into Fe^{III} and the resulting methaemoglobin

[152] S. Lang, *Arch. exp. Pathol. Pharmakol.*, 1894, **34**, 247.
[153] K. Lang, *Biochem. Z.*, 1933, **259**, 243.
[154] J. Schubert and W. A. Brill, *J. Pharmacol.*, 1968, **162**, 352.
[155] W. A. Himwich and J. P. Saunders, *Am. J. Physiol.*, 1948, **153**, 348.
[156] O. Schmiedeberg, *Arch. Heilk.*, 1867, **8**, 422.
[157] C. Fromageot and A. Royer, *Enzymologia*, 1945, **11**, 361.
[158] B. Vassel, R. Partridge, and M. L. Crossley, *Arch. Biochem.*, 1944, **4**, 59.
[159] R. T. Williams, 'Detoxication Mechanisms', Chapman and Hall, London, 1959, 2nd edn., pp. 390—396.
[160] K. K. Chen, C. L. Rose, and G. H. A. Clowes, *Am. J. Med. Sci.*, 1934, **188**, 767.

cannot transport O_2, but binds CN^- through its Fe^{III} iron to form the relatively non-toxic cyanomethaemoglobin complex. Administration of as much O_2 as possible to the poisoned victim is indispensible to this form of therapy. Combined nitrite–thiosulphate treatment is held to be synergistic, *i.e.* the effect of the combined therapy exceeds that of the sum of the separate effects, and since the cyanide–thiocyanate reaction is reversible, owing to thiocyanate oxidase,[161] the victim of CN^- poisoning ought to be carefully monitored. Although hydroxy-cobalamin (vitamin B_{12a}) complexes cyanide, its antidotal action is not as effective as that of the sodium nitrite–sodium thiosulphate treatment.[162]

In the case of fluoroacetate poisoning (section 3), the citric acid cycle in susceptible organs and tissues becomes blocked, and in Telodrin poisoning,[163–165] cerebral citric acid-cycle intermediates are syphoned-off at a rate which is in-commensurate with the normal functioning of the cycle. It will be seen that prompt administration of the respective intermediary metabolites, *viz.* of acetate or glutamate, would enhance the fueling of the citric acid cycle in the two cases, but that the resulting biochemical lesions, *viz.* aconitase inhibition in the case of fluoroacetate poisoning and marked glutamine synthesis in that of Telodrin poisoning, would remain. In the two cases, only a proportion of the poisoned animals which were given antidotal treatment in this way would be expected to survive intoxication, and this was indeed found to be the case. The phrase 'all or none effect' is used sometimes to describe such cases of intoxication.

Snake-bite constitutes a fine example, where the venom acts as a non-competitive antagonist at one or more receptor sites. It ought to be explained that antibodies can be raised to the various snake-venom antigens in mammals, usually in the horse. Antidotal procedure includes the prompt intravenous infiltration of a dilute solution of the appropriate horse anti-serum to form precipitin(s) in the circulating blood with unchanged venom antigen(s).[166] Lethal amounts of venom can sometimes be removed immediately after the bite by incision and suction. As the effects caused by the venom of the many different snakes vary dramatically, medical care in envenomation is essential.

6 Unspecific Toxicants, where there is No Obvious Receptor Implication

As has been argued previously (chapter 4), volatile general anaesthetics are a class of drug for which the drug-receptor concept seems to be inapplicable, and biological action depends on the thermodynamic activity; *i.e.* ΔG, the difference in Gibbs Free Energy between standard and biologically active states, is approximately the same for most compounds, irrespective of the absolute values of ΔG.

[161] F. Goldstein and F. Rieders, *Am. J. Physiol.*, 1953, **173**, 287
[162] C. L. Rose, R. M. Worth, K. Kikuchi, and K. K. Chen, *Proc. Soc. Exp. Biol. Med.*, 1965, **120**, 780.
[163] D. E. Hathway and A. P Mallinson, *Biochem. J.*, 1964, **90**, 61.
[164] D. E. Hathway, A. Mallinson, and D. A. A. Akintonwa, *Biochem. J.*, 1965, **94**, 676.
[165] D. E. Hathway, *Arch. Environ. Health.*, 1965, **11**, 380.
[166] J. H. Brown, 'Toxicology and Pharmacology of Venoms from Poisonous Snakes,' Charles. C. Thomas, Springfield, Illinois, 1973.

Furthermore, application of this principle to a wide range of bromochlorofluoroalkanes led to the discovery of halothane, $CF_3CHClBr$, undoubtedly the best anaesthetic known. As the individual substances (cyclopropane, ethanol, diethyl ether, chloroform, 1,1,2-trichloroethylene, halothane, as well as Xe, N_2O, *etc.*) represent whole classes of aliphatic and inorganic compounds, it follows that the toxicity of the paraffins, alcohols, dialkyl ethers, halogenoalkanes, and chloroalkenes is also unspecific, and the c.n.s. symptoms, which are found tend to support this supposition.

For other compounds, such as the industrial solvents (including the chloromethanes, -ethanes and -benzenes), together with the industrial alcohols, esters and ketones, the same unspecific principle seems to hold. Narcosis increases following the substitution pattern: alkanes < alcohols < dialkyl ethers < halogenoalkanes. Cyclopropane, chloroform, and 1,1,2-trichloroethylene ('Trilene') have been used extensively as anaesthetics. Anaesthetic potency and toxicity parallel one another. Whilst the liver and/or kidneys may be affected in the resulting states of anaesthesia, no single action relates to the drug-receptor category. Certain rough rules emerge, and in the case of the halogenoalkanes, toxic effects seem to depend on the ionisation of the C—X bond, and this suggests that there is perhaps some movement away from the entirely unspecific concept. In the case of petroleum, the n-hexane component is oxidized *in vivo* in the $(\omega-1)$ position to yield hexan-2-ol, and such substances would afford c.n.s. effects *via* the corresponding ketones.

A third group of unspecific substances comprise the lung irritants.[167] There are highly water-soluble compounds such as NH_3, HCl, formaldehyde, S_2Cl_2, and acrolein, which affect the eyes, larnyx, and trachea, less water-soluble ones such as the acyl chlorides, Cl_2, Br_2, SO_2, and bisisocyanates, which act on the bronchae and bronchioles, and the sparingly water-soluble NO_2, O_3, CdO, $CoCl_2$, *etc.*, which injure the bronchioles and alveoli at the base of the lungs. Irritation leads respectively to coughing, bronchial spasm, grey cyanosed syndrome, and oedema of the lungs, in such regions of the respiratory tract as may be affected. Whilst corrosive injury can be very extensive, if exposure is severe the effects are diverse, and it is in fact unlikely that these are receptor phenomena. In this case, the array of irritants in question seem to utilize such of the available physiological and pathological mechanisms as are consistent with their physico-chemical properties.

7 Concluding Remarks

Where there is receptor involvement, many toxicants act as antagonists: (i) the uncouplers of oxidative phosphorylation; (ii) fluoroacetate affording fluorocitrate, which interferes with the normal functioning of the citric acid cycle; (iii) organophosphates, and (iv) carbamates, which antagonize AChE; (v) 4-hydroxycoumarins such as dicoumarol and warfarin, which antagonize the

[167] D. Henschler, in 'Allgemeine und spezielle Pharmakologie und Toxikologie,' ed. W. Forth, D. Henschler, and W. Rummel, Bibliographisches Institut, Mannheim, Wien and Zürich, 1975, pp. 525—595.

flavoprotein, vitamin K reductase; (vi) CN^-, and (vii) HS^-, which by completely inhibiting the cytochrome a + a_3 complex, effectively stop cellular respiration; (viii) CO, which interferes with gas transport; (ix) heavy metals, (x) mercurials, and (xi) dithiocarbamates, which react with biologically functional groups; and (xii) the case of O_2-toxicity *vis-à-vis* sensitive enzymes.

The evidence for this is confirmed by kinetic studies and the discovery of antidotes. Thus, (i) in the case of organophosphates and carbamates, oximes such as pralidoxime iodide effectively compete with the action of the toxicants at the receptors; (ii) in that of NO_2^- or aniline-induced methaemoglobinaemia, phenothiazine dyes such as Methylene Blue facilitate the reduction of methaemoglobin; (iii) in that of CO poisoning, O_2 replaces CO at the haemoglobin prosthetic site; and (iv) in that of warfarin poisoning, treatment with vitamin K antagonizes the anticoagulative effect.

Where antagonism is non-competitive and biochemical lesions are formed, as in the case (i) of CN^-, $S_2O_3^{2-}$ and methaemoglobin Fe^{III} react with unchanged CN^- *in vivo*. In the case (ii) of fluoroacetate and (iii) of Telodrin pesticides, administration respectively of either acetate or glutamate enhances the fueling of the citric acid cycle in sensitive organs, and enables a proportion of the poisoned animals to survive. (iv) In the case of snake-bite, appropriate horse anti-serum forms precipitin(s) with unchanged venom antigen(s).

The foregoing arguments about toxicants and antagonism seem to be reasonably correct and, in a very old example,[168] alloxan acts specifically on the β cells of the islets of Langerhans in dogs, producing severe diabetes.

Many other toxicants, for example paraffins such as cyclopropane, the halogenoalkanes such as chloroform and halothane, the chloroethenes, vinyl chloride, vinylidene dichloride, trichloroethylene, and perchloroethylene, aliphatic esters, CS_2, Xe, N_2O, which represent whole groups of substances that contain some volatile general anaesthetics, are entirely unspecific. Another such group consists of the industrial solvents, including chloro-methanes, -ethanes, and -benzenes, as well as the industrial alcohols, esters, and ketones. A third group of unspecific toxicants makes up the lung irritants and includes highly water-soluble NH_3, HCl, formaldehyde, S_2Cl_2, and acrolein, the less water-soluble acyl chlorides, Br_2, Cl_2, SO_2, and bis-isocyanates, and the sparingly soluble N_2O, O_3, CdO, $CoCl_3$, *etc*. Whilst the irritation and corrosive injury may be extensive, the effects are diverse and do not seem to correspond in any way to receptor phenomena.

Thus, in comparison with drugs, toxicants behave either unspecifically or as antagonists. By corollary, it is unlikely that a toxicant would play the role of an agonist. In fact, for a toxicant to behave in this way, it would have to masquerade as a natural physiological agonist and, as far as the present writer is aware, synthetic diethylstilboestrol, which acts at the oestrogen receptor, is a unique example. Whilst paraquat (chapter 9) undoubtedly simulates some of the properties of naturally occurring polyamines such as cadaverine and putrescine, and is absorbed into the lungs by a mechanism which it shares with these substances, its toxicity is unrelated to their normal functioning. On the other

[168] J. S. Dunn, H. L. Sheehan, and N. G. B. McLetchie, *Lancet*, 1943, **i**, 484.

hand methacrylate, which is used industrially as a monomer, is an intermediary metabolite *per se*, and is consequently non-toxic.

It ought perhaps to be said that in this extension of simple theory to toxicology no reference has been made to the action of carcinogens, as this is considered (chapters 11 and 12) to be a very special case in which an active metabolite reacts with a receptor nucleic acid of the target-organ concerned in such a way as to modify its normal functioning in the affected cells of that organ.

Part III

Metabolism

Chapter 6 Metabolic Pathways for Industrial Chemicals and Pesticides

1 Introduction

Many of the industrial chemicals and pesticides, discussed in this chapter, are relatively lipophilic with the result that renal excretion would represent an inefficient eliminative route for them, as they would be reabsorbed into the plasma by the tubules of the kidneys. However, mammals possess a complement of enzyme systems with the capacity to transform lipophilic compounds into more polar metabolites, which are more readily excretable by the tubular mechanisms. Such a biotransformation, which seems to be the physiological function of these drug-metabolizing enzymes, is essentially a chemical process. But because metabolism occurs within a physiological situation, in the hepatocytes, in the cells of the adrenal cortex, kidneys, lungs, and placenta, and in the epithelial cells of the gastro-intestinal tract, it is influenced by such parameters as the physiological status and the sex, species, and strain of the animal(s) concerned (and some of these factors are considered in Part IV).

The late R. T. Williams[1] pointed out a general pattern for the metabolism of foreign compounds, which are transformed or degraded by oxidation, reduction, and/or hydrolysis in an initial stage that corresponds to catabolism in intermediary metabolism. More soluble conjugates, such as glucuronides, sulphate esters, mercapturic acids, and amino-acid derivatives, are synthesized subsequently from the resulting primary products of metabolism in a second

[1] R. T. Williams, in 'Symposium on Biological Approaches to Cancer Chemotherapy,' Academic Press, London, 1960, p. 21.

stage, which corresponds to anabolism in intermediary metabolism. Whilst enzymes responsible for foreign-compound metabolism occur variously in the cellular cytosol, mitochondria, and smooth endoplasmic reticulum (SER), the 'mixed function oxidases' associated with the SER have been studied most intensively during the last two decades. These systems depend on terminal oxidases, the cytochromes P-450, molecular O_2, and NADPH for their activity, and unit reaction might be represented by the expression in equation 1.

$$RH + O_2 + NADPH + H^+ \longrightarrow ROH + H_2O + NADP^+ \quad (1)$$

Thus, 1 mol of O_2 is utilized/mol of substrate, and only a single O atom appears in the new metabolite, ROH, the other one being reduced to water. (Numerous reductases and some transferases, concerned with conjugating reactions, are also associated with the SER.) In addition, in oxidative reaction processes, the cytosolic molybdenum hydroxylases play a role, which differs from that of the cytochrome P-450 mixed function oxidases. In the former case, nucleophilic attack by OH^- introduces oxygen into the substrate molecule, and, in this way, the entering O atom originates from water, not from molecular O_2 as in the latter case.

In those examples where the industrial chemical and pesticide molecules contain substituted aromatic or heteroaromatic nuclei as residues, readily metabolizable substituent groups provide sites for metabolic attack in the parent molecules. Thus, whilst *prima facie* evidence suggests that in general these nuclei are unmetabolized, this is not necessarily true for other compounds in which the same nuclei may be present in the form of unsubstituted residues, and in those compounds, these nuclei may represent the sites most susceptible to metabolic attack. Such features as this become apparent from metabolic studies with relatively complicated foreign compounds.

It is impossible in a short chapter such as this to deal with the metabolism of the vast array of industrial chemicals and pesticides which have been investigated. Accordingly, some ten or so individual compounds or classes of compound have been selected for discussion from each of the catagories of industrial chemicals, herbicides, and insecticides, together with three or so fungicides. The substances are important commercially and scientifically *per se*, and the corresponding metabolic studies, both singly and collectively, would appear to shed light on the possible predictability of biotransformation in mammals.

2 Industrial Chemicals

n–Hexane.—Biotransformation of paraffins might be illustrated by that of n-hexane, which was studied for toxicological reasons. The fact that n-hexane (1) and butyl methyl ketone (3) both cause peripheral neuropathy in rats suggests that the hexane-2,5-dione (5) metabolite (*v. infra*) or its dehydration product, 2,5-dimethylfuran (6), may be responsible. ($\omega-1$) oxidation of (1) in rats gives hexan-2-ol (2), which is oxidized to (3), whence further ($\omega-1$) oxidation yields

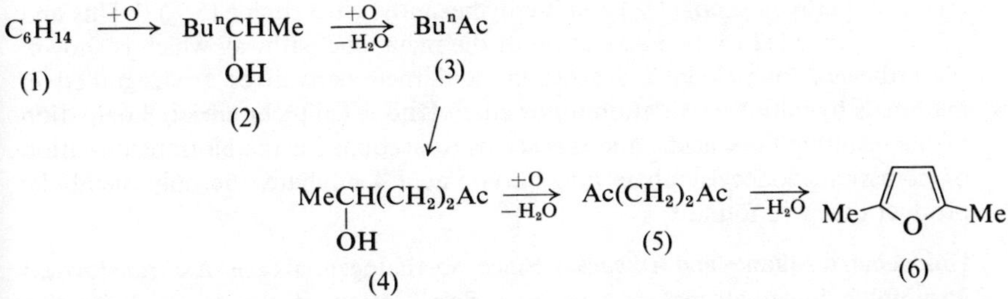

5-hydroxyhexan-2-one (4), which affords (5) and (6).[2–4] Excretion of [^{14}C]-norleucine in the urine of rats dosed [methyl-^{14}C]-(3) was traced to α oxidation leading to 1-hydroxyhexan-2-one, followed by transamination of that intermediate.[3] Moreover, whilst guinea-pigs metabolized respectively ethyl methyl ketone and isobutyl methyl ketone into 3-hydroxybutan-2-one and 4-hydroxy-4-methylpentan-2-one by ($\omega-1$) oxidation,[2] the absence of neurotoxicity was paralleled by that of (5). Further work[5–9] supports these results.[2–4] Thus, other metabolites, such as hexan-1-[5,6] and -3-ol,[7] do not lie on the neurotoxic pathway, and the onset of neuropathy in rats dosed any one out of the neurotoxic metabolites (3), hexane-2,5-diol, and (5), is related to urinary output of (5).[8] Whilst (3) was rapidly absorbed by dogs and man, ^{14}C-elimination from [1-^{14}C]-(3) was slow, suggesting that repeated administration of high doses of (3), and by implication of (1), may result in prolonged exposure to neurotoxic metabolites.[9]

Before leaving this subject, it is worthwhile considering the metabolic fate of alkyl chains as exemplified by two detergents. In rats, the major excretory products of the 2-ethylhexyl sulphate (7) were unchanged original substance (60%) and 2-ethyl-2,3-dihydroxyhexanoic acid (8) (30%); minor metabolites

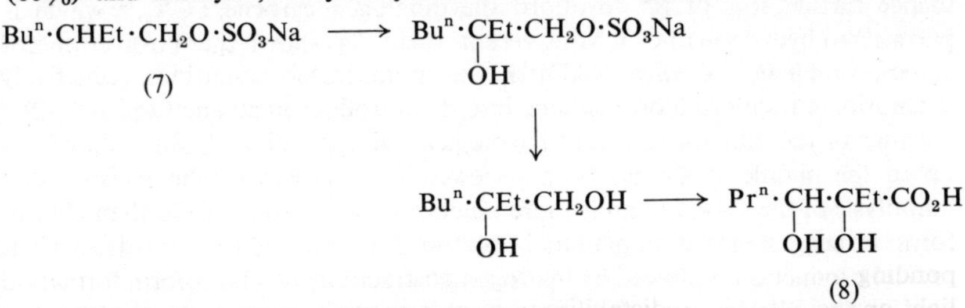

2 G. D. Di Vencenzo, C. J. Kaplan, and J. Dedinas, *Toxicol. Appl. Pharmacol.*, 1976, **36**, 511.
3 G. D. Di Vencenzo, M. L. Hamilton, C. J. Kaplan, and J. Dedinas, *Toxicol. Appl. Pharmacol.*, 1977, **41**, 547.
4 M. S. Abdel-Rahman, L. B. Hetland, and D. Couri, *Am. Ind. Hyg. Assoc. J.*, 1976, **37**, 95.
5 L. Perbellini, D. De Grandis, F. Semenzato, N. Rizzuto, and A. Simonati, *Toxicol. Appl. Pharmacol.*, 1978, **46**, 421.
6 P. Dolara, F. Franconi, D. Basoni, and G. Moneti, *Pharmacol. Res. Commun.*, 1978, **10**, 503.
7 L. Perbellini, F. Brugnone, G. Pastorello, and Grigolini, *Int. Arch. Occup. Environ. Health*, 1979, **42**, 349.
8 A. Aben, W. Flucke, F. Mihail, J. Thyssen, and G. Kimmerle, *Ecotoxicol. Environ. Saf.*, 1979, **3**, 204.
9 G. D. Di Vincenzo, M. L., Hamilton, C. J. Kaplan, W. J. Krasavage, and J. L. O'Donoghue *Toxicol. Appl. Pharmacol.*, 1978, **44**, 593.

included 2-ethylhexanol (1 %) and 2-ethylhexanoyl glucuronide (5 %).[10] This and other evidence led to the postulation of the metabolic pathway which is shown. Nevertheless, long-chain hydrocarbons and their derivatives are degraded in mammals by initial ω oxidation followed by Knoop (mitochondrial) β oxidation of the resulting fatty acids, and this seems to account for the biotransformation of potassium dodecylsulphate into butyric acid 4-sulphate, the only metabolic product that was found.[11]

Halogenated Alkanes and Alkenes.—Since polyhalogenoalkanes are transformed into polyhalogenoalkenes *in vivo*, any classification of the material for this subsection in terms of substituted alkanes and alkenes may be confusing. Accordingly, despite some difficulties, the subject-matter has been organized into C_1 compounds, C_2 compounds *etc.*

C_1 *Compounds.* Freons (Arctons) containing no hydrogen would be expected to be much more resistant to metabolism than the ones which do, and this is true for the evidence relating to trichlorofluoromethane. Thus, 97 % of a single dose was expired unchanged in 6 h from rats,[12] and no dichlorofluoromethane was formed when trichlorofluoromethane was incubated with liver microsomes, prepared from guinea-pigs, hamsters, mice, or rats, pre-treated with phenobarbitone.[12] However, the apparent binding with endoplasmic protein in experiments with rat-liver microsomes and NADPH[13] would seem to result from cytochrome P-450 'bioactivation'; this is reductive in the case of trichlorofluoromethane and CC_4 and oxidative for chloroform. Under anaerobic reducing conditions, rat-liver cytochrome P-450 converts various polyhalogenomethanes including trichlorofluoromethane, but not methylene dichloride, into CO. Possible attack might involve initial reductive removal of one halogen atom to give CX_3^- and thence further loss of X^- to afford the dihalogenocarbene, $:CX_2$,[14] which is known[15] to hydrolyse to CO. More recent work[16] has shown that rat-liver microsomes, supplemented with NADPH, under anaerobic conditions reductively dechlorinate trichlorofluoromethane into dichlorofluoromethane[16] (*cf.* ref. 12).

Much of the biochemical and toxicological evidence for CCl_4 and chloroform up to the middle 1970s has been reviewed by Hathway,[17] who stressed that homolysis of the C—Cl bond is more kinetically favoured for CCl_4 than chloroform; he suggested that, in mammals, biotransformation of CCl_4 involves $\cdot CCl_3$ radical production, followed by hydrogen abstraction and chloroform formation plus radical dimerization leading to some hexachloroethane, and thereafter complete oxidative dechlorination of chloroform with CO_2 production, in which $\cdot CCl_2$ is believed to be a key intermediate. Since that time, spin-trapping agents

[10] J. B. Knaak, S. J. Kozbelt and L. J. Sullivan, *Toxicol. Appl. Pharmacol.*, 1966, **8**, 369.
[11] W. H. B. Denner, A. H. Olavesen, G. M. Powell, and K. S. Dodgson, *Biochem. J.*, 1969, **111**, 43.
[12] P. J. Cox, L. J. King, and D. V. Parke, *Biochem. J.*, 1973, **130**, 13P.
[13] I. G. Sipes, G. Krishna, and J. R. Gillette, *Life Sci.*, 1977, **20**, 1541.
[14] G. Bonse and D. Henschler, *Crit. Rev. Toxicol.*, 1976, **4**, 395.
[15] C. R. Wolf, D. Mansuy, W. Nastainczyk, G. Deutschmann and V. Ullbrick, *Mol. Pharmacol.*, 1977, **13**, 698.
[16] C. R. Wolf, L. J. King, and D. V. Parke, *Chem.-Biol. Interact.*, 1978, **21**, 277.
[17] D. E. Hathway, *Arzneim.-Forsch*, 1974, **24**, 173.

have been used in studies[18,19] of CCl_4 metabolism *in vitro*. Claims [18,19] that the $\cdot CCl_3$ radical was trapped by these agents, as evidenced by e.s.r. monitoring, have been challenged.[20] Model experiments were implemented, and the 'preferred' interpretation of the e.s.r. spectra and hyperfine splitting by R. P. Mason *et al.*[21] is that the e.s.r. signals, recorded by all three groups of workers,[18–20] are due to a carbon-centred dienyl lipid radical adduct. The toxicological significance of the $\cdot CCl_3$ radical has been discussed.[11] It has been found[22] that irreversible binding of CCl_4 metabolites to testicular microsomal lipid occurs in rats within 3 h of dosage, and that covalent binding of CCl_4 metabolites to rat-liver microsomal protein is antagonized by the m.f.o. inhibitor, diethyldithiocarbamate, which prevents CCl_4 hepatotoxicity in rats.[23]

In just the same way as Hathway[17] had explained the formation of the major metabolite chloroform and of hexachloroethane from CCl_4 (*v. supra*), so that of precisely the same metabolites from bromotrichloromethane has also been attributed to initial $\cdot CCl_3$ radical production.[24] Unexpected minor metabolites, CCl_4 and bromodichloromethane, are formed, probably through reaction of the $\cdot CCl_3$ radical with the parent compound to give the bromodichloro radical.

$$\cdot CCl_3 + BrCCl_3 \longrightarrow CCl_4 + \cdot CBrCl_2 \xrightarrow[-R]{+RH} CHBrCl_2$$

Early work on the metabolism of chloroform has been reviewed,[17] and it has also been found[25] that, in human subjects and using $^{13}CHCl_3$, CO_2 was the only detectable metabolite. Thus, in an 8-h pulmonary excretion, unchanged chloroform accounted for up to 70% of a single i.g. dose, and CO_2 for up to 51%. No methylene dichloride and no 1,1,2,2-tetrachloroethane was excreted, and it was considered most unlikely that intial metabolic attack would involve homolysis of a C—Cl bond with expulsion of a Cl radical.[25] Mansuy *et al.*[26] have shown that phosgene is a chloroform metabolite in rat-liver microsomes: the condensation product with cysteine was identified as 4-carboxythiazolidin-2-one (9). This finding is of great importance to the toxicity of chloroform, as phosgene

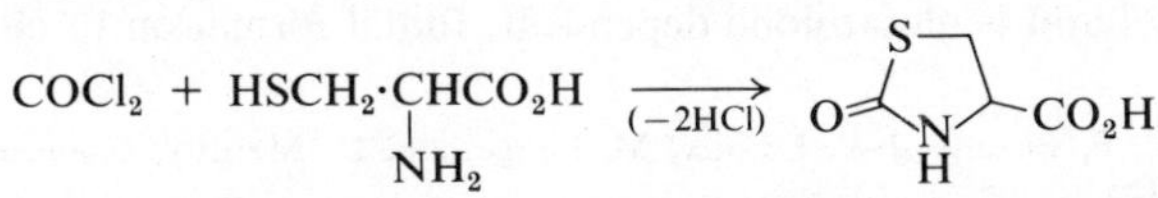

(9)

18 J. L. Poyer, R. A. Floyd, P. B. McCay, E. G. Janzen, and E. R. Davis, *Biochim. Biophys. Acta*, 1978, **539**, 402.
19 A. Ingall, K. A. K. Lott, T. F. Slater, S. Finch, and A. Stier, *Biochem. Soc. Trans.*, 1978, **6**, 962.
20 B. Halyanaraman, R. P. Mason, E. Perez-Reyes, C. F. Chignell, C. R. Wolf, and R. M. Philpot, *Biochem. Biophys. Res. Commun.*, 1979, **89**, 1065.
21 R. P. Mason, *Rev. Biochem. Toxicol.*, 1979, **1**, 151.
22 E. G. D. Toranzo, M. C. Villarruel, and J. A. Castro, *Toxicology*, 1978, **10**, 39.
23 C. P. Siegers, J. G. Filser, and H. M. Bolt, *Toxicol. Appl. Pharmacol.*, 1978, **46**, 709.
24 A. Bini, G. Vecchi, G. Vivoli, V. Vannini, and C. Cessi, *Pharmacol. Res. Commun.*, 1975, **7**, 143.
25 B. J. Fry, T. Taylor, and D. E. Hathway, *Arch. Int. Pharmacodyn.*, 1972, **196**, 98.
26 D. Mansuy, P. Beaune, T. Cresteil, M. Lange, and J.-P. Leroux, *Biochem. Biophys. Res. Commun.*, 1977, **79**, 513.

is a potential cross-linking agent in respect of nucleophilic protein and DNA constituents.[27] Pohl *et al.*[28] who, independently, identified phosgene as a metabolite of chloroform *in vitro*, have now shown that a deuterium isotope effect of *ca.* 2.1 is observed in the metabolism of $CDCl_3$ in rats.[29] This demonstrates unequivocally that initial metabolism of chloroform involves attack at the C—H bond, and in this respect chloroform differs from both bromoform and iodoform which, by contrast, afford CO as the major metabolite, *in vitro* and *in vivo*.[30,31]

Once it had been found that human subjects, who had been exposed to methylene dichloride, had high levels of carboxyhaemoglobin,[32,33] confirmatory experiments in rats showed[34–36] that other dihalogenomethanes were also metabolized into CO.[34,35] Proof of drug derivation was obtained from animal experiments using $^{13}CH_2Cl_2$ and $^{14}CH_2Cl_2$,[36] and in fact $^{14}CO_2$ was detected as well. The extent of the metabolic transformation of methylene dichloride is small, as over 90% of an i.p. dose (900 mg kg^{-1}) in rats was exhaled unchanged in 24 h. *In vitro* experiments[35] showed CO formation to be catalysed by rat-liver microsomal P-450, with dependence upon O_2 and NADPH. It appeared that the CO originated from formyl chloride, which is stable only at low temperatures, and which affords CO by spontaneous dismutation. In a biological situation, competing reactions would be its hydrolysis to formic acid and its reaction, as a strong electrophile, with nucleophilic sites in proteins and nucleic acids. When methylene dichloride was incubated with rat-liver microsomes plus NADPH in the presence of $^{18}O_2$, $C^{18}O$ was produced,[37,38] and an isotope effect ($k_H/k_D = 4$) was found when CD_2Cl_2 was used instead of normal methylene dichloride suggesting that, in oxidative metabolism, fission of the C—H bond of the molecule would be rate-limiting.[37] All this evidence is consistent with putative hydroxylation, followed by spontaneous loss of HCl with transient formation of formyl chloride, and dismutation to CO and HCl.
Attempted trapping of formyl chloride with 3,4-dimethylaniline in an experiment *in vitro* failed but, in a stannous phosphate model oxidation system, a small amount of formylated amine was identified.[38]

The other known pathway for methylene dichloride metabolism occurs in the cytosol and is glutathione dependent. Initial formation of chloromethyl-

[27] T. Cresteil, P. Beaune, J.-P. Leroux, M. Lange, and D. Mansuy, *Chem.-Biol. Interact.*, 1979, **24**, 153.
[28] L. R. Pohl, B. Bhooshan, N. F. Whittaker, and G. Krishna, *Biochem. Biophys. Res. Commun.*, 1977, **79**, 684.
[29] L. R. Pohl, J. W. George, J. L. Martin, and G. Krishna, *Biochem. Pharmacol.*, 1979, **28**, 561.
[30] A. E. Ahmed, V. L. Kubic, and M. W. Anders, *Drug Metab. Dispos.*, 1977, **5**, 198.
[31] M. W. Anders, J. L. Stevens, R. W. Sprague, Z. Shaath, and A. E. Ahmed, *Drug Metab. Dispos.*, 1978, **6**, 556.
[32] R. D. Stewart, T. N. Fisher, M. J. Hosko, J. E. Petersen, E. D. Baretta, and H. C. Dodd, *Science*, 1972, **176**, 295; *Arch. Environ. Health*, 1972, **25**, 342.
[33] R. S. Ratney, D. H. Wegman, and H. B. Elkins, *Arch. Environ. Health*, 1974, **28**, 223.
[34] V. L. Kubic, M. W. Anders, R. R. Engel, C. H. Barlow, and W. S. Caughey, *Drug. Metab. Dispos.*, 1974, **2**, 53.
[35] V. L. Kubic and M. W. Anders, *Drug Metab. Dispos.*, 1975, **3**, 104.
[36] G. D. Di Vincenzo and M. L. Hamilton, *Toxicol. Appl. Pharmacol.*, 1975, **32**, 385.
[37] V. L. Kubic and M. W. Anders, *Pharmacologist*, 1975, **17**, 184.
[38] V. L. Kubic and M. W. Anders, *Biochem. Pharmacol.*, 1978, **27**, 2349.

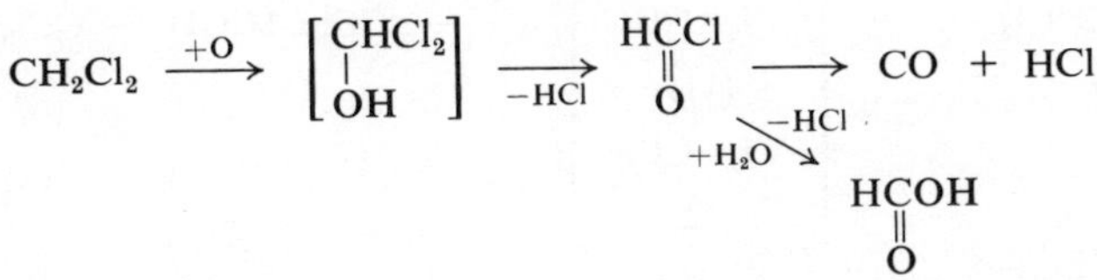

glutathione is followed by its ready hydrolysis to yield the unstable hydroxymethylglutathione, which decomposes to regenerate glutathione and to afford formaldehyde.

$$CH_2Cl_2 + GSH \xrightarrow{\text{transferase}} GSCH_2Cl + Cl^-$$

$$\downarrow +H_2O,\ -HCl$$

$$[GSCH_2OH] \longrightarrow GSH + CH_2O$$

In the presence of NAD^+, such incubations afford formic acid in place of formaldehyde.[39]

The outstanding toxicological problem posed by methylene dichloride is discussed in chapter 11.

Although methyl chloride metabolism does not appear to have been investigated intensively, the fact that operatives, who have been overcome by the vapour, suffer from alcoholic intoxication, suggests that methyl chloride is hydrolysed *in vivo*.

C_2 *Compounds*. A decade ago, Yllner[40–42] made product analyses following the murine metabolism of various halogenoethanes. In the case of pentachloroethane (10), trichloroethanol (13) and trichloroacetic acid (14) were the major urinary metabolites, and trichloroethylene (11) and tetrachloroethylene (12) were the pulmonary ones: the exhaled air contained large amounts of unchanged original substance.[40] In that of 1,1,2,2-tetrachloroethane (15), dichloroacetic acid (16), trichloroethanol (13), trichloroacetic acid (14), glyolylic acid (17), glycine (18), and oxalic acid (19) were excreted in the urine, and drug-related CO_2 (up to one-half of the dose) was expired in the exhaled air, which contained none of the original substance.[41] Yllner suggested that in the case of both (10) and (15), (13) and (14) originated from trichloroethylene (11), but this was not established. The major metabolite of 1,1,1,2-tetrachloroethane (20) was (13) and the minor one was (14):[42] a large proportion of a dose of (20) was expired unchanged.

Since halogenoalkanes can be metabolized into alkylcysteines, the corresponding nucleoside analogues and olefins, it might be appropriate to discuss glutathione mediated reactions in respect of halogenoethanes. Thus, whilst the presence of 2-chloroethanol in the blood of rats dosed 1,2-dichloroethane[43] provides strong evidence for chloroacetaldehyde formation, which would account for the mutagenicity of this halogenoethane (chapter 11), it is also

[39] A. E. Ahmed and M. W. Anders, *Biochem. Pharmacol.*, 1978, **27**, 2021.
[40] S. Yllner, *Acta Pharmacol. Toxicol.*, 1971, **29**, 481
[41] S. Yllner, *Acta Pharmacol. Toxicol.*, 1971, **29**, 499.
[42] S. Yllner, *Acta Pharmacol. Toxicol.*, 1971, **29**, 471.
[43] M. G. Kokarovtseva and N. I. Kiseleva, *Farmakol. Toksikol.*, 1978, **41**, 118.

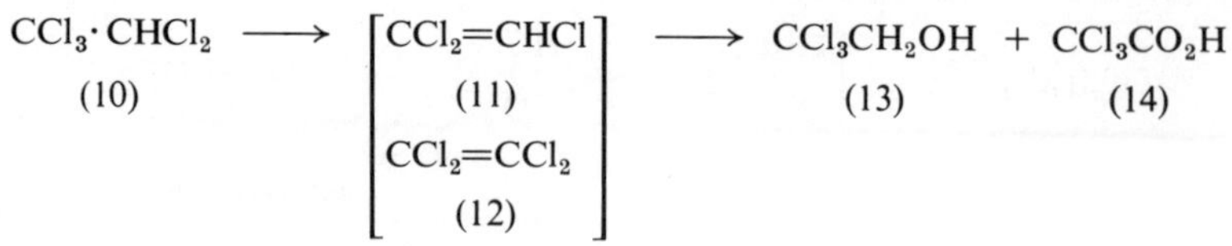

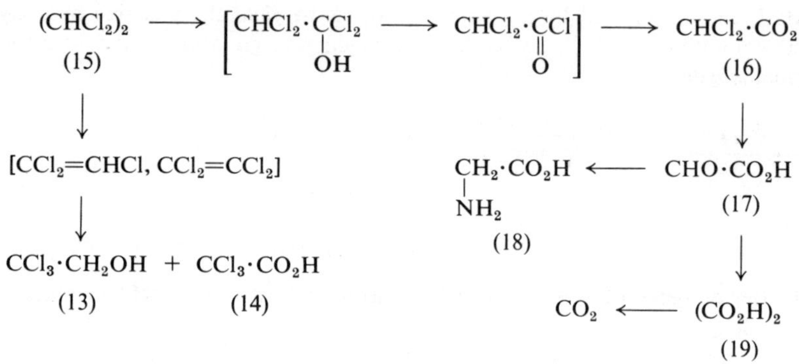

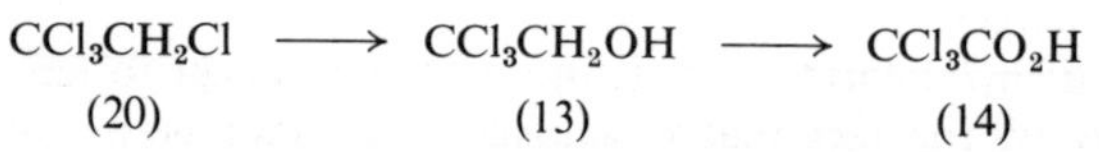

feasible that *S*-(2-chloroethyl)cysteine and/or 2-chloroethylmercapturic acid, formed by initial attack by thiols, may be involved,[44] and of course even 2-chloroethylglutathione is a 'sulphur mustard' (see Green and Hathway[45]) *per se*. If this were in fact so, then it would exemplify a mechanism of toxicity mediated by glutathione. However, the compounds $RSCH_2CH_2Cl$ would serve also as substrates for glutathione transferases, and the products, $RSCH_2SG$, would be self-protecting. Ethylene (22) is formed both in the metabolism of 1,2-dibromoethane (21) and in that of 1,2-dichloroethane, but the reaction is much slower in the latter case.[46]

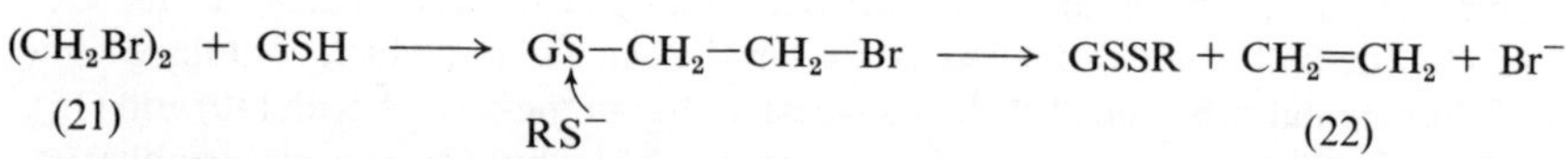

Dependent upon the method for stabilizing major vinyl chloride metabolites, either esters of *N*-acetyl-*S*-(2-hydroxyethyl)cysteine,[23] the authentic metabolite,[45] or of *N*-acetyl-*S*-(2-chloroethyl)cysteine,[24] a chemically related artefact,[47] were isolated from the urine of treated animals. If the Fischer–Speier reaction with methanol were used, the *O*-methyl ester of (24) was obtained, whereas the *O*-methyl ester of (23) was produced with diazomethane.[45] Since (i) treatment of the *O*-methyl ester of (23) with methanolic HC1 gave a mixture of the *O*-methyl esters of (24) and *S*-(2-chloroethyl)cysteine, and (ii) hydrolysis of the *O*-methyl ester of (24) yielded the *O*-methyl ester of (23), it was considered that the reversible

44 U. Rannug and B. Beije, *Chem.-Biol. Interact.*, 1979, **24**, 265.
45 T. Green and D. E. Hathway, *Chem.-Biol. Interact.*, 1977, **17**, 137.
46 J. C. Livesey and M. W. Anders, *Drug Metab. Dispos.*, 1979, **7**, 199.
47 T. Green and D. E. Hathway, *Chem.-Biol. Interact.*, 1975, **11**, 545.

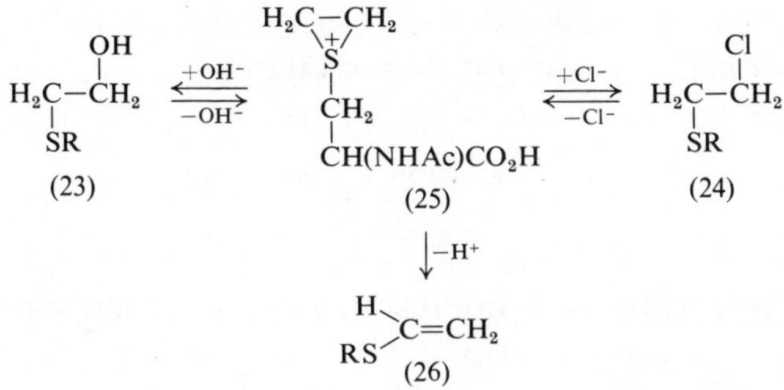

reaction processes involving (23) and (24) were modulated through the intermediacy of the episulphonium ion (25) and, for example, formation of (25) would be rate-determining in respect of the hydrolysis of (24).[45] It was predictable that nucleophilic attack of OH^- on (25) would give olefin through β-elimination,[48] and, in fact, a small amount of such a substance, *N*-acetyl-*S*-vinylcysteine (26), was recovered from the urine of animals treated with vinyl chloride, whenever diazomethane esterification was used for protecting the *S*-containing metabolites.[45]

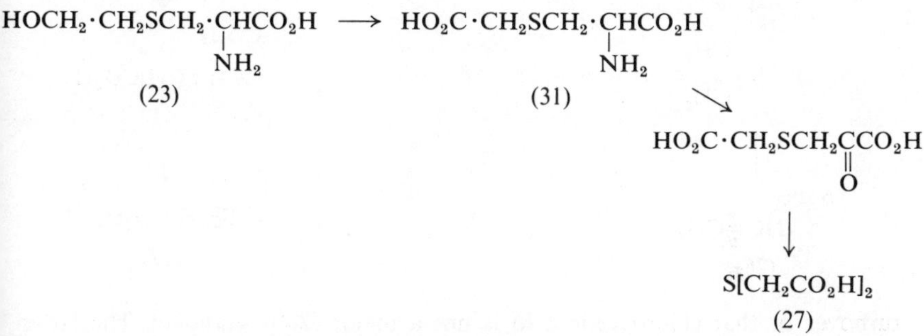

The fact that rats dosed *S*-(2-hydroxyethyl)cysteine afforded 0.5% of thiodiglycolic acid (27), taking into consideration the extreme instability of the initial substance under gentle reaction conditions, provided a clue to the biogenesis of the other major vinyl chloride metabolite, *viz.* (27). Biotransformations undoubtedly concerned involved end-group oxidation, transamination, and oxidative decarboxylation, and suggested other sources for (27) formation. The fact that high yields of (27) were obtained in animals treated separately with chloroacetaldehyde (30), chloroacetic acid, or *S*-carboxymethylcysteine (31) implied that these compounds might be on a common metabolic pathway linking vinyl chloride (28) with (27) and possibly with the other *S*-containing metabolites, (23) and (26). However, other evidence excluded chloroacetic acid: (i) <0.1% of the dose had ever been detected as chloroacetic acid in the body fluids of any of the (28)-treated rats, thereby implying either a high rate of

[48] A. G. Ogston, E. R. Holiday, J. S. L. Philpot, and L. A. Stocken, *Trans. Faraday Soc.*, 1948, **44**, 45.

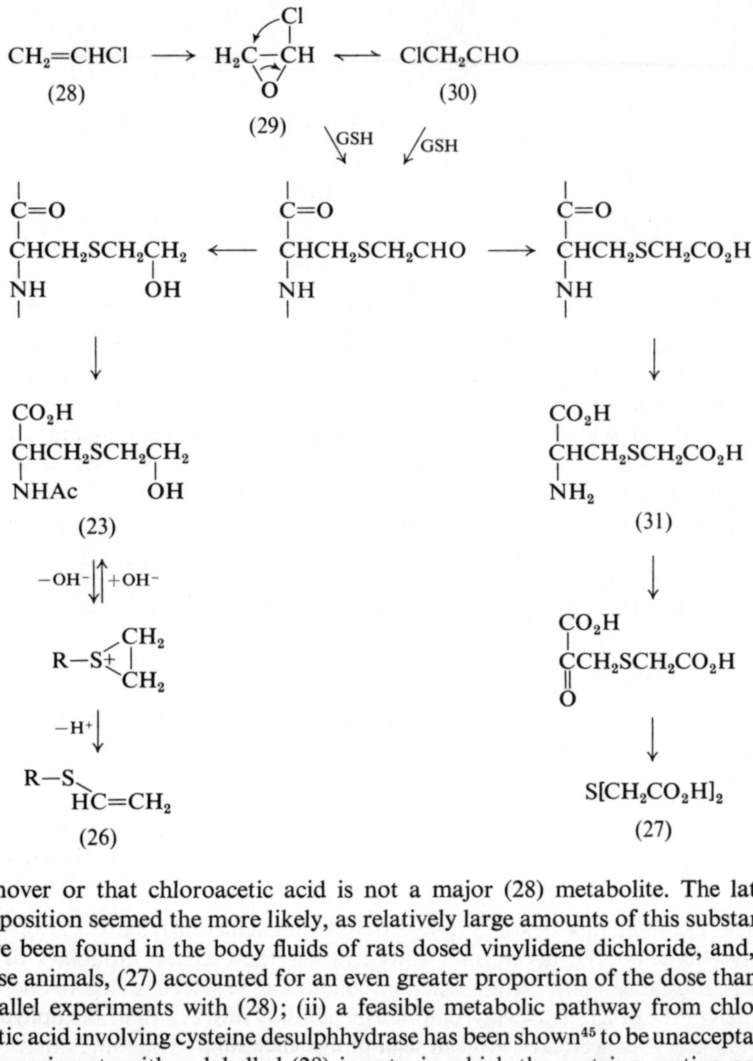

turnover or that chloroacetic acid is not a major (28) metabolite. The latter supposition seemed the more likely, as relatively large amounts of this substance have been found in the body fluids of rats dosed vinylidene dichloride, and, in those animals, (27) accounted for an even greater proportion of the dose than in parallel experiments with (28); (ii) a feasible metabolic pathway from chloroacetic acid involving cysteine desulphhydrase has been shown[45] to be unacceptable in experiments with unlabelled (28) in rats, in which the cysteine–cystine pools had been labelled adequately with ^{14}C. The formation of labelled (27) showed that a part of the C-skeleton must be derived in fact from cysteine; (iii) in rats dosed (22), the presence of (23) and (27), but not of chloroacetic acid, amongst the urinary metabolites was established by stringent mass fragmentometric methods.

Hence, there is a strong supposition that in rats, chloroethylene oxide (29) is formed from (28),[49] and is transformed spontaneously into (30)[50] and there

[49] B. L. Van Duuren, *Ann. N. Y. Acad. Sci.*, 1975, **246**, 258.
[50] H. Gross and J. Freiburg, *J. prakt. Chem.*, 1969, **311**, 506.

is supporting evidence[51–53] for vinyl chloride epoxidation *in vitro*. The biological relationship of glutathione *S*-epoxide transferase and substrate epoxide is well-known, and the fact that (30) affords *in vivo* both (23) and (27) infers that (28) metabolism involves a reaction between glutathione and (29) and (30).[45] This supposition is confirmed by the identification of *S*-carboxymethylcysteine (31) amongst the hydrolytic products, isolated from an hepatic extract, prepared from animals treated with vinyl chloride.[45] Again, since (29) and (30) are mutagens of *S. typhimurium* strains[54–56] and in Chinese hamster V79 cells,[57] both these substances may contribute substantially to vinyl chloride carcinogenicity in mammals. Thus, the foregoing arguments provide convincing evidence for a metabolic pathway, involving chloroethylene oxide and chloroacetaldehyde, for vinyl chloride in the living mammal. Finally, chloroethylene oxide is in fact formed from vinyl chloride *in vivo*, because precisely the same nucleoside analogues, *viz.* 9-(β-D-2′-deoxyribofuranosyl)imidazol[2,1-*i*]purine (etheno deoxyadenosine) and 1-(β-D-2′-deoxyribofuranosyl)imidazol[1,2-*c*]pyrimidin-2(1*H*)-one (ethenodeoxycytidine), which are formed when chloroacetaldehyde or chloroethylene oxide reacts with calf-thymus DNA *in vitro*, are formed in the liver DNA of living animals (rats) exposed chronically to vinyl chloride in their drinking water.[58] Thus the metabolic pathway, tentatively put forward for vinyl chloride, is entirely valid.

On general grounds, some similarities would be expected in the biotransformations of vinylidene dichloride and vinyl chloride. In fact, thiodiglycolic acid (40) is a major metabolite of both chloroethylenes, and more *S*-carboxymethylcycteine (39) is formed from vinylidene chloride than from vinyl chloride. These facts are reconcilable with a metabolic pathway for vinylidene dichloride (32) where chloroacetic acid (35) occupies a key position, in which case, (39) and (40) would be representatives of a sequence of degradation products, derived from the detoxification of (35) through the enzyme-catalysed reaction with glutathione and the resulting product, carboxymethylglutathione (37). Previous work[45] had established the biotransformation of (39) and (40) (*v. supra*), and, in work on the fate of (32),[59] some evidence was found for the intermediary lactic and pyruvic acids. As in the case of vinyl chloride,[45] a part of the C-skeleton of (40) must be derived from cysteine, as labelled (40) resulted from experiments with unlabelled (32) in rats in which the cysteine–cystine pools had been labelled adequately with ^{14}C:[59,60] this evidence invalidates any cysteine desulphydrase (EC4.4.1.1) participation. A great deal of evidence suggests a route (Scheme 1)

[51] A. G. Salmon, *Cancer Lett.*, 1976, **2**, 109.
[52] A Barbin, H. Bresil, A. Croisy, P. Jacquignon, C. Malaveille, R. Montesano, and H. Bartsch, *Biochem. Biophys. Rev. Commun.*, 1975, **67**, 596.
[53] H. Bartsch and R. Montesano, *Mutat. Res.*, 1975, **32**, 93.
[54] H. Bartsch, C. Malaveille, and R. Montesano, *Int. J. Cancer*, 1975, **15**, 429.
[55] C. Malaveille, H. Bartsch, A. Barbin, A. M. Camus, R. Montesano, A. Croisy, and P. Jacquignon, *Biochem. Biophys. Res. Commun.*, 1975, **63**, 363.
[56] J. McCann, V. Simon, D. Streitwieser, and B. N. Ames, *Proc. Nat. Acad. Sci.*, 1976, **72**, 3190.
[57] E. Huberman, H. Bartsch, and L. Sachs, *Int. J. Cancer*, 1975, **15**, 539.
[58] T. Green and D. E. Hathway, *Chem.-Biol. Interact.*, 1978, **22**, 211.
[59] B. K. Jones and D. E. Hathway, *Chem.-Biol. Interact.*, 1978, **20**, 27.
[60] G. H. Walker and D. E. Hathway, *Biochem. J.*, 1977, **167**, 505.

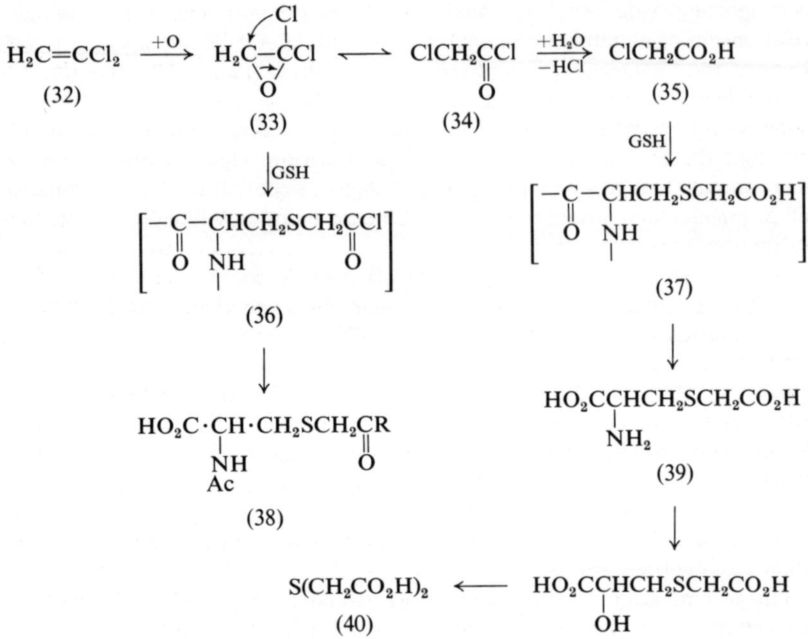

Scheme 1

for vinylidene dichloride (32) metabolism, which is economical in primary biotransformations in the R. T. Williams-sense (*v. supra*). Irrespective of whether [1-^{14}C]dichloroethylene or [1-^{14}]chloroacetic acid was administered to rats, one molecular proportion of the resulting [^{14}C]-(40) gave one equivalent of $^{14}CO_2$ in the microscale Kolbe electrolysis reaction.[61] This evidence is entirely consistent with the transformation of (32) into (35), which involves migration of one Cl atom and the loss of the other one. Hence, the metabolic pathway [(32)→(35), (35)→(40)], which was tentatively proposed for the biotransformation of (32) into (40) (*v. supra*), does in fact operate in the living mammal. On account of the established metabolic pathway for (40), the formation of the other major metabolite, *viz.* the *N*-acetyl-*S*-cysteinylacetyl derivative (38) of (32), but not of (35),[59] must mean that this derivative arises from an earlier (32) metabolite than (35). The work[59] suggests, but does not prove, that (38) may be formed from 1,1-dichloroethylene oxide (33) through the agency of glutathione *S*-epoxide transferase [EC4.4.1.7], the resulting *S*-glutathione acetyl chloride (36), and its subsequent reactions. This supposition is important, as the reactivity shown by (33) may apply too in the case of the possible interaction of reactive (32) metabolites with mouse-kidney DNA.[62,63]

The interesting feature of trichloroethylene (41) metabolism is that in man, as far as is known hitherto, spontaneous rearrangement of the epoxide affords

[61] H. Kolbe, *Annalen*, 1849, **69**, 257.
[62] S. Yllner, *Acta Pharmacol. Toxicol.*, 1971, **30**, 69.
[63] C. Maltoni, G. Cotti, L. Morisi, and P. Chieco, *Med. Lav.*, 1977, **68**, 241.

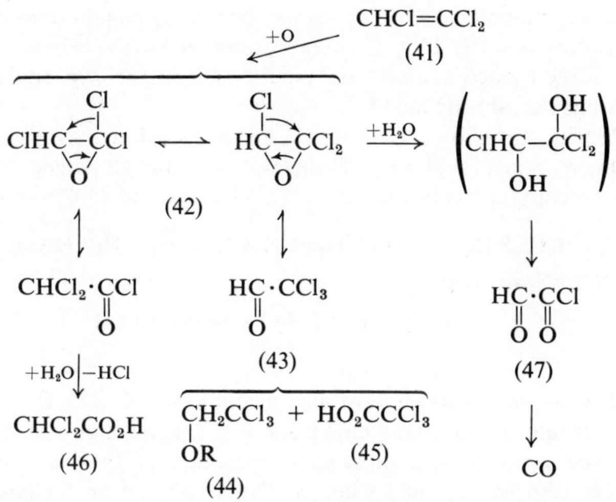

chloral (43) which has been identified in the blood,[64] and which gives rise to the urinary products,[65,66] *viz.* trichloroethanol *O*-glucuronide (44; R = $C_6H_9O_6$) and trichloroacetic acid (45). No dichloroacetic acid (46) has ever been detected in the body fluids of treated animals and man.[67] The foregoing evidence is utterly consistent with the relative harmlessness of this bulk chemical (41), which has been produced for one-half of a century. Nevertheless, data derived from studies with vinylidene dichloride (32) and (41) suggest that similar mutagenic and tumourogenic properties in mice may be attributable to rearrangement of 1,1-dichloroethylene oxide (33) and 1,1,2-trichloroethylene oxide (42) respectively into chloroacetyl chloride and dichloroacetyl chloride.[68] Identification in mice of the new (41) metabolite, (46) [in addition to (45)] strongly supports this supposition. The small proportion of (46) in relation to (45) in the urine of the treated mice is consistent with the spill-over model, suggested by Hathway[68] for (41) metabolism in these animals. Rat-liver microsomes prepared from animals pre-treated with phenobarbitone or benzopyrene convert (41) into CO and this process, which is dependent on NADPH–O_2, seems to be mediated by cytochrome P-450.[69] It is feasible that CO production might involve intermediate formation of glyoxyl chloride (47).

The epoxide of tetrachloroethylene (perchloroethylene) can rearrange only in one way, and this solvent affords trichloroethanol and trichloroacetic acid as major metabolites.[70]

[64] W. J. Cole, R. G. Mitchell, and R. F. Salamonsen, *J. Pharm. Pharmacol.*, 1975, **27**, 167.
[65] T. C. Butler, *J. Pharmacol.*, 1949, **97**, 84.
[66] J. W. Daniel, *Biochem. Pharmacol.*, 1963, **12**, 795.
[67] G. Bonse, Th. Urban, D. Reichert, and D. Henschler, *Biochem. Pharmacol.*, 1975, **24**, 1829.
[68] D. E. Hathway, *Cancer Lett.*, 1980, **8**, 263.
[69] P. S. Traylor, W. Nastainczyk, and V. Ullrich, in 'Microsomes and Drug Oxidations,' eds. V. Ullrich, I. Roots, A. Hildebrandt, R. W. Estabrook, and A. H. Conney, Pergamon, Oxford, 1977, p. 615.
[70] W. H. Braun, *J. Chromatogr.*, 1978, **150**, 212.

C_3-*Compounds*. Epichlorohydrin appears to be rapidly metabolized in mammals, and in rats approximately 20% of a dose was excreted in the exhaled air as CO_2.[71] The urine of the treated animals contained *S*-(2,3-dihydroxypropyl)mercapturic acid and a bis-mercapturic acid.[72]

Alkyl chloride, bromide, or iodide (48) injected s.c. into rats was metabolized into alkylmercapturic acid (49), *S*-allylcysteine, *S*-allylcysteine *S*-oxide, and *S*-(3-hydroxypropyl)mercapturic acid (50).[73] Compound (50) was considered[73]

$$CH_2{=}CHCH_2X \longrightarrow CH_2{=}CH{\cdot}CH_2SCH_2{\cdot}CH(NHAc)CO_2H$$

(48; X = Cl, Br, or I) (49)

$$HOCH_2[CH_2]_2SCH_2CH(NHAc)CO_2H$$

(50)

to be formed by mercapturation of allyl alcohol (48; X = OH), as it was produced also in rats, administered allyl alcohol.[74] This reaction was considered to have involved acrolein, and subsequent reduction of the aldehyde group to CH_2OH. No (50) was formed when *S*-allylglutathione or *S*-allylcysteine was injected into rats.[73]

Methanol.—Mammals metabolize methanol into CO_2 through formaldehyde and formic acid, and it is the accumulation of these intermediates which is considered to account for the response in those species (chapter 8) that are susceptible to methanol poisoning.[75–77]

Carbon Disulphide.—Early work[78] with $C^{35}S_2$ in rats showed that 50% of an injected dose was excreted in the exhaled air and the remainder in the urine mainly as $^{35}SO_4^{2-}$ and, on general grounds, it might be surmised that CO_2 and SO_4^{2-} would represent the ultimate products of oxidation although a great deal of a dose of CS_2 would be expected to be excreted unchanged from mammals. Thus, (i) 2-mercapto-2-thiazolin-5-one (51) and thiourea (52) were isolated from the urine of workers, who had been exposed to CS_2,[79] and (ii)

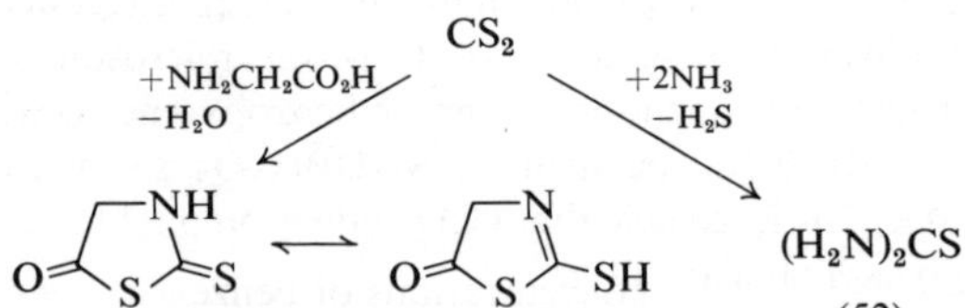

(51) (52)

[71] W. W. Weigel, H. B. Plotnick, and W. L. Conner, *Res. Commun. Chem. Path. Pharmacol.*, 1978, **20**, 275.
[72] G. Fakhouri and A. R. Jones, *Aust. J. Pharm. Sci.*, 1979, **8**, 11.
[73] C. M. Kaye, J. J. Clapp, and L. Young, *Xenobiotica*, 1972, **2**, 129.
[74] C. M. Kaye and L. Young, *Biochem. J.*, 1970, **119**, 53P.
[75] T. R. Tephly, *Fed. Proc.*, 1977, **36**, 1627.
[76] A. B. Makar and T. R. Tephly, *J. Toxicol. Environ. Health*, 1976, **2**, 1201.
[77] K. E. McMartin, G. Martin-Amat, P. E. Noker, and T. R. Tephly, *Biochem. Pharmacol.*, 1979, **28**, 645.
[78] M. Jakubowski, *Med. Pr.*, 1971, **22**, 195.
[79] M. Pergal, N. Vukojevic, N. Cinn-Popov, D. Djuric, and T. Bojovic, *Arch. Environ. Health*, 1972, **25**, 38, 42.

$^{14}CS_2$ was oxidized in rats to $^{14}CO_2$ in quantities proportional to the activity of liver cytochrome P-450.[80] None of this work had revealed a reactive metabolite consistent with the well-known hepatotoxicity of CS_2, and a new approach in this direction was initiated when Neal *et al.*[81,82] identified COS as an intermediate in the oxidation of CS_2 to CO_2 *in vitro*. Both reaction stages are NADPH-dependent and mediated by cytochrome P-450, and the common by-product,

$$CS_2 \xrightarrow{+O} COS + S$$

$$COS \xrightarrow{+O} CO_2 + S$$

atomic sulphur, is involved with the inhibition of cytochrome P-450 by CS_2 and COS. Irreversible binding of ^{35}S to the microsomes was shown by means of $C^{35}S_2$, and singlet S atoms, themselves powerful electrophiles, would appear to have been involved. Half of the bound sulphur was released from rat-liver microsomes on treatment with CN^-, giving $^{35}SCN^-$, and this evidence suggests[83] in fact that part of the sulphur was bound as $RS^{35}SH$. (Similar labelling of rat-liver microsomes resulted with [^{35}S]parathion, which contains $\rangle P \rightarrow S$ linkage.) Dalvi and Neal[84] showed conclusively that rats dosed $^{14}CS_2$ by inhalation excreted COS and CO_2 in the exhaled air, thereby demonstrating that COS is a CS_2 metabolite *in vivo*. The fact that cytochrome P-450 induction would have enhanced CO_2 production and correspondingly diminished COS may have mitigated against its recognition in previous animal experiments.

Aromatic Hydrocarbons.—Relatively little benzene (1—2% of a dose) is oxidized to CO_2 and excreted in the exhaled air of treated animals (and of man), but one-quarter of the dose was excreted as conjugates of phenol in the urine, together with small amounts of pyrocatechol, quinol and hydroxyquinol conjugates, about 1% as phenylmercapturic acid, and 1.5% as *trans,trans*-muconic acid.[85] Glucuronide and sulphate contributed to the phenol conjugates, but sulphate accounted for those of the hydroxyphenols.[85] The possibility that damage to the haematopoietic system and development of leukaemia may arise through biotransformations of benzene in bone marrow has given impetus to metabolic study, but the concentrations of glucuronide and sulphate conjugates of benzene metabolites found in bone marrow were the same as those in the liver of exposed animals.[86] However, when the concentrations of benzene, phenol, pyrocatechol, and quinol, resulting from inhalational exposure of rats to benzene, were

[80] F. de Matteis and A. S. Seawright, *Chem.-Biol. Interact.*, 1973, **7**, 375.
[81] R. R. Dalvi, R. E. Poore, and R. A. Neal, *Life Sci.*, 1974, **14**, 1785.
[82] R. R. Dalvi, A. L. Hunter, and R. A. Neal, *Chem.-Biol. Interact.*, 1975, **10**, 349.
[83] G. L. Catignani and R. A. Neal, *Biochem. Biophys. Res. Commun.*, 1975, **65**, 629.
[84] R. R. Dalvi and R. A. Neal, *Biochem. Pharmacol.*, 1978, **27**, 1608.
[85] R. T. Williams, 'Detoxication Mechanisms,' Chapman and Hall, London, 1959, pp. 188—236.
[86] R. Snyder, L. S. Andrews, E. W. Lee, C. M. Witmer, M. Reilly, and J. J. Kocsis, in 'Biological Reactive Intermediates,' eds. D. J. Jollow, J. J. Kocsis, R. Snyder, and H. Vainio, Plenum Press, New York, 1977, p. 286.

measured in the blood and bone marrow,[87] phenol was found to be the main metabolite in bone marrow at the beginning of exposure, but concentrations of pyrocatechol and quinol built up subsequently and persisted both in the blood and bone marrow of the animals for at least 9 h after exposure had ended. Evidence obtained from binding studies in microsomal systems suggested[88] that a product of the further metabolism of phenol was responsible for the binding, and not a primary metabolite of benzene *per se*. The possibility that primary metabolites of benzene may originate through epoxidation (*v. infra*) was considered briefly by Williams[85] nearly 25 years ago, and during the last two decades this concept has been accepted. However, consideration of the metabolism of benzene hydrocarbon homologues features attack on readily metabolizable substituent alkyl groups, in agreement with the argument used in the Introduction (*v. supra*). On that account such aromatic nuclei appear to be largely unmetabolized.

PhEt (53) ⟶ PhCHOHMe (54) ⟶ COMePh (55) ⟶ $Ph{\cdot}CO{\cdot}CH_2OH$ (56)

(56) ↙ $Ph{\cdot}CHOH{\cdot}CH_2OH$ (57) ⟶ $Ph{\cdot}CHOH{\cdot}CHO$ (58) ⟶ $Ph{\cdot}CHOH{\cdot}CO_2H$ (59)

(56) ↓ $Ph{\cdot}CO{\cdot}CHO$ (60) ⟶ $Ph{\cdot}CO{\cdot}CO_2H$ (61)

Stereoselective biotransformation of ethylbenzene (53) into (−)-mandelic acid (59) has been studied in rats by means of large numbers of metabolites and possible intermediates.[89] (−)-(59) was obtained from the metabolism of both (+)- and (−)-methyl phenyl carbinol (54), acetophenone (55), and ω-hydroxyacetophenone (56), and the stereoselective step must occur during oxidation or reduction of (56). Either pathway is feasible, as the oxidation product, phenylglyoxal (60) and the reduction product, phenylethylene glycol (57) both give (−)-(59) stereoselectivity. Benzoylformic acid (61) was a by-product in all these feeding experiments, but no (−)-(59) resulted from the metabolism of (61) and *vice versa*. Large amounts of (+)-(59) were obtained from (+)-(57), but only very small amounts from (−)-(57), and so the reduction of (56) to glycol (57) is very highly stereoselective; however other steps might also be important.

Hydroxylation of the methyl group in *p*-xylene (62) occurred in experiments with rat-liver or -lung microsomes *in vitro*, and the resulting *p*-methylbenzyl alcohol (63) was converted into *p*-toluic acid (65) by the hepatic cytosolic fraction.[90] Endogenous glycine was rate-limiting with regard to the rate of excretion of methylhippuric acid (66), the terminal metabolite of (62).[91] After a

87 D. E. Rickert, T. S. Baker, J. S. Bus, C. S. Barrow, and R. D. Irons, *Toxicol. Appl. Pharmacol.*, 1979, **49**, 417.
88 A. Tunek, K. L. Platt, P. Bentley, and F. Oesch, *Mol. Pharmacol.*, 1978, **14**, 920.
89 H. R. Sullivan, W. M. Miller, and R. E. McMahon, *Xenobiotica*, 1976, **6**, 49.
90 C. Harper, *Fed. Proc.*, 1975, **34**, 785.
91 V. Rühimaeki, *Scand. J. Work Environ. Health*, 1979, **5**, 135.

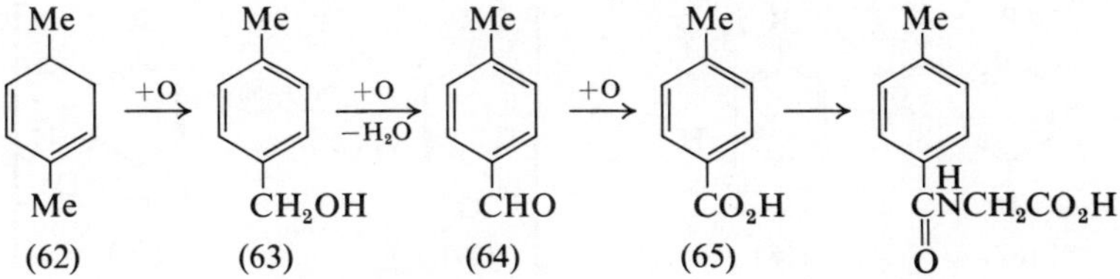

(62) (63) (64) (65) (66)

single injection of (62), rats lost 65% of their pulmonary *p*-xylene hydroxylase activity, and experiments showed that the inactivation of cytochrome P-450 by (62) was brought about by tolualdehyde (64), which required NADPH to inactivate the enzyme system.[92]

Halogeno Benzenoid Compounds.—Before discussing specific compounds, it is worthwhile recapitulating that in the general case, arene oxides, formed from monosubstituted benzenes: (i) react with nucleophilic sites of proteins and nucleic acids; (ii) rearrange through NIH shift into phenols; (iii) undergo ring-fission with epoxide hydratase to give *trans*-1,2-dihydroxydihydrobenzenes; (iv) form with glutathione *S*-epoxide transferase, 1-glutathionyl-2-hydroxy-1,2-dihydrobenzenes (Scheme 2). It might be said that NIH shift in the *p*-hydroxylation of many monosubstituted benzenes (*in vitro* and *in vivo*) has been confirmed

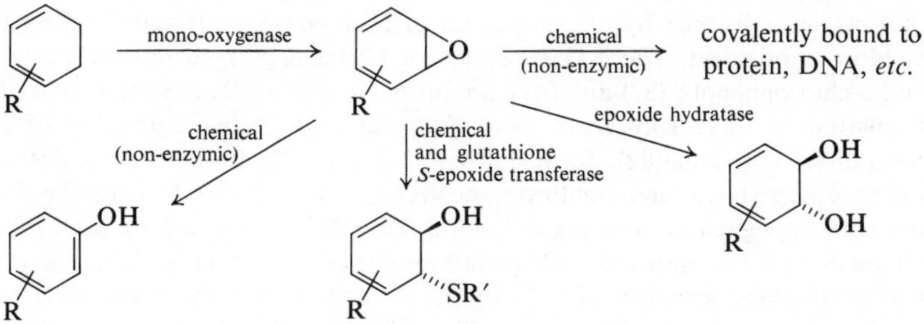

Scheme 2

by labelling the *p*-position with D or ^{3}H, and determining the proportion of label retained in the phenol produced by migration into the *m*-position. If *p*-hydroxylation occurred exclusively by NIH shift, then the D or ^{3}H in the phenols (71) and (72), derived from labelled monosubstituted benzenes (67), would reflect only a kinetic isotope-effect of 3—10 in the enolisation of the keto tautomer (70), which is formed by quantitative migration of the label on (68), probably through the zwitterion (69) and not by concerted rearrangement of (68). Whilst retention of label, for example, for phenylalanine is almost quantitative, that for many other monosubstituted benzenes is somewhat less, and the corresponding phenols must be formed (or partly formed) by alternative reactions, involving direct loss of label from the zwitterion (69).[93]

[92] J. M. Patel, C. Harper, and R. T. Drew, *Drug Metabol. Dispos.*, 1978, **6**, 368.
[93] J. W. Daly, D. M. Jerina, and B. Witkop, *Experientia*, 1972, **28**, 1129.

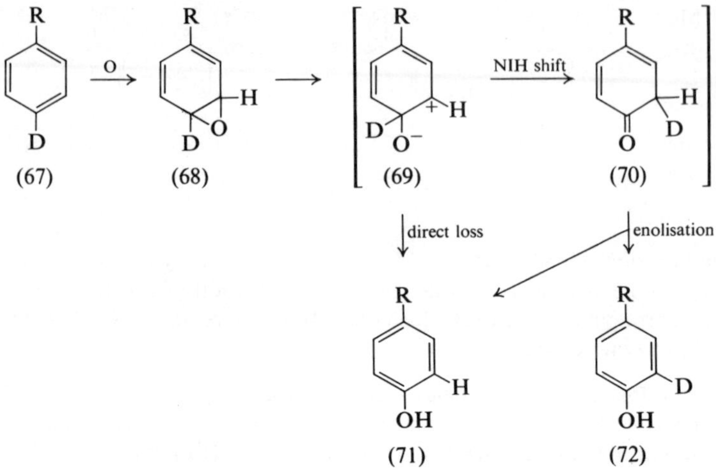

The metabolism of [U-^{14}C]chlorobenzene revealed an array of products,[94] of which those that were known already were formed in the same proportions as had been reported previously.[95–97] All of the products in the recent work[94] can be derived theoretically from the two arene oxides, (74) and (75). The substantial amount of *m*-chlorophenol (88) found suggests that its keto tautomer (80), which is formed by rearrangement of both epoxides, is stabilized by the β-chloro substituent. Those keto tautomers, (79) and (81), corresponding to *o*- and *p*-chlorophenols, (87) and (89), are probable intermediates in the respective formation of these substances from (74) and (75). Dehydrogenation of the *trans*-diols, (78) and (82), formed from (74) and (75) by epoxide hydratase, yields respectively 3- and 4-chloropyrocatechol, (91) and (92). Finally, the three chlorophenylmercapturic acids (85), (86), and (90), are formed through initial interaction of the epoxides with glutathione to give (76), (77), (83), and (84). Chlorobenzenes, labelled with D in the 3- and 4-positions, were used[93] to confirm that formation of *m*- and *p*-chlorophenol, (88) and (89), did involve an NIH shift.

1,4-Dibromobenzene (93) was metabolized in pigs[98] and rabbits[99] into two phenols, (95) and (96), themselves derivable from a single arene oxide intermediate.

Rabbits dosed separately 1,2,3-, 1,2,4-, and 1,3,5-trichlorobenzenes and 1,2,3,4- and 1,2,3,5-tetrachlorobenzenes excreted in the urine phenols, which had been produced by NIH shift.[100] Some of the corresponding tri- and tetra-bromobenzenes also gave phenols by rearrangement in rabbits.[99]

[94] J. R. Lindsay-Smith, B. A. J. Shaw, and D. M. Foulkes, *Xenobiotica*, 1972, **2**, 215.
[95] J. N. Smith, B. Spencer, and R. T. Williams, *Biochem. J.*, 1950, **47**, 284.
[96] W. H. Azouz, D. V. Parke, and R. T. Williams, *Biochem. J.*, 1952, **50**, 702.
[97] D. V. Parke and R. T. Williams, *Biochem. J.*, 1955, **59**, 415.
[98] J. Kohli and S. Safe, *Chemosphere*, 1976, **5**, 433.
[99] L. O. Ruzo, S. Safe, and O. Hutzinger, *J. Agric. Food Chem.*, 1976, **24**, 291.
[100] J. Kohli, D. Jones, and S. Safe, *Can. J. Biochem.*, 1976, **54**, 203.

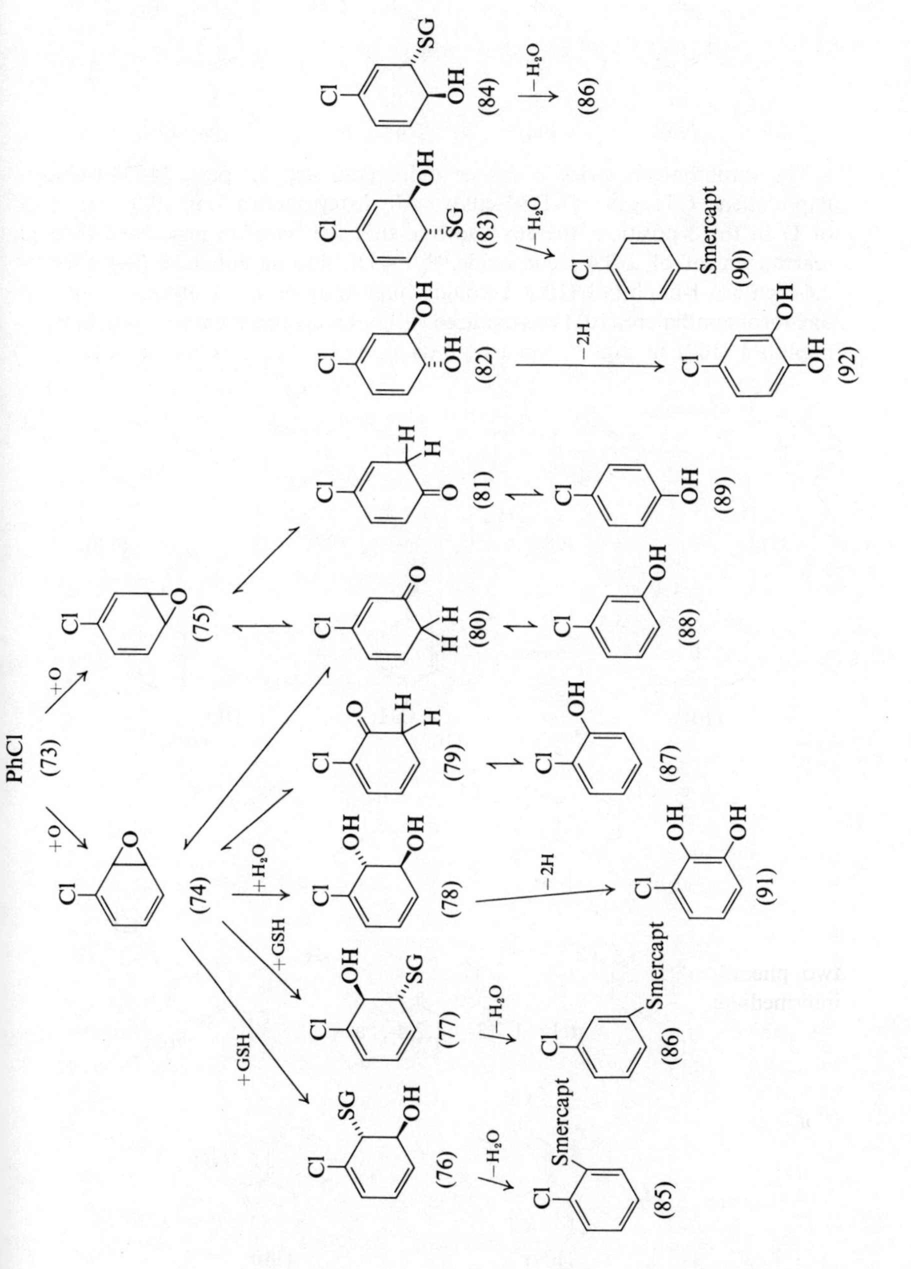
PhCl
(73)
+O
(74)
(75)
+H₂O
+GSH
(76)
(77)
(78)
(79)
(80)
(81)
(82)
(83)
(84)
−H₂O
−2H
(85)
(86)
(87)
(88)
(89)
(90)
(91)
(92)
Cl
OH
SG
Smercapt
H
O

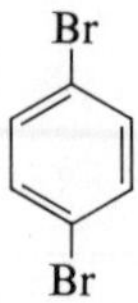
(93)

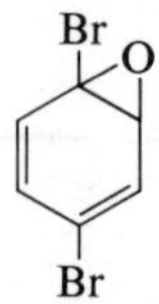
(94)

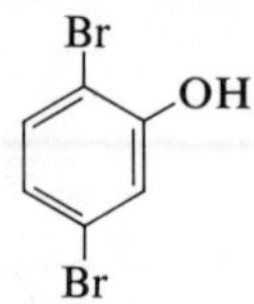
(95)

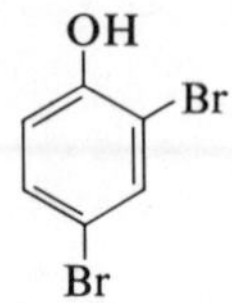
(96)

The naphthalene series is rather more complex. In pigs, [4-D]-1-chloronaphthalene (97) gave [3-D]-1-chloro-4-hydroxy-naphthalene (98) with 18% of D in the 3-position, thereby showing that the reaction proceeded through rearrangement of a 3,4-arene oxide.[101] 1,4-Dichloronaphthalene (99) afforded 2,4-dichloro-1-naphthol (100) through migration of a Cl atom,[101] but 1,2-dichloronaphthalene (101) was oxidized without rearrangement to 3,4-dichloro-1-naphthol (102) in pigs[101] and to 5,6-dichloro-1,2-dihydroxynaphthalene (103)

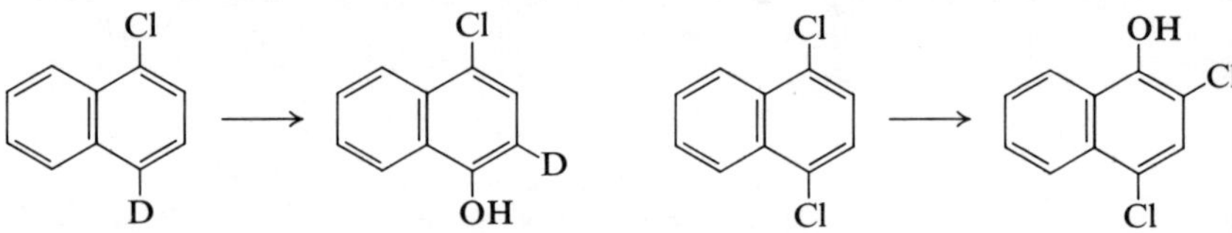
(97) (98) (99) (100)

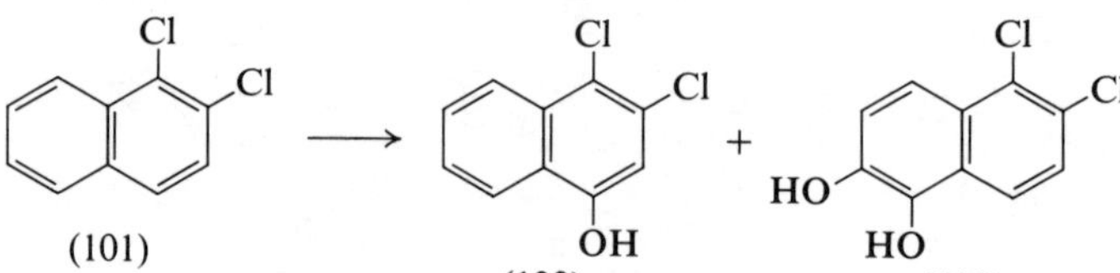
(101) (102) (103)

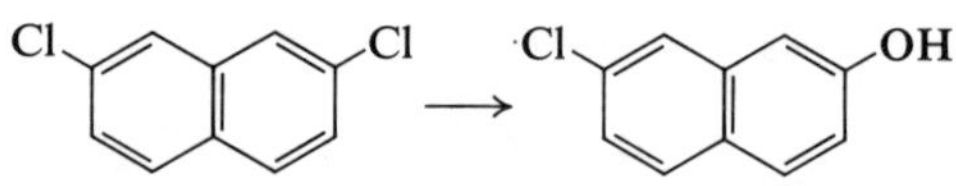
(104) (105)

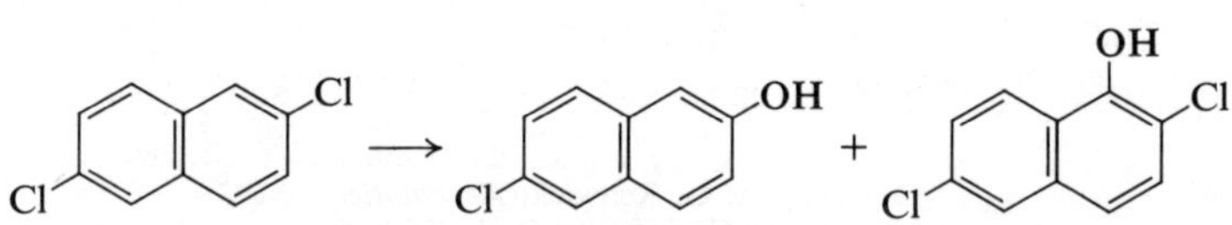
(106) (107) (108)

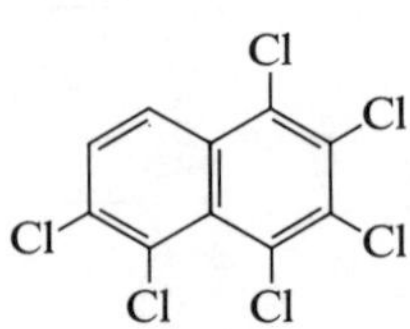
(109)

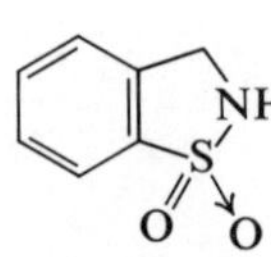
(110)

[101] L. O. Ruzo, D. Jones, S. Safe, and O. Hutzinger, *J. Agric. Food Chem.*, 1976, **24**, 581.

in rats.[102] 2,7-Dichloronaphthalene (104) was metabolized into 7-chloro-2-naphthol (105) in rats by a dechlorination reaction,[102] and the 2,6-isomer (106) was metabolized by rats[102] and rabbits[103] into the products (107) and (108), thereby suggesting the intermediacy of an arene oxide. In pigs, 1,2,3,4,5,6-hexachloronaphthalene (109) was unmetabolized;[101] 1,4-dibromonaphthalene was metabolized into 2,4-dibromo-1-naphthol.[98]

Phenol.—In most of the animals which have been studied,[104] conjugation with glucuronic acid and sulphate predominates over primary metabolism into quinol, which becomes similarly conjugated. Phenol toxicity in species like cats, which are poor conjugators, is due to conversion of free quinol into *p*-benzoquinone, itself a powerful inhibitor of mitochondrial respiration.

Saccharin.—Very thorough investigation has shown conclusively[105,106] that pure saccharin is entirely unmetabolized both in human subjects and in animals: no drug-related CO_2, HCO_3^-, or 2-sulphamoylbenzoic acid were formed. However, the metabolic fate of a number of impurities, present in commercial saccharin, has also been studied.[107–110] Toluene-*o*- and -*p*-sulphonamides and 2- and 4-sulphamoylbenzoic acids[107,108] did not yield any surprising metabolites, which might have caused tissue accumulation. Whilst the metabolism of BIT, benzo[d]isothiazoline 1,1-dioxide (110), in man is readily accounted for in terms of saccharin, 2- sulphamoylbenzoic acid, and 2-sulphamoylbenzyl alcohol, in rats, an unidentified labile urinary metabolite is also produced.[109] Hence, the bladder cancer produced by carcinogenicity testing might be associated feasibly with this labile conjugate.[110] In rats, two other impurities of commercial saccharin, *viz.* 5-chlorosaccharin and 3-amino[d]isothiazole 1,1-dioxide, were rapidly excreted unchanged.[110]

Hindered Phenolic Antioxidants.—Mention is made here of the mammalian metabolism of the hindered phenolic antioxidants,[111–120] which provide the possibility for free radical reactions in biological circumstances, and which

[102] I. Chu, D. C. Villeneuve, V. Secours, and A. Viau, *J. Agric. Food Chem.*, 1977, **25**, 881.
[103] I. Chu, V. Secours, and A. Viau, *Chemosphere*, 1976, **5**, 439.
[104] I. D. Capel, M. R., French, P. Millburn, R. L. Smith, and R. T. Williams, *Xenobiotica*, 1972, **2**, 25.
[105] J. L. Byard, E. W. McChesney, L. Golberg, and F. Coulston, *Food Cosmet. Toxicol.*, 1974, **12**, 175.
[106] L. M. Ball, A. G. Renwick, and R. T. Williams, *Xenobiotica*, 1977, **7**, 189.
[107] L. M. Ball, R. T. Williams, and A. G. Renwick, *Xenobiotica*, 1978, **8**, 183.
[108] A. G. Renwick, L. M. Ball, D. L. Corina, and R. T. Williams, *Xenobiotica*, 1978, **8**, 461.
[109] A. G. Renwick and R. T. Williams, *Xenobiotica*, 1978, **8**, 475.
[110] A. G. Renwick, *Xenobiotica*, 1978, **8**, 487.
[111] D. E. Hathway, *Adv. Food Res.*, 1967, **15**, 1.
[112] A. S. Wright, R. S. Crowne, and D. E. Hathway, *Biochem. J.*, 1965, **95**, 98.
[113] J. C. Dacre, F. A. Denz, and T. H. Kennedy, *Biochem. J.*, 1956, **64**, 777.
[114] B. D. Astill, D. W. Fassett, and R.-L. Roundabush, *Biochem. J.*, 1960, **75**, 543.
[115] W. S. Golder, A. J. Ryan, and S. E. Wright, *J. Pharm. Pharmacol.*, 1962, **14**, 268.
[116] A. S. Wright, D. A. A. Akintonwa, R. S. Crowne, and D. E. Hathway, *Biochem. J.*, 1965, **97**, 303.
[117] A. S. Wright, R. S. Crowne, and D. E. Hathway, *Biochem. J.*, 1966, **99**, 146.
[118] A. S. Wright, R. S. Crowne, and D. E. Hathway, *Biochem. J.*, 1967, **102**, 351.
[119] J. W. Daniel, J. C. Gage, and D. I. Jones, *Biochem. J.*, 1968, **106**, 783.
[120] L. I. Wiebe, J. R. Mercer, and A. J. Ryan, *Drug Metabol. Dispos.*, 1978, **6**, 296.

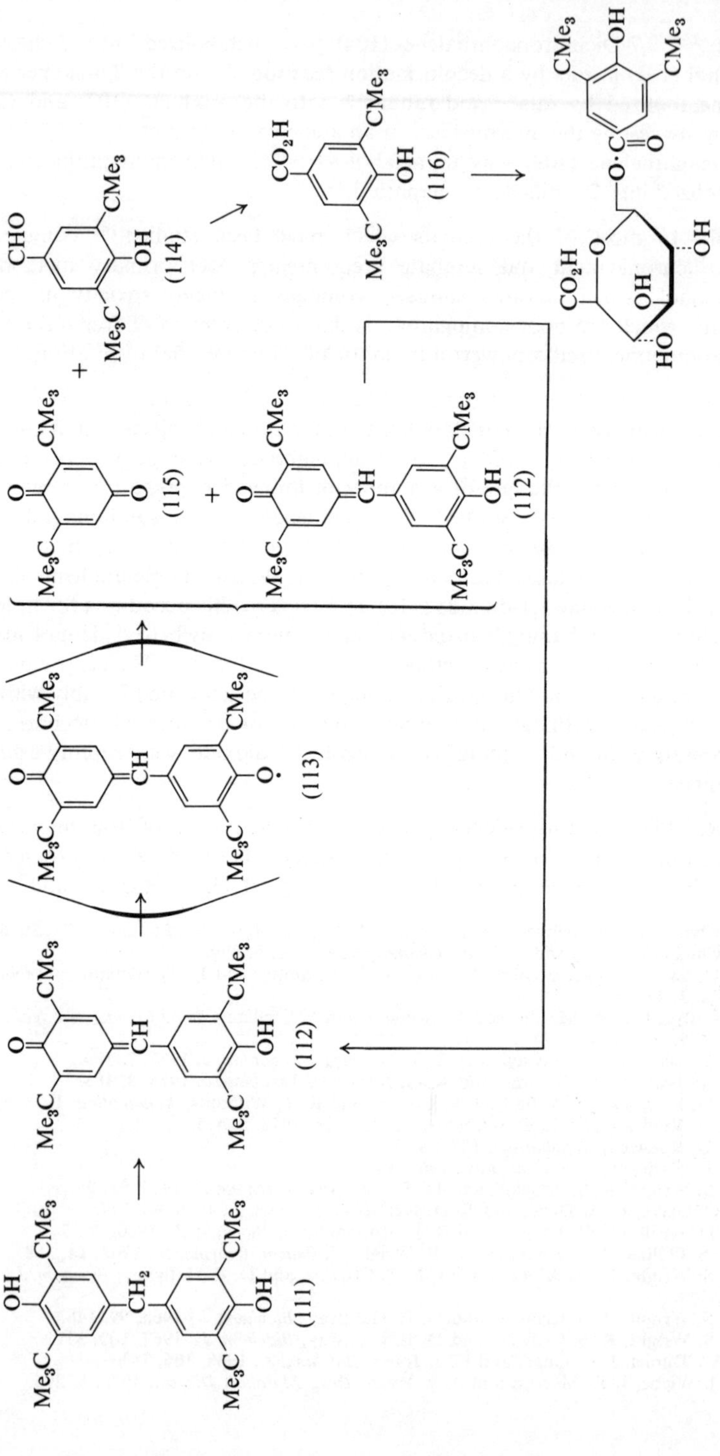

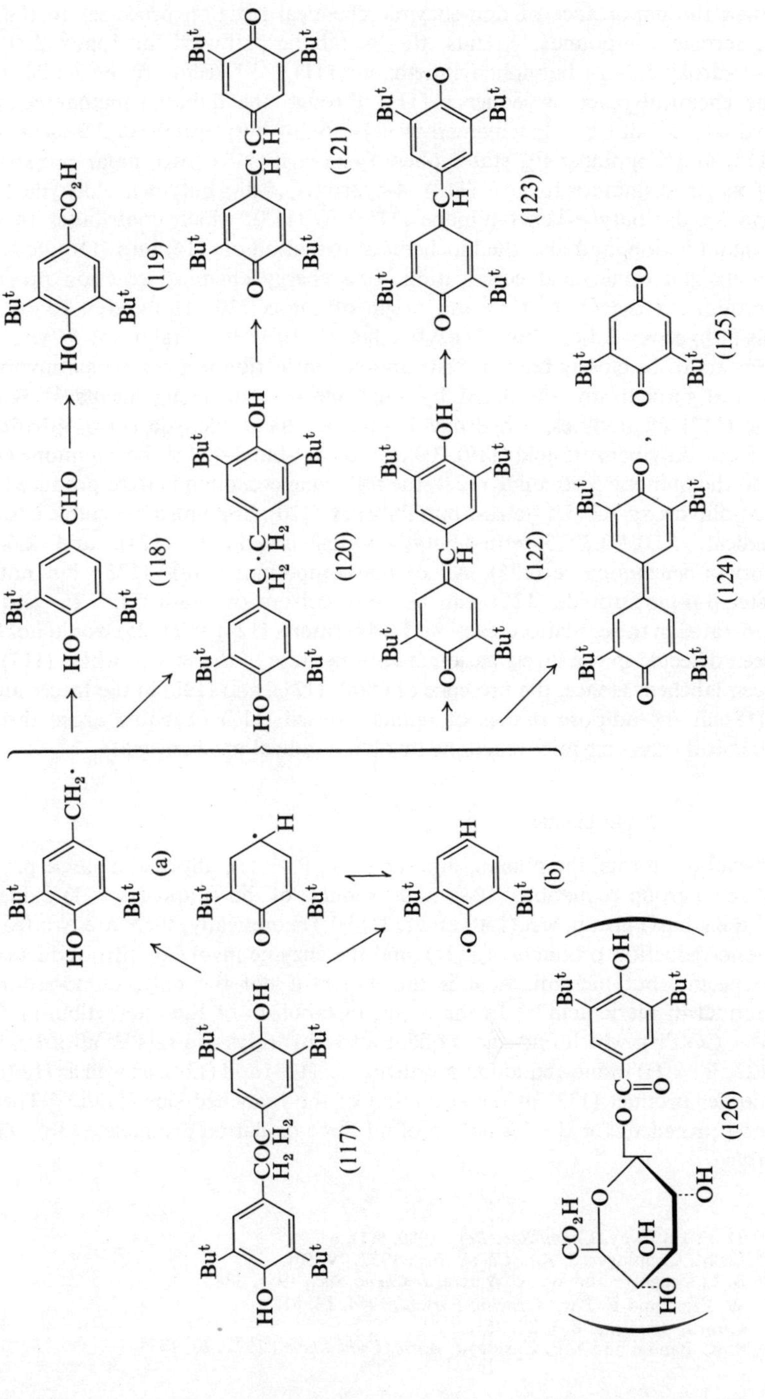

stress the importance of non-enzymic chemical reaction processes to the fate of foreign compounds.[121] Thus, the 'metabolic pathway' for Ionox 220, bis-(4-hydroxy-3,5-di-t-butylphenyl)methane (111),[111,117] seems to be made up of the chemical reaction sequence (111) through the quinone methanide, 4-(4-hydroxy-3,5-di-t-butylphenylmethylene)-2,6-di-t-butylcyclohexa-2,5-dien-1-one (112) and Coppinger's[122] stable phenoxy radical (113) [two molar proportions of which dismutate to give (112), 4-hydroxy-3,5-di-t-butylbenzaldehyde (114), and 2,6-di-t-butyl-*p*-benzoquinone (115)] to (115), which contributes to anti-oxidant action, and also the biochemical oxidation of (114) into (116), followed by its glucuronic acid conjugation. Low-energy chemical reaction processes account for the orientation and origin of Ionox 220 metabolites. Ionox 201, bis-(4-hydroxy-3,5-di-t-butylbenzyl) ether (117),[111,118] metabolism *in vivo* also appears to be closely related to its antioxidant action *in vitro*, which involves a radical mechanism, simulated by single-electron oxidizing agents.[118] Besides the (117) metabolites, 4-hydroxy-3,5-di-t-butylbenzaldehyde (118), 4-hydroxy-3,5-di-t-butylbenzoic acid (119), 3,3′,5,5′-tetra-t-butyl-4,4′-stilbenequinone (121), and the quinone methanide (122), the following compounds were produced, *viz.* 4,4′-dihydroxy-3,3′,5,5′-tetra-t-butylbibenzyl (120), Coppinger's[122] stable phenoxy radical (123), 3,3′5,5′-tetra-t-butyl-4,4′-diphenoquinone (124), and 2,6-di-t-butyl-*p*-benzoquinone (125). All of the compounds (118)—(125), but not the ester β-D-glucuronide (126), can be derived from two radicals,[123] (a) and (b), generated in the oxidation reaction. Furthermore, (124) and (125) would not have been detected in the investigation *in vivo*, because of the way in which (117) had been labelled. Hence, the presence of (118), (121), and (122) in the faeces and of (118) in the adipose tissues of animals dosed (117) probably arose through chemical (non-enzymic) reactions involving radical mechanisms.

3 Herbicides

Phenols.—In rats, the phenol, dinoseb (127; R = H), afforded a single product of nitro-group reduction, (128), and products of the ω and (ω − 1) oxidation of the s-butyl group, *viz.* (130) and (131).[124] Theoretically, there are two feasible mono-reduction products of (127), and the enzyme involved, nitro-reductase, is unspecific, but picramic acid is the major, if not the only, mono-reduction product of picric acid.[125] In the event, metabolism of the ester, dibuton (127; R = CO_2Pr^i), which undergoes quantitative hydrolysis in rats,[126] afforded both (127; R = H) mono-reduction products, *viz.* (128) and (129), as well as (130) and another product (132) of the oxidation of the branched side-chain.[126] There is good precedent for the formation of all three oxidation products, (130)—(132), *in vivo*.

[121] D. E. Hathway, *Chem. Soc. Rev.*, 1980, **9(1)**, 63.
[122] G. M. Coppinger, *J. Am. Chem. Soc.*, 1957, **79**, 501.
[123] S. L. Cosgrave and W. A. Waters, *J. Chem. Soc.*, 1951, 388.
[124] W. Ernst and F. Bär, *Arzneim.-Forsch.*, 1964, **14**, 81.
[125] Girard, *Annalen*, 1853, **88**, 261.
[126] S. K. Bandal and J. E. Casida, *J. Agric. Food Chem.*, 1972, **20**, 1235.

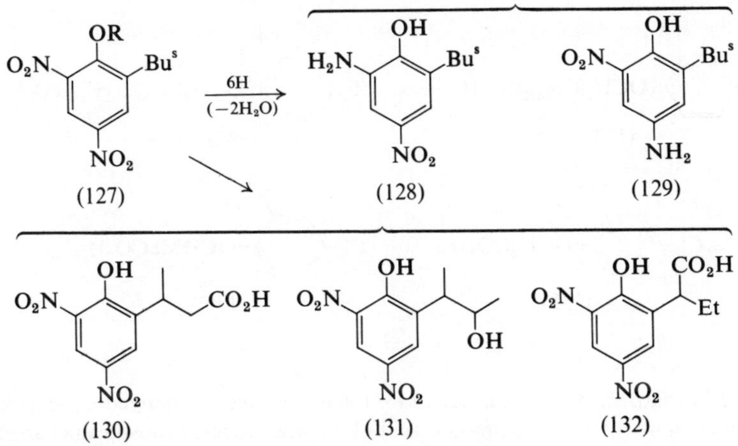

(127) (128) (129)

(130) (131) (132)

Phenoxyacetic Acids.—In general, the halogenophenoxyacetic acids are practically unmetabolized by mammals. Thus, in man and dogs,[127,128] rabbits and rats,[129] and sheep,[130] 2,4-D (2,4-dichlorophenoxyacetic acid) was excreted unchanged: 96% of an oral dose in 72 h in sheep[130] and up to 100% in 6 days in rats.[131] No trace of any 2,4-D metabolite was found in either of the quantitative studies,[130,131] but later, small amounts of the glycine and taurine conjugates were identified in rats;[132] not apparently in human subjects.[133] At least 95% of the dose of 2,4,5-T was excreted unchanged in pregnant rats,[134] and the remainder appears to be made up of 2,4,5-T conjugates including the glycine[132,135] and taurine[132] ones. Unchanged herbicide had been detected previously[136] in the urine of dairy cows, treated with 2,4,5-T. In guinea-pigs, the major metabolite of 4-(2,4-dichlorophenoxy)butyric acid (133) is the β-oxidation product, *viz.* 2,4-D (135),[137] and 4-(2,4,5-trichlorophenoxy)butyric acid is metabolized rapidly into 2,4,5-T and 2,4,5-trichlorophenol.[132,137] Methyl substituents of 4-chloro-2-methyl-phenoxyacetic (135)[138,139] and Silvex (136)[140,141] were unmetabolized in

[127] M. Nencki and P. Giacosa, *Z. physiol. Chem.*, 1880, **4**, 337.
[128] H. Thierfelder and E. Schempp, *Arch. ges. Physiol.*, 1917, **167**, 280.
[129] S. Levey and H. B. Lewis, *J. Biol. Chem.*, 1947, **168**, 213.
[130] D. E. Clark, J. E. Young, R. L. Younger, L. M. Hunt, and J. K. McLaran, *J. Agric. Food Chem.*, 1964, **13**, 43.
[131] S. Khanna and S. C. Fang, *J. Agric. Food Chem.*, 1966, **14**, 500.
[132] W. Grunow and C. Böhme, *Arch. Toxicol.*, 1974, **32**, 217.
[133] J. D. Kohli, R. N. Khanna, B. N. Gupta, M. M. Dhar, J. S. Tandon, and K. P. Sircar, *Xenobiotica*, 1974, **4**, 97.
[134] S. C. Fang, E. Fallin, M. L. Montgomery, and V. H. Freed, *Toxicol. Appl. Pharmacol.*, 1973, **24**, 555.
[135] W. Grunow, C. Böhme, and B. Budczies, *Food Cosmet. Toxicol*, 1971, **9**, 667.
[136] L. E. St John, D. G. Wagner, and D. J. Lisk, *J. Dairy Sci.*, 1964, **47**, 1267.
[137] C. H. van Peteghem and A. M. Heyndrickx, *Bull. Environ. Contamin. Toxicol.*, 1975, **14**, 632.
[138] H. Elo, *Acta Pharmacol. Toxicol.*, 1976, **39**, 58.
[139] P. Fjelstad and A. Wannag, *Scand. J. Work Environ. Health*, 1977, **3**, 100.
[140] M. W. Sauerhoff, W. H. Braun, and J. E. Le Beau, *J. Toxicol. Environ. Health*, 1977, **2**, 605.
[141] M. W. Sauerhoff, M. B. Chenoweth, R. J. Karbowski, W. H., Braun, J. C. Ramsey, P. J. Gehring, and G. E. Blau, *J. Toxicol. Environ. Health*, 1977, **3**, 941.

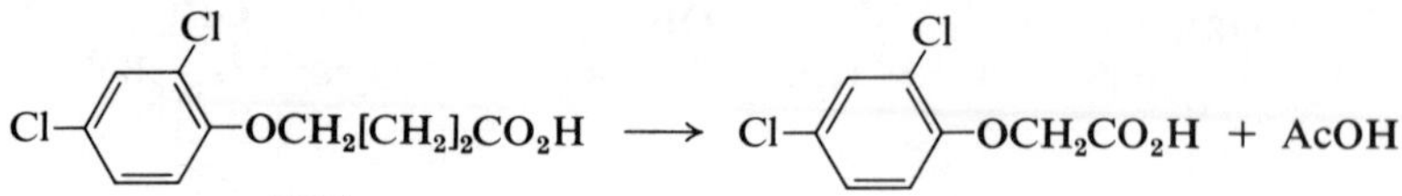

(133) (134)

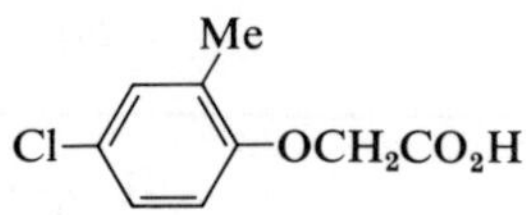

(135)

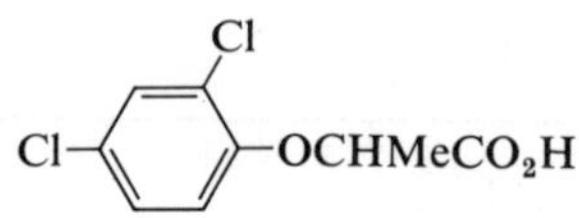

(136)

rats and in man. In human subjects, (135) was excreted unchanged or as (135) conjugates in 48 h.[139] The propionic acid (136) was excreted mostly unchanged and conjugates that may have been formed were unidentified.[140,141] Great interest is associated with a teratogenic by-product, 2,3,7,8-tetrachlorodibenzo-

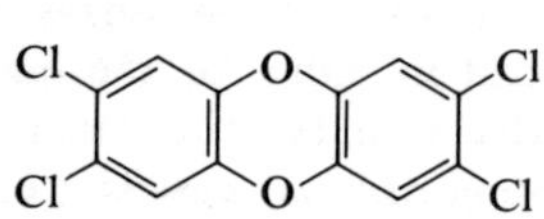

(137)

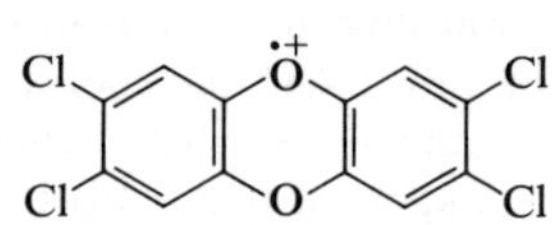

(138)

p-dioxin (137) in 2,4,5-T synthesis. Whilst (137) accumulated in the liver microsomes of chronically dosed rats,[142,143] binding was reversible, as dioxin residues were excreted from the animals when dosing ended. No (137) metabolites have been identified. The fact that microsomal binding of (137) increased in induced animals suggests that a cytochrome P-450 oxidative process occurs, possibly involving production of the cation radical (138).[144] Thus, nuclear uptake and binding of (137) seems to be mediated by a cytosol receptor, and such binding would be essential to induction of mono-oxygenase activity.[145]

Carbamates and Thiocarbamates.—In rats, the *p*-hydroxylation product (145) is the most important metabolite of chloropropham (139). Hydroxylation of the isopropyl residue accounted for about one-third of (139) metabolism, and approximately four times as much of the monohydroxy compounds, (140) and (146), as of the dihydroxy compound (142) was produced. Further oxidation of (140) gave the 1-carboxyethyl derivative (141). Besides *m*-chloroaniline, (139)

[142] J. R. Allen, J. P. Van Miller, and D. H. Norback, *Food Cosmet. Toxicol.*, 1975, **13**, 501.
[143] W. C. Dauterman and W. Muecke, *Pestic. Biochem. Physiol.*, 1974, **4**, 212.
[144] J. O. Nelson, R. E. Menzer, P. C. Kearney, and J. R. Plimmer, *Bull. Environ. Contamin. Toxicol.*, 1977, **18**, 9.
[145] W. F. Greenlee and A. Poland, *J. Biol. Chem.*, 1979, **254**, 9814.

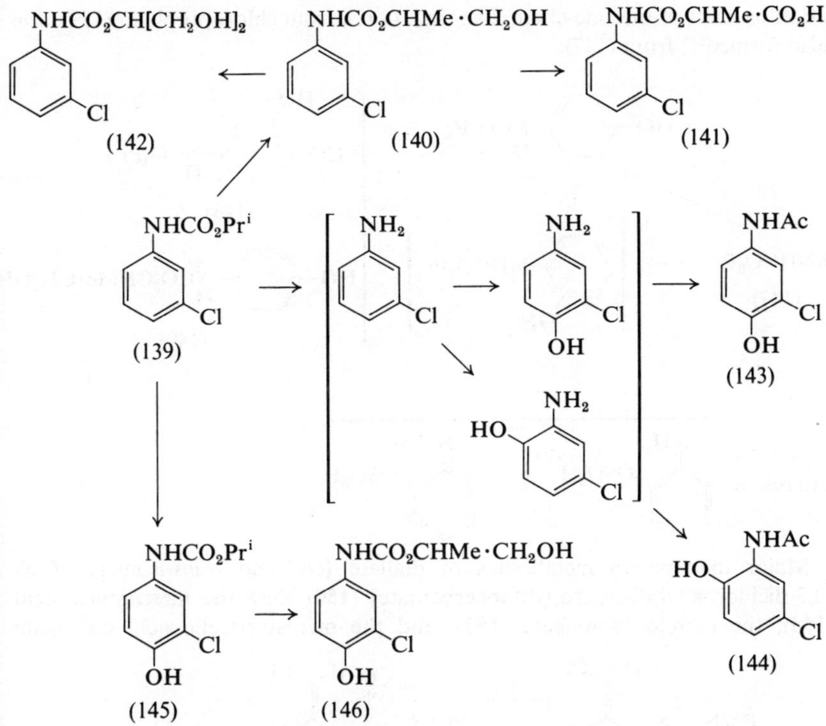

hydrolysis gave CO_2 and isopropyl alcohol, which was oxidized to acetone and CO_2. The *m*-chloroaniline liberated was hydroxylated to give 4- and 6-hydroxy-3-chloroacetanilide (143) and (144).[146–151]

o- and *p*-Hydroxylation products preponderated in the metabolism of propham (147) in rats and goats, and included the doubly hydroxylated derivatives, (148) and (149), where the side-chain oxidized product (149) of (147) corresponded to that, (146), of chloropropham. Preferential hydrolysis of the *o*-hydroxy compounds may have occurred, as both *o*-hydroxyaniline and *o*-hydroxy acetanilide were identified as the sulphates[152] (*cf.* ref. 153). A double hydroxyl-

146 L. G. Aleksandrova and M. A. Klisenko, *Gig. i Sanit.*, 1971, **36**, 108.
147 L. G. Aleksandrova and M. A. Klisenko, in 'Proceedings of the 2nd All-Union Conference on the Studies on Residues of Pesticides and Prevention of their Pollution of Human and Animal Food and of the Environment,' ed. O. M. Tamm, Research Institute Epidemiological and Microbiological Hygiene, Tallinn, 1971, pp. 127–130.
148 C. Böhme and W. Grunow, *Food Cosmet. Toxicol.*, 1969, **7**, 125.
149 S. C. Fang, E. Fallin, M. L. Montgomery, and V. H. Freed, *Pestic. Biochem. Physiol.*, 1974, **4**, 1.
150 W. Grunow, C. Bohme, and B. Budczies, *Food Cosmet. Toxicol.*, 1970, **8**, 277.
151 S. A. Kosyan, in 'Proceedings of the Conference on Toxicology and Hygiene of Mineral Oil Distillation Products,' Yaroslavl Medical Institute, Yaroslavl, 1971, vol. 2, pp. 110—115.
152 G. D. Paulson, A. M. Jacobsen, R. G. Zaylskie, and V. J. Feil, *J. Agric. Food. Chem.*, 1973, **21**, 804.
153 G. M. Holder and A. J. Ryan, *Nature*, 1968, **220**, 77.

ation product of the side-chain, like that, (142), from chloropropham (139), was also formed[149] from (147).

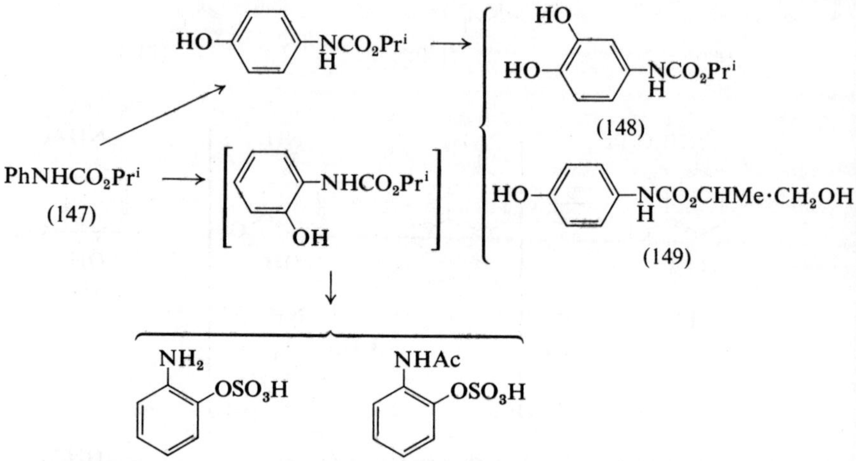

Major mammalian metabolites of diallate [*cis*- and *trans*-isomers of *S*-(2,3-dichloroallyl)di-isopropylthiocarbamate] (150) were the mercapturic acid (155), the cysteine conjugate (153), and the mercaptoacetic acid conjugate

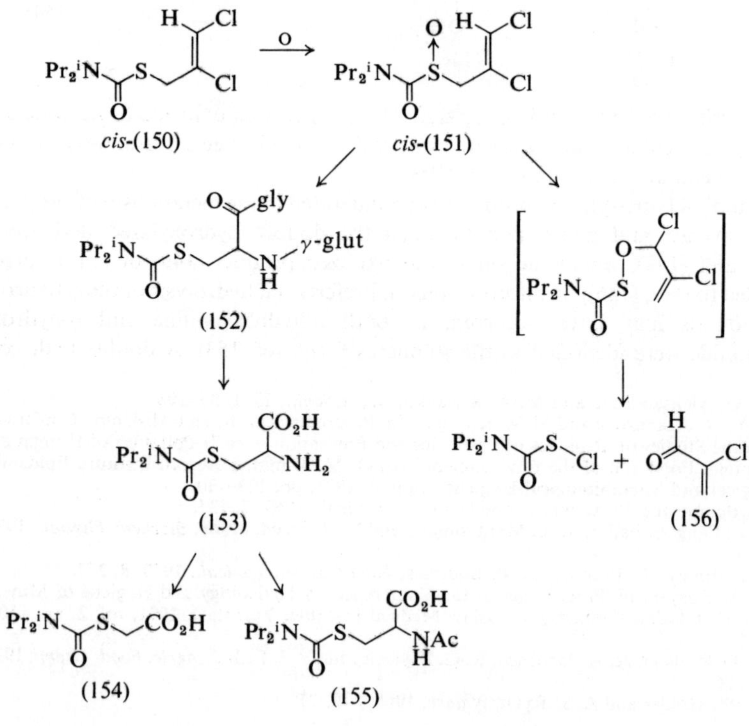

(154),[154] but none of these metabolites were formed *in vitro*. However, large amounts of the glutathione conjugate (152), formed from (150) sulphoxide (151), was detected in incubations to which glutathione had been added.[154] In addition, the mutagenic metabolite 2-chloroacrolein (156) of (150) was shown [155,156] to be formed through successive [2,3]-sigmatropic rearrangement and 1,2-elimination.

Diphenyl Ethers.—Diphenyl ethers are predominantly lipid-soluble, and their metabolic fate illustrates, in some cases, accumulation by adipose tissues and the faecal excretion of unchanged biocide, and in others, rapid metabolism and excretion. The diphenyl ether linkage presents varying degrees of resistance to hydrolysis.

In rats, 75% of a dose of GOAL, 2-chloro-1-(3-ethoxy-4-nitrophenoxy)-4-trifluoromethylbenzene (157) was excreted unchanged in the faeces.[157] (157) features nitro-group reduction and oxidative *O*-dealkylation, and affords (158)—(161) as major metabolites in the faeces.[157] The chlorinated ring was unattacked.

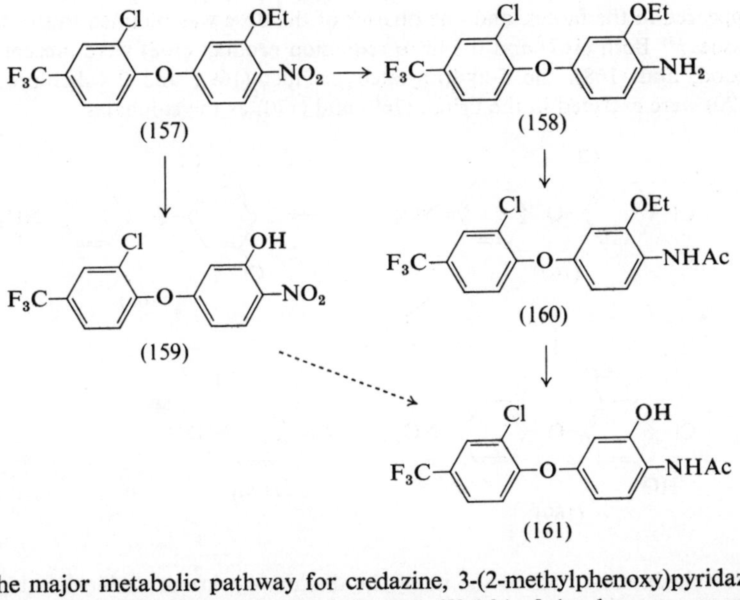

The major metabolic pathway for credazine, 3-(2-methylphenoxy)pyridazine (162) involved oxidation of the methyl group:[158] 2% of the dose was excreted as the alcohol (163), 43% as the carboxylic acid (164), and 38% as its hydrolytic fission product, pyridazin-3-one (165). Hydroxylation of (162) also occurred, and the sulphate ester of the phenol (166) accounted for 5% of the dose. The major microsomal product *in vitro* was (163).

[154] Y. S. Chen, I. Schuphan, and J. E. Casida, *J. Agric. Food Chem.*, 1979, **27**, 709.
[155] I. Schuphan, J. D. Rosen, and J. E. Casida, *Science*, 1979, **205**, 1013.
[156] I. Schuphan and J. E. Casida, *Tetrahedron Lett.*, 1979, **841**.
[157] I. L. Alder, B. M. Hones, and J. P. Wargo, *J. Agric. Food Chem.*, 1977, **25**, 1339.
[158] M. Nakagawa and M. Audo, *Agric. Biol. Chem. (Jpn)*, 1977, **41**, 1975.

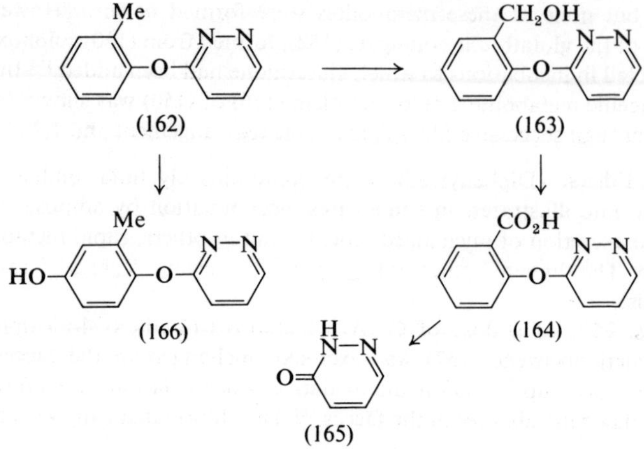

In sheep, excretion of nitrofen (167) is slow (76% in 99 h); much of this appeared in the faeces, and one-quarter of the dose was retained in the adipose tissues.[159] Both (167) and the nitro reduction product (168) were present in the blood, and (168), the 5-hydroxylated product (169), and 2,4-dichlorophenol (170) were excreted in the urine; (169) and (170) as the sulphates.

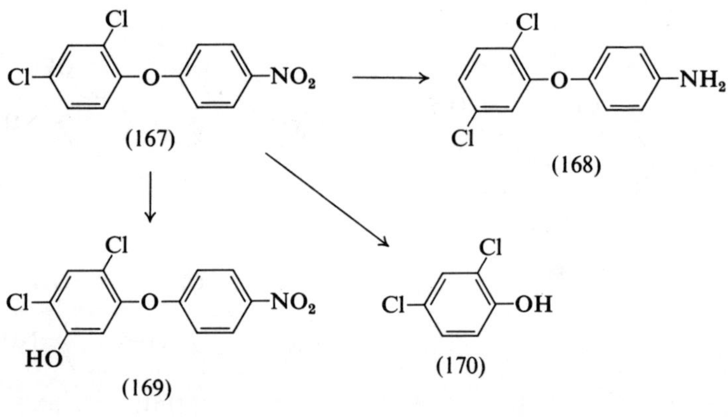

***s*-Triazines.**—In all of the many 2,6-diamino-*s*-triazine herbicides that have been investigated, the *s*-triazine ring is unmetabolized and biotransformations are confined to the 2,4,6-substituents. Oxidative *N*-dealkylation is a common metabolic pathway. The purpose of this discussion is served by the 2-chloro derivatives, which illustrate most of the metabolic features. Out of the mammalian metabolites of atrazine, 2-chloro-4-ethylamino-6-isopropylamino-*s*-triazine (171), which gave all three *N*-dealkylation products, *viz*. (172), (173), and (176), and two further oxidation products, (174) and (175), compounds (172),

[159] L. M. Hunt, W. F. Chamberlain, B. N. Gilbert, D. E. Hopkins, and A. R. Gingrich, *J. Agric. Food Chem.*, 1977, **25**, 1062.

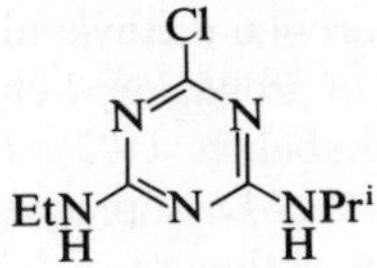

(171)

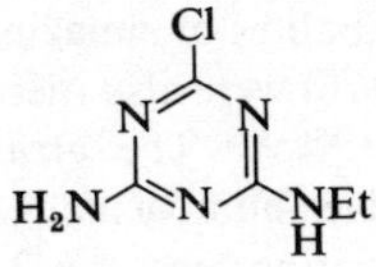

(172)

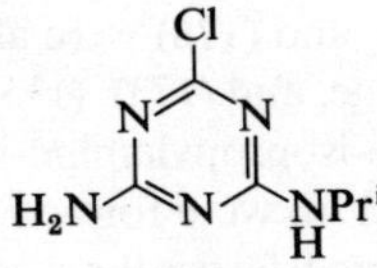

(173)

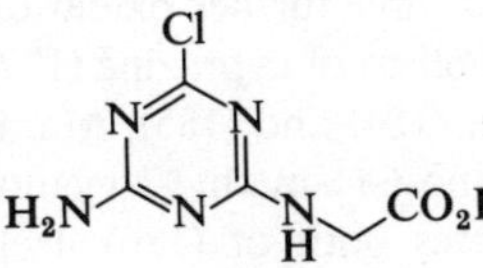

(174)

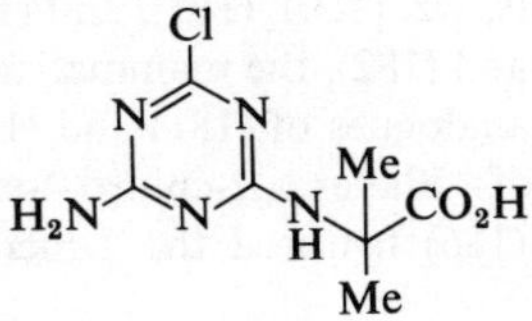

(175)

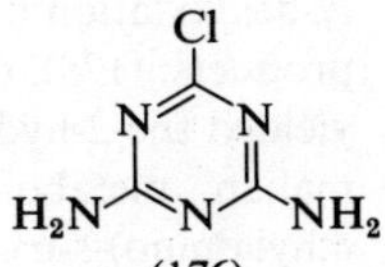

(176)

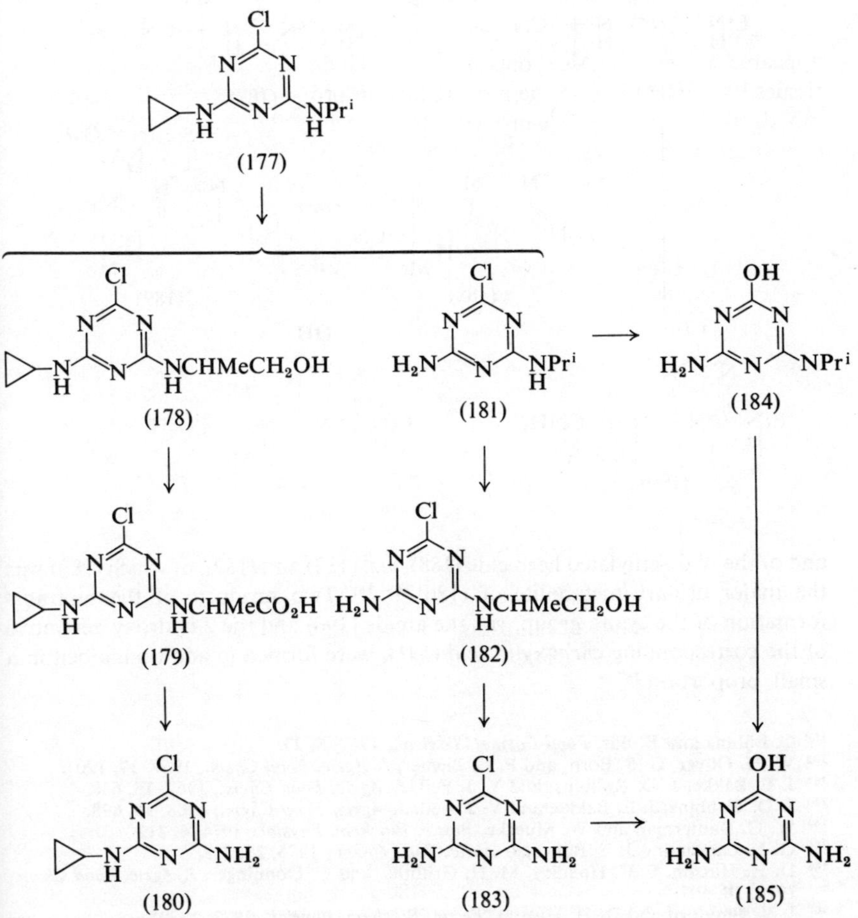

(174), and (176) were also metabolites of simazine, 2-chloro-4,6-diethylamino-*s*-triazine, and (173), (175), and (176) were also metabolites of propazine, 2-chloro-4,6-di-isopropylamino-*s*-triazine.[160–163] The atrazine metabolites (172), (173), and (176) were formed by rat-liver homogenates *in vitro*.[164] *N*-Deisopropylation occurred faster than *N*-de-ethylation, and the 2-hydroxy analogues of (171)—(173) and (176) were found not to be (171) metabolites.[164] Besides the three *N*-dealkylation products, *viz.* (180), (181), and (183) and three further oxidation products, (178), (179), and (182), the mammalian metabolism of cyprazine (177) yielded the 2-hydroxy analogues of (181) and (183), *viz.* (184) and (185), Mammalian metabolism of Bladex, 2-chloro-4-ethylamino-6-(1-methyl-1-cyano-ethylamino)-*s*-trizaine (186) featured the 2-mercapturates both of (186) itself

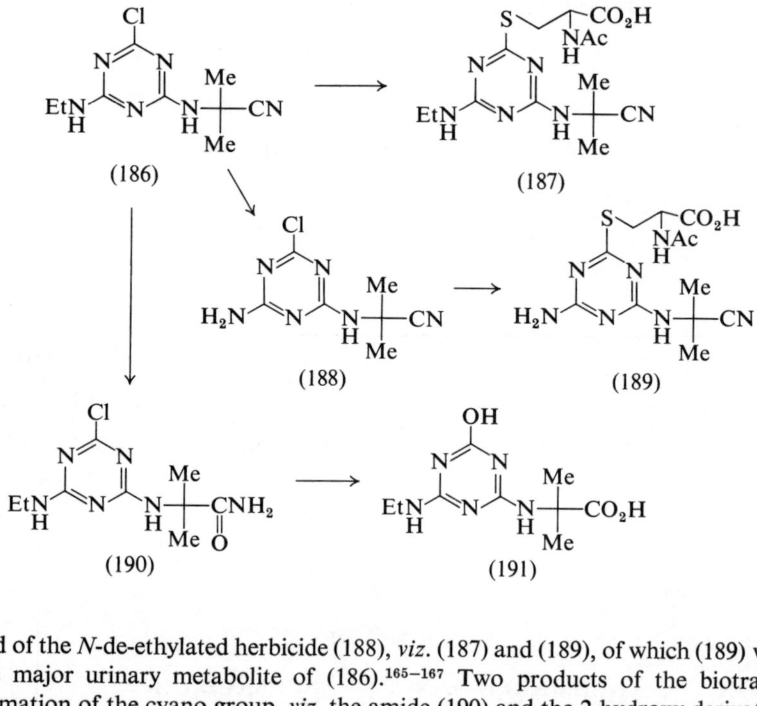

and of the *N*-de-ethylated herbicide (188), *viz.* (187) and (189), of which (189) was the major urinary metabolite of (186).[165–167] Two products of the biotransformation of the cyano group, *viz.* the amide (190) and the 2-hydroxy derivative of the corresponding carboxylic acid (191), were formed in addition, albeit in a small proportion.[167]

[160] C. Böhme and F. Bär, *Food Cosmet. Toxicol.*, 1967, **5**, 23.
[161] W. H. Oliver, G. S. Born, and P. L. Ziemer, *J. Agric. Food Chem.*, 1969, **17**, 1207.
[162] J. E. Bakke, J. D. Robbins, and V. J. Feil, *J. Agric. Food Chem.*, 1967, **15**, 628.
[163] J. D. Robbins, J. E. Bakke, and V. J. Feil, *J. Agric. Food Chem.*, 1968, **16**, 698.
[164] W. C. Dauterman and W. Muecke, *Pestic. Biochem. Physiol.*, 1974, **4**, 212.
[165] G. L. Larsen and J. E. Bakke, *J. Agric. Food Chem.*, 1975, **23**, 388.
[166] D. H. Hutson, E. C. Hoadley, M. H. Griffiths, and C. Donninger, *J. Agric. Food Chem.*, 1970, **18**, 507.
[167] J. V. Crayford and D. H. Hutson, *Pestic. Biochem. Physiol.*, 1972, **2**, 295.

4 Insecticides

Organophosphates and Organothiophosphates.—This is one of the oldest groups of insecticides, and it has been used widely for more than three decades. The fact that biotransformation of organophosphates sometimes results either in bioactivation or in detoxification seems to have divided the subject-matter. Dethionation of P(S) compounds to P(O) compounds constitutes the principal activation reaction, and others include hydroxylation, which is restricted to phosphoramides, thioether oxidation, and cyclization. All four activation reactions take place in insects, and the first three occur also in plants. In contrast, detoxification of organophosphates is brought about theoretically by hydrolysis. Thus, phosphatase-catalysed reactions afford the following fission:

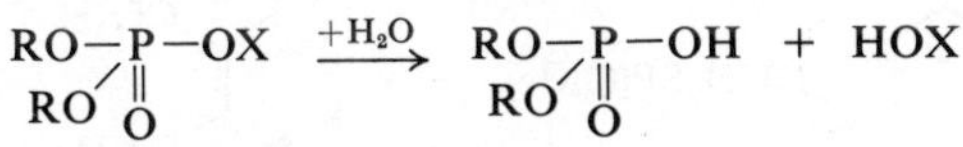

and this route is analogous to AChE inhibition. Alternatively the following type of reaction also takes place widely:

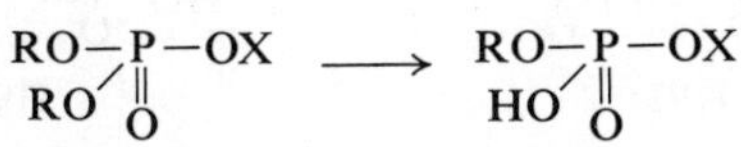

This second metabolic pathway has been regarded as another hydrolytic reaction,[168] and biotransformation of chlorfenvinphos, 2-chloro-1-(2,4-dichlorophenyl)vinyl diethyl phosphate into 2-chloro-1-(2,4-dichlorophenyl)vinyl ethyl hydrogen phosphate in dogs[169] illustrates this. But, in this case, two explanations for the reaction have been established, one of them[170] involving oxidative *O*-dealkylation, and the other,[171] glutathione alkyl transferase. An essentially similar reaction is probably the *O*-demethylation of bidrin, dimethyl 3-hydroxy-*N*,*N*-dimethyl-*cis*-crotonamide phosphate (192). Other detoxification reactions involve carboxy-esterase action, for example, the metabolism of malathion[172,173] [equation (2)], amidase action, for example, the biotransformations of dimethoate into dimethoate acid[174] [equation (3)], and of imidan into phthalamic acid[175] [equation (4)], and oxidative *N*-dealkylation, for example, bidrin (192) to give Azodrin, dimethyl 3-hydroxy-*N*-methyl-*cis*-crotonamide phosphate (194) (*v. infra*).[176]

[168] F. W. Plapp and J. E. Casida, *J. Econ. Entomol.*, 1958, **51**, 800.
[169] D. H. Hutson, D. A. A. Akintonwa, and D. E. Hathway, *Biochem. J.*, 1967, **102**, 133.
[170] C. Donninger, D. H. Hutson, and B. A. Pickering, *Biochem. J.*, 1967, **102**, 26P.
[171] D. H. Hutson, B. A. Pickering, and C. Donninger, *Biochem. J.*, 1967, **106**, 20P
[172] J. B. Knaak and R. D. O'Brien, *J. Agric. Food Chem.*, 1960, **8**, 198.
[173] R. D. O'Brien, W. C. Dauterman, and R. P. Neidermeier, *J. Agric. Food Chem.*, 1961, **9**, 39.
[174] T. Uchida, J. Zsintzsch, and R. D. O'Brien, *Toxicol. Appl. Pharmacol.*, 1966, **8**, 259.
[175] J. J. Menn and J. B. McBain, *J. Agric. Food Chem.*, 1964, **12**, 162.
[176] R. E. Menzer and J. E. Casida, *J. Agric. Food Chem.*, 1965, **13**, 102.

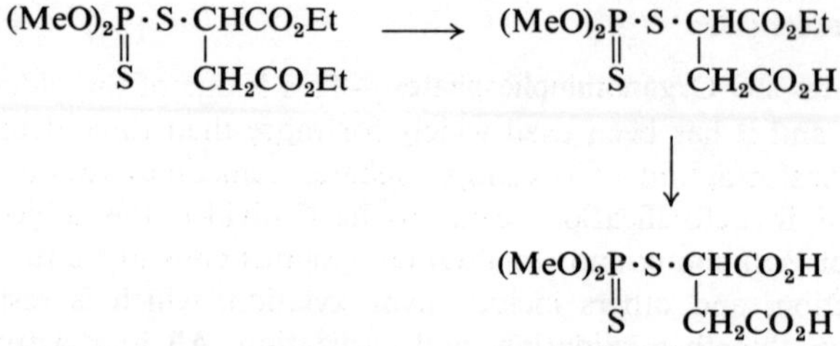

(2)

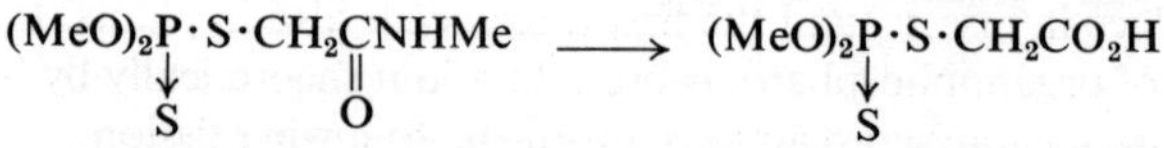

(3)

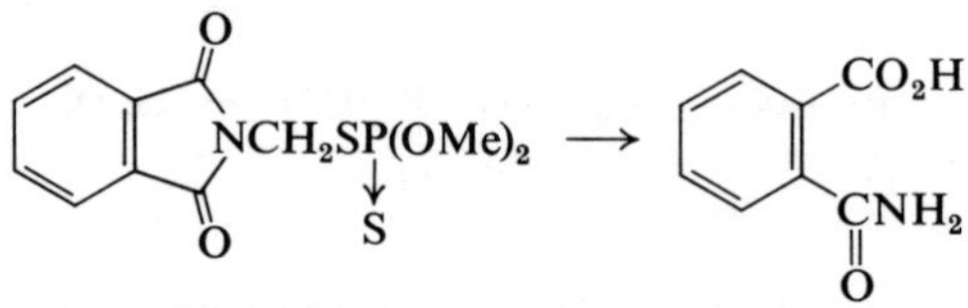

(4)

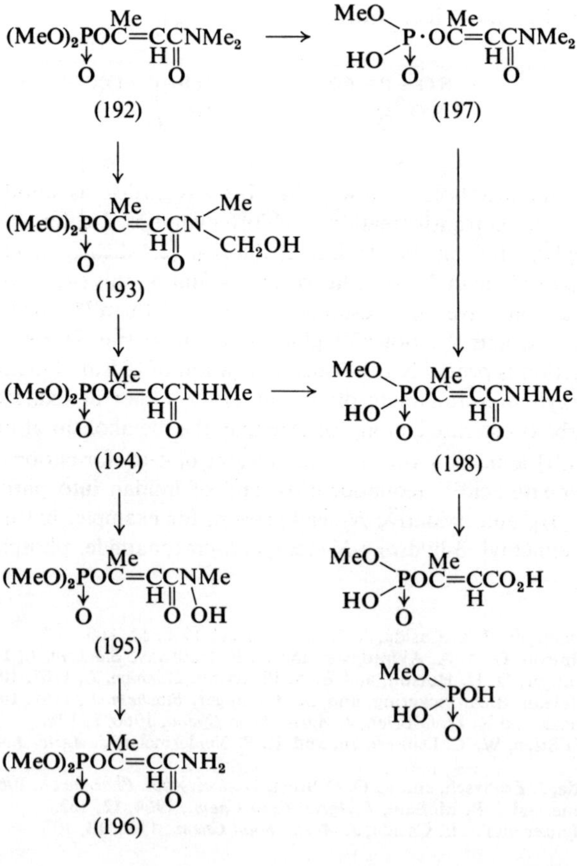

(192) (193) (194) (195) (196) (197) (198)

Bidrin (192) affords products of oxidative *N*-demethylation and hydrolytic *O*-demethylation.[176,177] In the *N*-demethylation process, small amounts of the methylolamide (193) are accompanied by larger amounts of the insecticide, Azodrin (194), which is further metabolized into dimethyl 3,*N*-dihydroxy-*N*-methyl-*cis*-crontonamide phosphate (195) and dimethyl 3-hydroxy-*cis*-crotonamide phosphate (196). Toxicity increases with *N*-demethylation. *O*-Demethylation products, (197) and (198), corresponding to (192) and (194), were metabolized further into methyl 3-hydroxy-*cis*-crotonic acid phosphate and methyl phosphate.

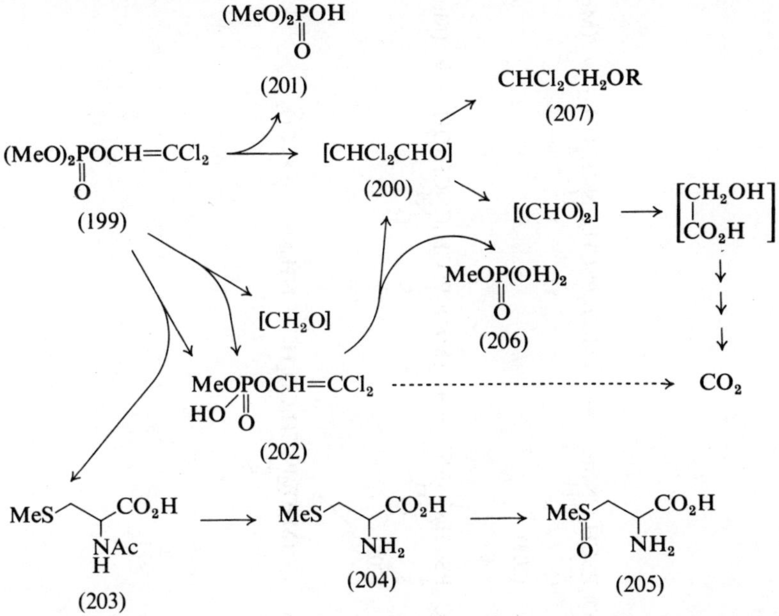

The metabolism of dichlorvos, 2,2-dichloroethenyl dimethyl phosphate (199), has been thoroughly investigated,[178–188] and initial biotransformation involves either hydrolysis into dichloroacetaldehyde (200) and dimethyl phosphate (201) or *O*-demethylation to demethyl-dichlorvos (202), which is mediated

177 D. L. Bull and D. A. Lindquist, *J. Agric. Food Chem.*, 1964, **12**, 310.
178 E. Hodgson and J. E. Casida, *J. Agric. Food Chem.*, 1962, **10**, 208.
179 J. E. Casida, L. McBride, and R. P. Niedermeier, *J. Agric. Food Chem.*, 1962, **10**, 370.
180 D. H. Hutson, D. Blair, E. C. Hoadley, and B. A. Pickering, *Toxicol. Appl. Pharmacol.*, 1971, **19**, 378.
181 A. C. Page, J. E. Loeffler, H. R. Hendrickson, C. K. Huston, and D. M. De Vries, *Arch. Toxicol.*, 1972, **30**, 19.
182 D. H. Hutson and E. C. Hoadley, *Arch. Toxicol.*, 1972, **30**, 9.
183 D. Blair, E. C. Hoadley, and D. H. Hutson, *Toxicol. Appl. Pharmacol.*, 1975, **31**, 243.
184 J. C. Potter, J. E. Loeffler, R. D. Collins, R. Young, and A. C. Page, *J. Agric. Food Chem.*, 1973, **21**, 163.
185 J. C. Potter, A. C. Boyer, R. L. Marxmiller, R. Young, and J. E. Loeffler, *J. Agric. Food Chem.*, 1973, **21**, 734.
186 D. H. Hutson and E. C. Hoadley, *Xenobiotica*, 1972, **2**, 107.
187 D. H. Hutson, E. C. Hoadley, and B. A. Pickering, *Xenobiotica*, 1971, **1**, 593.
188 L. Dicowsky and A. Morello, *Life Sci.*, 1971, **10(II)**, 1031.

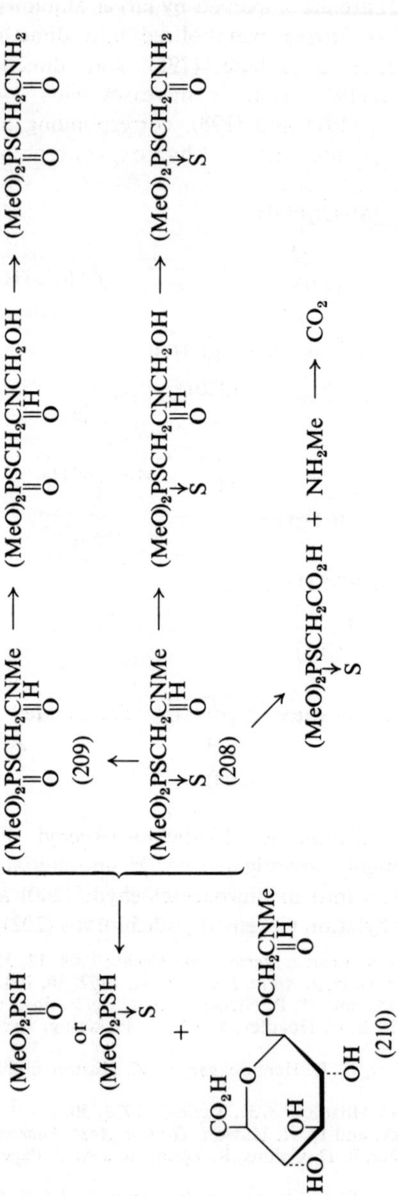

both by *S*-alkyl glutathione transferases and by cytochrome P-450. Tracer studies[186] showed the importance of hydrolytic cleavage, and they also detected the presence of the three sulphur-containing metabolites, (203)—(205). The demethyl derivative (202) is only partially excreted *per se*,[186] as it undergoes rapid hydrolysis to afford methyl phosphate (206) and more (200). Methyl glutathione and formaldehyde, the by-products of *O*-demethylation, both serve as substrates for CO_2 production *in vivo*. More dichloroethanol glucuronide (207; $R = C_6H_9O_6$) is formed by parenteral than by enteral administration. Finally, the metabolism of (199) has been discussed[189] in terms of soft and hard acids and bases.

In rats, oxidative dethionation of dimethoate (208), dimethyl *S*-(*N*-methylcarbamoylmethyl)phosphorodithioate occurs to give dimethoxon (209) which is responsible for the AChE inhibition of (208).[190] Carboxyamidase action cleaves the C—N bond of (208) with liberation of methylamine, which produces CO_2 by oxidative *N*-demethylation. Another major metabolic pathway involves esteratic fission of the S—C bond, with formation of dimethyl phosphorothioate from (209) and dimethyl phosphorodithioate from (208): the non-phosphorus residue is excreted in the urine of animals as the *O*-glucuronide (210).[190] Both

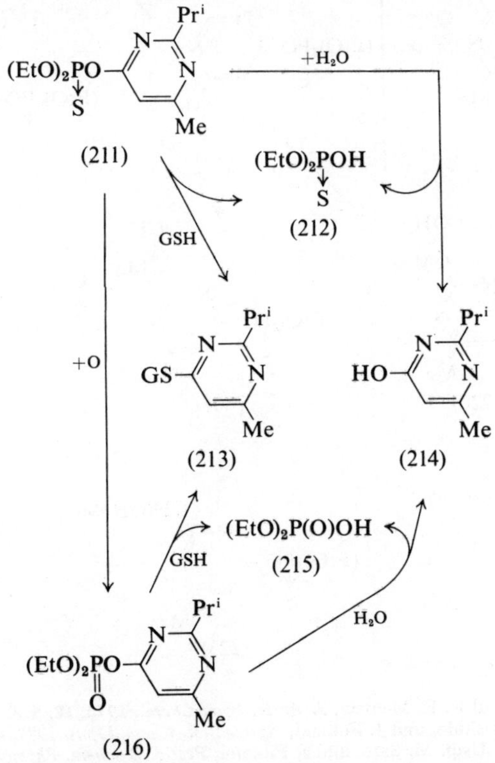

189 C. Bedford and J. Robinson, *Xenobiotica*, 1972, **2**, 307.
190 A. Hassan, S. M. A. D. Zayed, and M. R. E. Bahig, *Biochem. Pharmacol.*, 1969, **18**, 2429.

(208) and (209) formed methylolamides and underwent oxidative *N*-demethylation.[191] In this way, rats excreted 60% of a dose of (208) in the urine and exhaled air in 24 h.[190]

In vitro study of diazinon, diethyl 2-isopropyl-4-methylpyrimidin-6-yl thiophosphate (211), showed that it underwent oxidative dethionation to give diazoxon (216), and that both (211) and (216) were substrates for glutathione *S*-aryl transferase, which gave *S*-(2-isopropyl-4-methylpyrimidin-6-yl)glutathione (213) by loss respectively of diethyl phosphorothioate (212) and diethyl phosphate (215).[192–196] 2-Hydroxy-6-isopropyl-4-methylyprimidine (214) was formed by esteratic cleavage from (211) and from (216). It is problematical[194,195] whether the oxidative *O*-de-ethylation of (216) takes place. Animal experiments showed

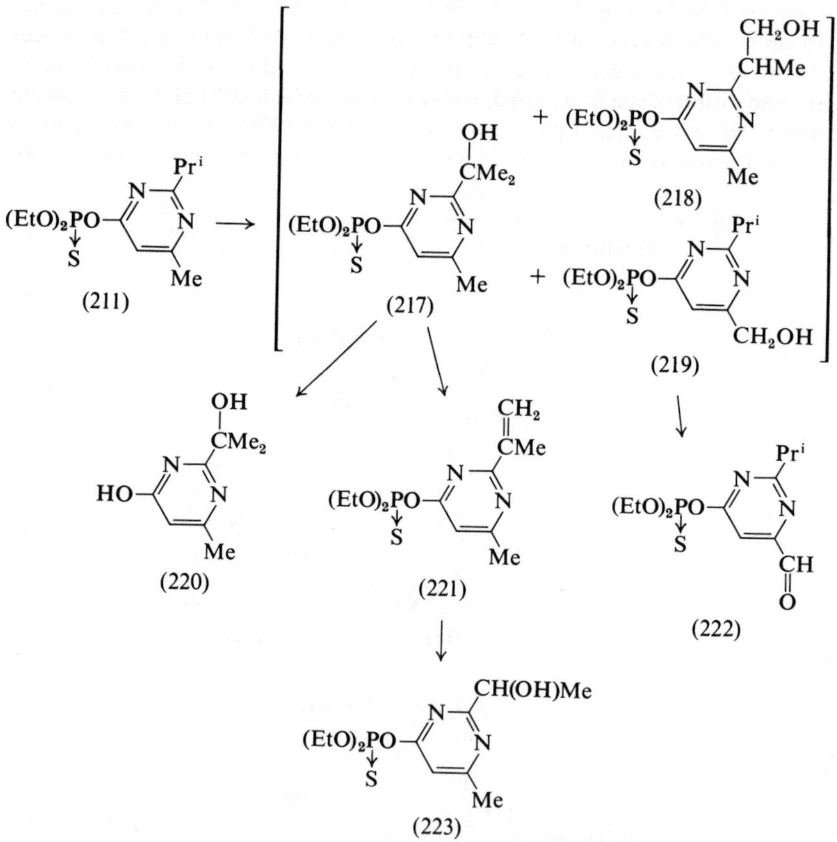

[191] G. W. Lucier and R. E. Mentzer, *J. Agric. Food Chem.*, 1970, **18**, 698.
[192] K. Usui, T. Schishido, and J. Fukami, *Agric. Biol. Chem. (Jpn)*, 1977, **41**, 2491.
[193] T. Shishido, K. Usui, M. Sato, and J. Fukami, *Pestic. Biochem. Physiol.*, 1972, **2**, 51.
[194] T. Shishido and J. Fukami, *Pestic. Biochem. Physiol.*, 1972, **2**, 39.
[195] T. Shishido, K. Usui, and J. Fukami, *Pestic. Biochem. Physiol.*, 1972, **2**, 27.
[196] R. S. H. Yang, E. Hodgson, and W. C. Dauterman, *J. Agric. Food Chem.*, 1971, **19**, 10.

that initial *C*-hydroxylation of (211) yielded all three monohydroxylation products, *viz.* (217)—(219), resulting from biotransformation of the two alkyl groups attached to the pyrimidine ring, as well as products, *viz.* (221)—(223), of the subsequent modification of the hydroxyalkyl side-chains in (217) and (219).[197,198] With their unchanged phosphorothionyl residues, each of the six metabolites, (217)—(219) and (221)—(223), would afford theoretically a range of metabolites corresponding to those, *viz.* (212)—(216), formed from (211).

Carbamates.—Biotransformation of carbaryl, 1-naphthyl *N*-methylcarbamate (224) by rat-liver microsomes afforded the methylolamide, 1-naphthyl *N*-hydroxymethylcarbamate (225), 5,6-dihydroxy-5,6-dihydro-1-naphthyl *N*-methylcarbamate (228), 5-hydroxy-1-naphthyl *N*-methylcarbamate (229), 4-hydroxy-1-naphthyl *N*-methylcarbamate (230),[199–202] and 1-naphthyl *N*-hydroxy-*N*-methylcarbamate (233).[203] When incubated with (224), human and rat-liver homogenates gave equal amounts of (229) and (230), but much of the parent (224) remained unchanged, and more (225) was produced by rat liver than by human liver:[204–206] in addition, some 1-naphthol was formed by hydrolysis.[199] Thus, epoxidation [(226) and (227)] is implicit from the identification of the (224) metabolites, (228), (229), and (230),[207] and the two mercapturates, *viz.* (231) and (232), as well as the glucuronide of (228) were identified[207,208] in the urine of treated rats. The (224) metabolite, (228),[209] and smaller amounts of compounds (224), (225), (230), and (234) have been identified[210–212] in the milk of cows, grazed on contaminated herbage.

DDT Groups.—In this context, only biotransformations of DDT, 1,1,1-trichloro-2,2-*bis*(*p*-chlorophenyl)ethane *per se* and of its *o,p'*-isomer are discussed. Absence of labelled material and of suitable chromatographic methods in the years following World War II hindered the resolution of the metabolism of DDT (see Scheme 3) in mammals, but a great deal of careful work throughout three

197 N. F. Janes, A. F. Machin, M. P. Quick, H. Rogers, D. E. Mundy, and A. J. Cross, *J. Agric. Food. Chem.*, 1973, **21**, 121.
198 B. Sekine, *Jpn Pestic. Inf.*, 1972, **10**, 77.
199 H. W. Dorough and J. E. Casida, *J. Agric. Food. Chem.*, 1964, **12**, 294.
200 H. W. Dorough, N. C. Leeling, and J. E. Casida, *Science*, 1963, **140**, 170.
201 A. Hassan, S. M. A. D. Zayed, and F. M. Abdel-Hamid, *Biochem. Pharmacol.*, 1966, **15**, 2045.
202 R. J. Kuhr and H. W. Dorough, 'Carbamate Insecticides: Chemistry, Biochemistry and Toxicology,' Chemical Rubber, Cleveland, Ohio, 1976, p. 109.
203 R. K. Locke, *J. Agric. Food Chem.*, 1972, **20**, 1078.
204 F. Matsumura and C. T. Ward, *Arch. Environ. Health*, 1966, **13**, 257.
205 A. Stother, *Biochem. Pharmacol.*, 1970, **19**, 2525.
206 A. Strother, *Toxicol. Appl. Pharmacol.*, 1972, **21**, 112.
207 J. R. Bend, G. M. Holder, E. Protos, and A. J. Ryan, *Aust. J. Biol. Sci.*, 1971, **24**, 535.
208 L. J. Sullivan, J. M. Eldridge, J. B. Knaak, and M. J. Tallant, *J. Agric. Food Chem.*, 1972, **20**, 980.
209 R. L. Baron, J. A. Sphon, J. T. Chen, E. Lustig, J. D. Doherty, E. A. Hansen, and S. M. Kolbye, *J. Agric. Food Chem.*, 1969, **17**, 883.
210 H. B. Camp, J. R. Buttram, K. L. Hays, and B. W. Arthur, *J. Econ. Entomol.*, 1963, **56**, 402.
211 H. W. Dorough, *J. Agric. Food Chem.*, 1967, **15**, 261.
212 W. E. Whitehurst, E. T. Bishop, F. E. Critchfield, G. G. Gyrisco, E. W. Huddleston, H. Arnold, and D. J. Lisk, *J. Agric. Food Chem.*, 1963, **11**, 167.

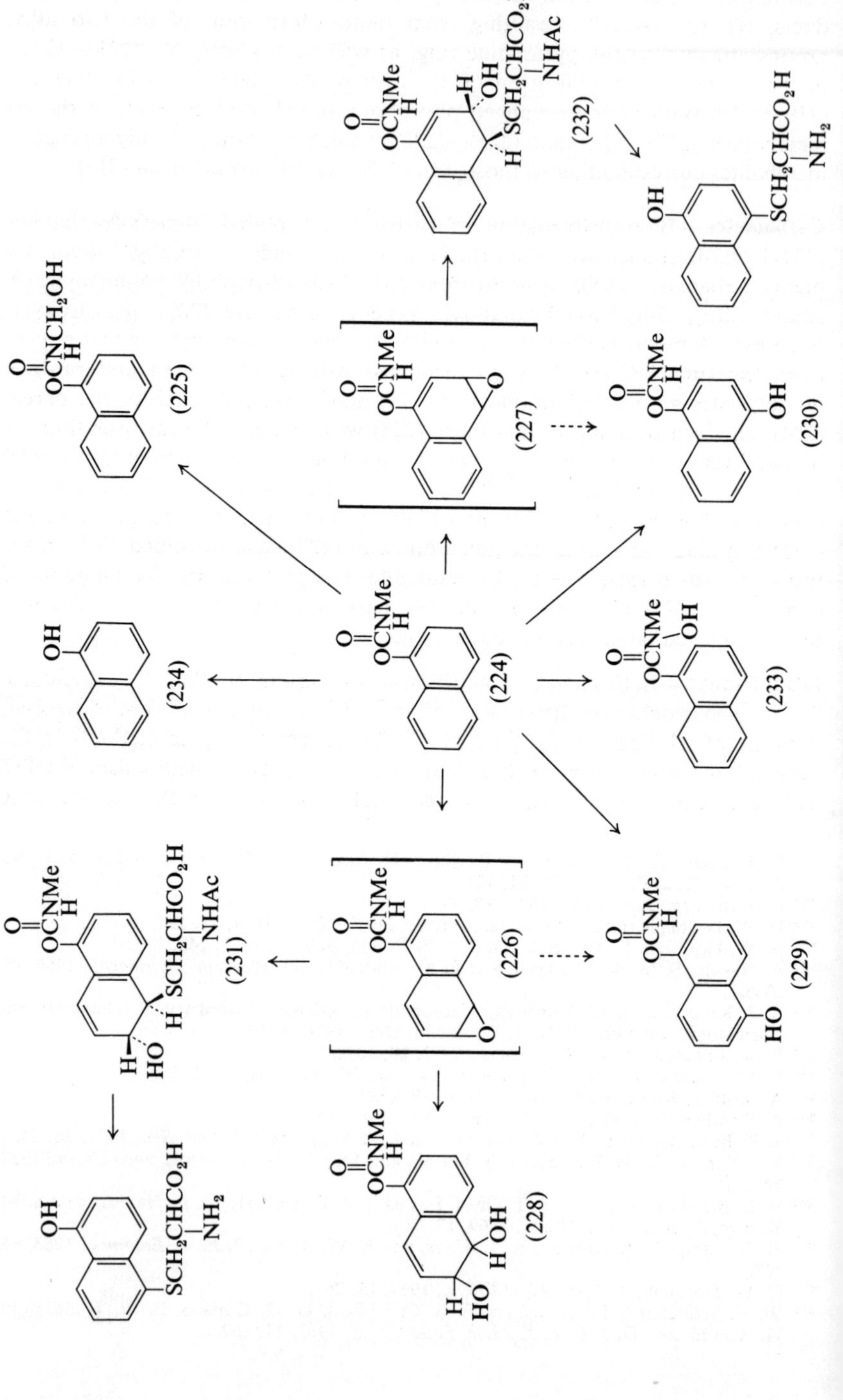
(224)
(225)
(226)
(227)
(228)
(229)
(230)
(231)
(232)
(233)
(234)

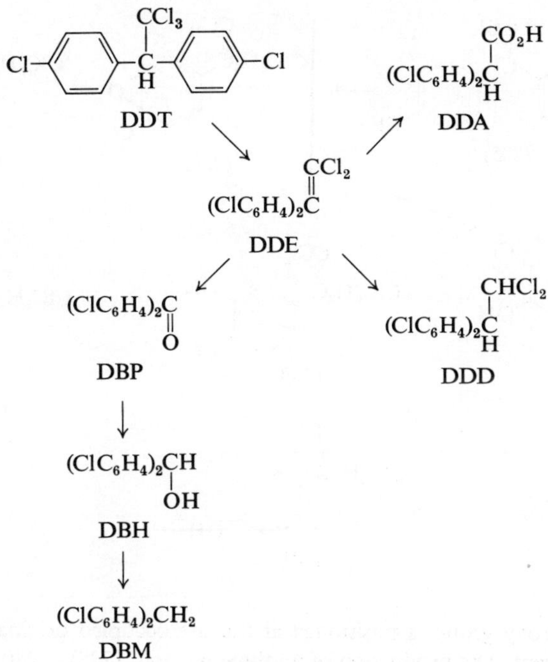

Scheme 3

decades,[213–219] much of it with unlabelled compounds, established eventually that the faecal metabolites of treated animals consisted of DDA, its conjugates with aspartic acid and serine, and a mixture of DDE, DBP, DBH, and DBM (see Scheme 3).[218,219] DDD had been shown[217] to be retained in the adipose tissues of rats treated with DDT. If it is assumed that biotransformation of DDT into DDA proceeds *via* DDE, although details of the reaction processes from DDE to DDA are still lacking, the relationship with the other DDT metabolites becomes clear[219] (*cf.* ref. 222). No phenols were detected in any of these studies,[213–219] and DDT was for a long time considered to be rather inert towards hydroxylation. However, the identification of two phenols with a *p,p′*-DDE structure in a field study involving seal faeces, stimulated a controlled investigation of DDE (235) in rats, which led to the identification of three phenols, *viz.* (238)—(240); two of these, (238) and (239), proved identical with the ones that had been isolated from seals.[220] It is apparent that in one metabolite, (238), the Cl atom has migrated into an adjacent position and that the

213 J. A. Jensen, C. Cueto, W. E. Dale, C. F. Rothe, G. W. Pearce, and A. M. Mattson, *J. Agric. Food. Chem.*, 1957, **5**, 919.
214 R. R. Ofner and H. O. Calvery, *J. Pharmacol.*, 1945, **85**, 363.
215 P. A. Neal, T. R. Sweeney, S. S. Spicer, and W. F. von Oettinger, *U.S. Public Health Reports*, 1946, **61**, 403.
216 W. C. White and T. R. Sweeney, *U.S. Public Health Reports*, 1945, **60**, 66.
217 W. P. McKinley and H. C.Grice, *J. Assoc. Off. Agric. Chem.*, 1960, **43**, 725.
218 J. D. Pinto, M. N. Camien, and M. S. Dunn, *J. Biol. Chem.*, 1965, **240**, 2148.
219 R. H. Bishara, G. S. Born, and J. E. Christian, *J. Pharm. Sci.*, 1972, **61**, 1912.
220 G. Sundström, B. Jansson, and S. Jenson, *Nature*, 1975, **255**, 627.

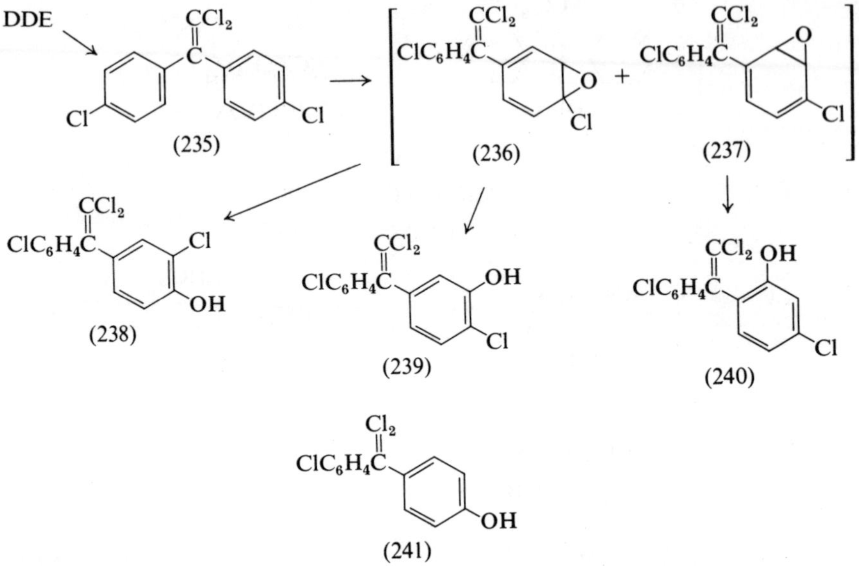

(235) (236) (237) (238) (239) (240) (241)

phenolic hydroxy group is positioned at the site occupied originally by the Cl atom substituent. The production of all three phenols, (238)—(240) is explicable mechanistically in terms of the formation of two intermediate arene oxides (236) and (237). Abundant evidence, gathered over 30 years, shows that the reductive dechlorination of DDT to DDD *in vitro* and *in vivo* proceeds at greater rates than oxidation, and this supposition is substantiated by further animal experiments. Thus, in pigs,[221] no phenols were formed directly from DDT, but a very small amount of (239), a known hydroxylation product of DDE, was excreted in the urine of these animals. In rats dosed DDT, (239) was again the major phenolic product, but careful scrutiny revealed in addition the presence of (238) and (240), as well as of 'a substitution product (241)'.

Metabolic study[223,224] of *o,p′*-DDT revealed the presence of the analogous *o,p′*-DDA, *o,p′*-DDD, and *o,p′*-DBH, but no *o,p′*-DDE, and of a number of phenolic metabolites, where the phenolic hydroxy group(s) was (were) substituted in the *o*-chlorophenyl residues, and this is borne out by study of *o,p′*-DDD,[225–227] which is used medicinally for the treatment of adrenal cortical carcinoma.

[221] G. Sundström, *J. Agric. Food Chem.*, 1977, **25**, 18.
[222] J. E. Peterson and W. H. Robinson, *Toxicol. Appl. Pharmacol.*, 1964, **6**, 321.
[223] V. J. Feil, C. J. H. Lamoureux, E. Styrvoky, R. G. Zaylskie, E. J. Thacker, and G. M. Holman, *J. Agric. Food Chem.*, 1973, **21**, 1072.
[224] M. F. Cranmer, *Bull. Environ. Contamin. Toxicol.*, 1972, **7**, 121.
[225] V. D. Reif and J. E. Sinsheimer, *Drug Metabol. Dispos.*, 1975, **3**, 15.
[226] V. D. Reif, J. E. Sinsheimer, J. C. Ward, and D. E. Schteingart, *J. Pharm. Sci.*, 1974, **63**, 1730.
[227] V. D. Reif, B. C. Littleton, and J. E. Sinsheimer, *J. Agric. Food Chem.*, 1975, **23**, 996.

Dieldrin-Aldrin Group.—This is a most important group of insecticides, which has sustained continuous biochemical and chemical investigation throughout two decades (1960—1980), but within the context of the present chapter, attention will be focused on dieldrin plus aldrin and endrin as pertinent representatives. Early studies[228–234] on the metabolism of aldrin and dieldrin in mammals underwent a surge forward (i) with 'the new numbering' for alicyclic structures in accordance with the accepted von Baeyer–IUPAC names,[235,236] with the penetrating thinking and structural studies of J. D. McKinney *et al.*,[237–239a] and with those of C. T. Bedford *et al.*[240–243] In rats and mice, *trans*-4,5-dihydroxy-4,5-dihydroaldrin (243) is a faecal metabolite and 4,5-*seco*-aldrin-4,5-dicarboxylic acid (245) is a urinary metabolite of dieldrin (242).[236,244] (243) had been reported

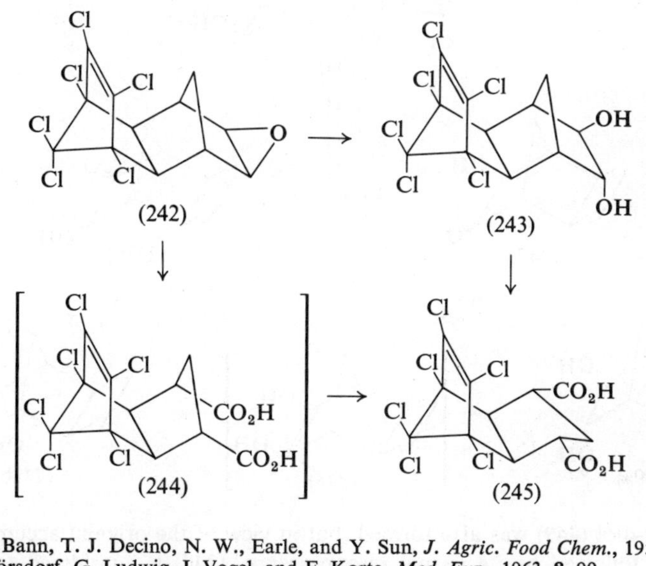

[228] J. M. Bann, T. J. Decino, N. W., Earle, and Y. Sun, *J. Agric. Food Chem.*, 1956, **4**, 937.
[229] K. Mörsdorf, G. Ludwig, J. Vogel, and F. Korte, *Med. Exp.*, 1963, **8**, 90.
[230] F. Korte and H. Arent, *Life Sci.*, 1965, **4**, 2017.
[231] A. K. Klein, J. D. Link, and N. F. Ives, *J. Assoc. Off. Analyt. Chemists*, 1968, **51**, 895.
[232] A. Richardson, M. K. Baldwin, and J. Robinson, *J. Sci. Food Agric.*, 1968, **19**, 524.
[233] R. D. Hedde, K. L. Davison, and J. D. Robbins, *J. Agric. Food Chem.*, 1970, **18**, 116.
[234] V. J. Feil, R. D. Hedde, R. G. Zoylskie, and C. H. Zachrison, *J. Agric. Food Chem.*, 1970, **18**, 120.
[235] W. R. Benson, *J. Assoc. Off. Analyt. Chemists*, 1969, **52**, 1109.
[236] C. T. Bedford, *Pestic. Sci.*, 1974, **5**, 473.
[237] J. D. McKinney, H. B. Matthews, and N. K. Wilson, *Tetrahedron Lett.*, 1973, **21**, 1895.
[238] J. D. McKinney, S. M. De Paul Palaszek, H. B. Matthews, and M. H. Behendale, in 'Pesticides and the Environment: A Continuing Controversy,' ed. W. B. Deichmann, Intercontinetal Medical Book Corp., New York, 1973, p. 103 *et seq.*
[239] J. D. McKinney, H. B. Matthews, and L. Fishbein, *J. Agric. Food. Chem.*, 1972, **20**, 597.
[239a] H. B. Matthews and J. D. McKinney, *Drug. Metabol. Dispos.*, 1974, **2**, 333.
[240] C. T. Bedford and R. K. Harrod, *Chemosphere*, 1972, **1**, 255.
[241] C. T. Bedford, and R. K. Harrod, *J. Chem. Soc., Chem. Commun.*, 1972, 735.
[242] C. T. Bedford, in 'Foreign Compound Metabolism in Mammals Vol. 3,' ed. D. E. Hathway, The Chemical Society, London, 1975, pp. 365—448.
[243] C. T. Bedford, and D. H. Hutson, unpublished data, mentioned in ref. 242.
[244] M. K. Baldwin, J. Robinson, and D. V. Parke, *Food Cosmet. Toxicol.*, 1972, **10**, 333.

previously[230] as a (242) urinary metabolite in sheep, but an improved synthesis was described,[240] and (245) is a new (242) metabolite, which was found also in the urine of rats dosed (243).[245] The conformational isomer of (245) with two Ψ-axial carboxy groups (244) has no free existence at room temperature,[242] and the compound is properly represented by the conformation, where the carboxy groups occupy Ψ-equatorial positions (245). McKinney *et al.*[237–239a] prepared the *cis*-diol, (*exo*)-*cis*-4,5-dihydroxy-4,5-dihydroaldrin (246) from (242) *in vitro*.

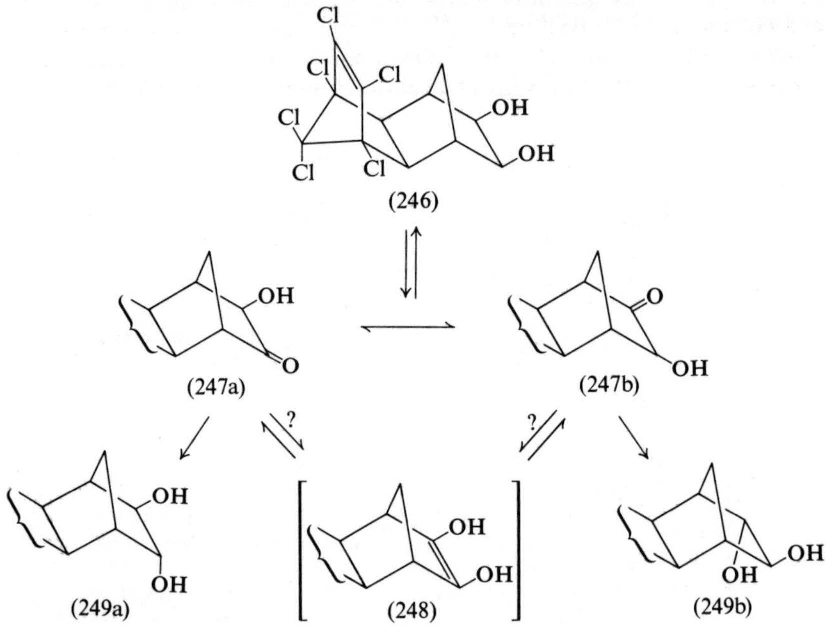

The *trans*-diol (249) was also formed, but in view of the original accumulation of (246), followed by its virtual disappearance, (246) is considered to be an obligatory intermediate in the generation of *trans*-diol, *viz.*(249). 5-*exo*-Hydroxy-4-oxo-4,5-dihydroaldrin (247a) or (247b) must be the intermediate in this biotransformation, formed by a complete or partially stereoselective dehydrogenation of (246), which upon reduction would give (249a) or (249b). The racemic ketol (247) with the enzyme system gave (246) plus (249). Interconversions between ketols and vicinal diols are reminiscent of the situation concerning the hydroxyoestrones *vis-à-vis* the oestriols,[246–249] of the transformation of 16-oxo-oestradiol-17β and 16β-hydroxyoestrone *via* 16-oxo-oestrone,[250] and of the structurally similar camphane-2,3-diols and the corresponding ketols.[251] The

[245] J. Oda and W. Müller, *Environ. Qual. Saf.*, 1972, **1**, 248.
[246] G. F. Marrian, K. H. Loke, E. J. D. Watson, and M. Panattoni, *Biochem. J.*, 1957, **65**, 12.
[247] D. S. Layne and G. F. Marrian, *Biochem. J.*, 1958, **70**, 244.
[248] J. B. Brown and G. F. Marrian, *J. Endocrinol.*, 1957, **15**, 307.
[249] H. Breuer and L. Nocke, *Biochim. Biophys. Acta*, 1959, **36**, 271.
[250] H. Breuer and R. Knuppen, *Acta Endocrinol.*, 1961, **36**, 393.
[251] H. Matthews and F. Matsumara, *J. Agric. Food Chem.*, 1969, **17**, 845.

foregoing complex situation relating to the dieldrin metabolites has been discussed at some length.[238,242] Structural assignment of (251) to *syn*-12-hydroxy-dieldrin,[236] a known rat faecal (242) metabolite[233,234] was confirmed by detailed spectroscopy and characterization,[239,244] and by total synthesis.[241] Bedford argues[242] (*cf.* ref. 238) that the radical intermediate (250), postulated to lead to (251), would also afford the bridged ketone, *viz.* 'dieldrin pentachloroketone' (255), which is a metabolite both of (242), and of photodieldrin (254).[231,232] Compound (250) was represented[242] as a radical and direction of it with hydroxy radical or its biological equivalent gave (251). Juxtaposition of the dichloroethylene grouping with C-12 in (250) makes intramolecular radical rearrangement

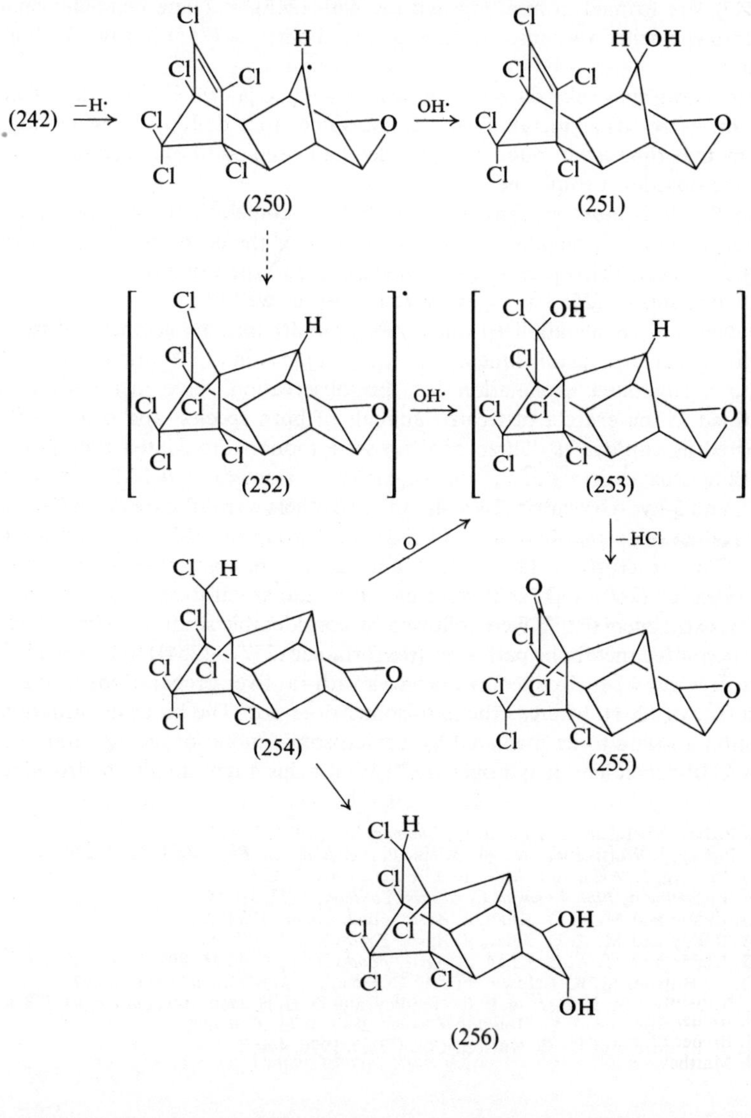

(250) (251) (252) (253) (254) (255) (256)

feasible and, if operative, would lead to the bridged radical (252). Reaction of hydroxy radical with (252) would then give the α-chlorohydrin (253), which would furnish (255) through the loss of HCl. In the event of glucuronic acid conjugation competing with the dehydrochlorination process, then such a glucuronide conjugate as would be formed from (253) would seem to be consistent with the polar metabolite of (242), which was reported[251] to have liberated (255) upon glucuronidase treatment.

4,5-*seco*-Aldrin-4,5-dicarboxylic acid (245) ought not to be considered to be a terminal metabolite of (242), as two pentachlorinated dicarboxylic acids, in both of which a Cl atom has been lost from the dichloromethylene position in (245), are formed in rats, injected i.v. with (245).[253] These pentachlorinated dicarboxylic acids were also detected as metabolites of (245) in rat-liver homogenates.[252]

After about six weeks' daily administrations of [^{14}C]aldrin[254] or [^{14}C]dieldrin,[255] each rat excreted, as metabolites, ^{14}C equivalent to a daily dose, which means that by that time a saturated body burden had been established, commensurate with the dose-level employed.

Finally, it is now established[256,257] that photodieldrin (254) gives rise to several mammalian metabolites. The major one is the corresponding *trans*-diol (256),[258] which is also present as its glucuronide in the urine of treated rabbits. Small amounts of (255) (*v. supra*) were formed as well.[258]

Endrin (257) is metabolized much more rapidly than its geometrical isomer, dieldrin (242), and detailed metabolic study of (257) in rats[259] and rabbits[260] has led to a suggested explanation for this observation. Five metabolites were identified in the excreta of treated animals of both species, and some of them occurred as conjugates. Three of them were monohydroxylated products, *viz.* *syn*-12-hydroxyendrin (258), its geometrical isomer, *anti*-12-hydroxyendrin (259), and 3-hydroxyendrin (260) and the two others were 12-oxoendrin (261) and the product of formal hydration of the epoxy group of (257), *viz.* the *trans*-diol (262). The structures of (258), (259), and (261) were confirmed by synthesis,[264] and those of (260) and (262) were based on the spectral data. Moreover, the animal experiments[259,260] were followed by considerable studies *in vitro*,[261] which have permitted metabolic pathways [see formulae (257)—(264)] to be specified.[262] Thus, free *syn*-12-hydroxyendrin behaves with rat-liver preparations as the true precursor of (261), whereas the *anti*-isomer does not. The biotransformation in question appears to be mediated by a microsomal mono-oxygenase and not by an NADP-dependent dehydrogenase.[261] Whilst this might involve hydroxylation

[252] J. P. Lay, W. Klein, and F. Korte, *Chemosphere*, 1974, **3**, 193.
[253] J. P. Lay, I. Weisgerber, and W. Klein, *Pestic. Biochem. Physiol.*, 1975, **5**, 226.
[254] G. Ludwig, J. Weis, and F. Korte, *Life Sci.*, 1964, **3**, 123
[255] K. L. Davison, *Bull. Environ. Contamin. Toxicol.*, 1973, **10**, 16.
[256] G. Reddy and M. A. Q. Khan, *J. Agric. Food. Chem.*, 1974, **22**, 910.
[257] G. Reddy and M. A. Q. Khan, *J. Agric. Food Chem.*, 1975, **23**, 861.
[258] G. Reddy and M. A. Q. Khan, *J. Agric. Food Chem.*, 1978, **26**, 292.
[259] D. H. Hutson, M. K. Baldwin, and E. C. Hoadley, *Xenobiotica*, 1975, **5**, 697.
[260] C. T. Bedford, R. K. Harrod, E. C. Hoadley, and D. H. Hutson, *Xenobiotica*, 1975, **5**, 485.
[261] D. H. Hutson and E. C. Hoadley, *Chemosphere*, 1974, **3**, 205.
[262] C. T. Bedford and D. H. Hutson, *Chem. Ind.*, 1976, 440.

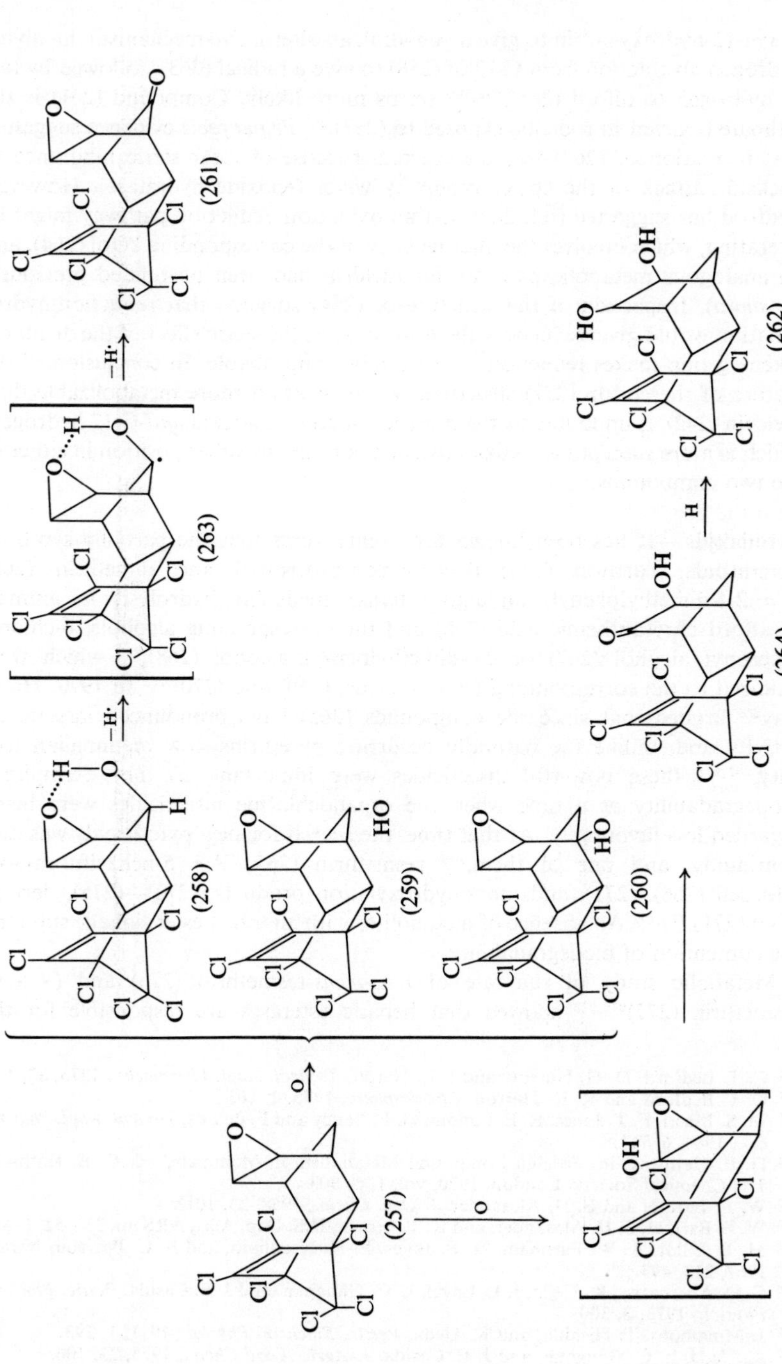
(257)
(258)
(259)
(260)
(261)
(262)
(263)
(264)

of *syn*-12-hydroxyendrin to give a *gem*-diol, an alternative mechanism, involving hydrogen abstraction from C-12 of (258) to give a radical (263), followed by loss of hydrogen to afford (261),[259,260] seems more likely. Compound (261) is the ultimate toxicant in rodents, exposed to (257).[263] *Prima facie* evidence suggested that formation of (262) was unexpected, because of clear steric hindrance to backside attack of the epoxy group by water (epoxide hydratase). However, Bedford has suggested (ref. 262) that an oxidation–reduction pathway might be operating, which involves the intermediacy of the corresponding ketol (264), and an analogous metabolic pathway for dieldrin had been postulated previously (*v. supra*). Inspection of the structure of (264) suggests that reduction/hydrogenation would give exclusively the *trans*-diol, as the steric effect of the dichloroalkene group makes reduction to the *cis*-diol improbable. In conclusion,[262] the feature of the endrin (257) structure, which makes it more metabolizable than dieldrin (242), is undoubtedly the presence of an unhindered *anti*-C-12 hydrogen, which is more susceptible to oxidative attack than any other position in either of the two compounds.

Pyrethroids.—It has been known for twenty years that the partially synthetic pyrethroids, barthrin (265; R = 6-chloropiperonyl) and dimethrin (265; R = 2,4-dimethylphenyl) undergo esterase mediated hydrolysis in animals to afford chrysanthemic acid (266) and the corresponding alcohols, 6-chloropiperonyl alcohol (267) or 2,4-dimethylbenzyl alcohol (268),[265] which were oxidized to the corresponding benzoic acids, (269) and (270).[265] In 1970, Hathway[266] argued that since the compounds (265) have pronounced insecticidal activity and, unlike the naturally occurring pyrethrins, low mammalian toxicity,[267,268] these powerful insecticides were important, as they exemplified biodegradability at a time when the organochlorine insecticides were being regarded less favourably. At that time, the search for new pyrethroids was also continuing, and one of them,[269] resmethrin (265; R = 5-benzylfuran-3-yl) afforded (266), (271), and monohydroxylation products, (272)—(275), derived from (271).[270,271] An absence of metabolites with an intact ester linkage supports the contention of biodegradability.

Metabolic study of the fate of (+)-*trans*-resmethrin (276) and (+)-*cis*-resmethrin (277)[272,273] showed that hepatic esterases are responsible for the

[263] C. T. Bedford, D. H. Hutson, and I. L. Natoff, *Toxicol. Appl. Pharmacol.*, 1975, **33**, 115.
[264] C. T. Bedford and R. K. Harrod, *Chemosphere*, 1973, **2**, 163.
[265] M. S. Masri, F. T. Jones, R. E. Lundin, G. F. Bailey and F. de Eds, *Toxicol. Appl. Pharmacol.*, 1964, **6**, 711.
[266] D. E. Hathway, in 'Foreign Compound Metabolism in Mammals,' ed. D. E. Hathway, The Chemical Society, London, 1970, vol. **1**, p. 303.
[267] W. F. Barthel and B. H. Alexander, *J. Org. Chem.*, 1958, **23**, 1012.
[268] W. F. Barthel, B. H. Alexander, and R. T. Brown, U.S. Dep. Agr., ARS no. 33—51, 1—13.
[269] M. E. Elliot, A. W. Farnham, N. F. Jones, P. H. Needham, and B. C. Pearson, *Nature*, 1967, **213**, 493.
[270] C. O. Abernathy, K. Ueda, J. L. Engel, L. C. Gaughan, and J. E. Casida, *Pestic. Biochem. Physiol.*, 1973, **3**, 300.
[271] J. Mujamoto, T. Nishida, and K. Ueda, *Pestic. Biochem. Physiol.*, 1971, **1**, 293.
[272] K. Ueda, L. C. Gaughan, and J. E. Casida, *J. Agric. Food Chem.*, 1975, **23**, 106.
[273] K. Ueda, L. C. Gaughan, and J. E. Casida, *Pestic. Biochem. Physiol.*, 1974, **5**, 280.

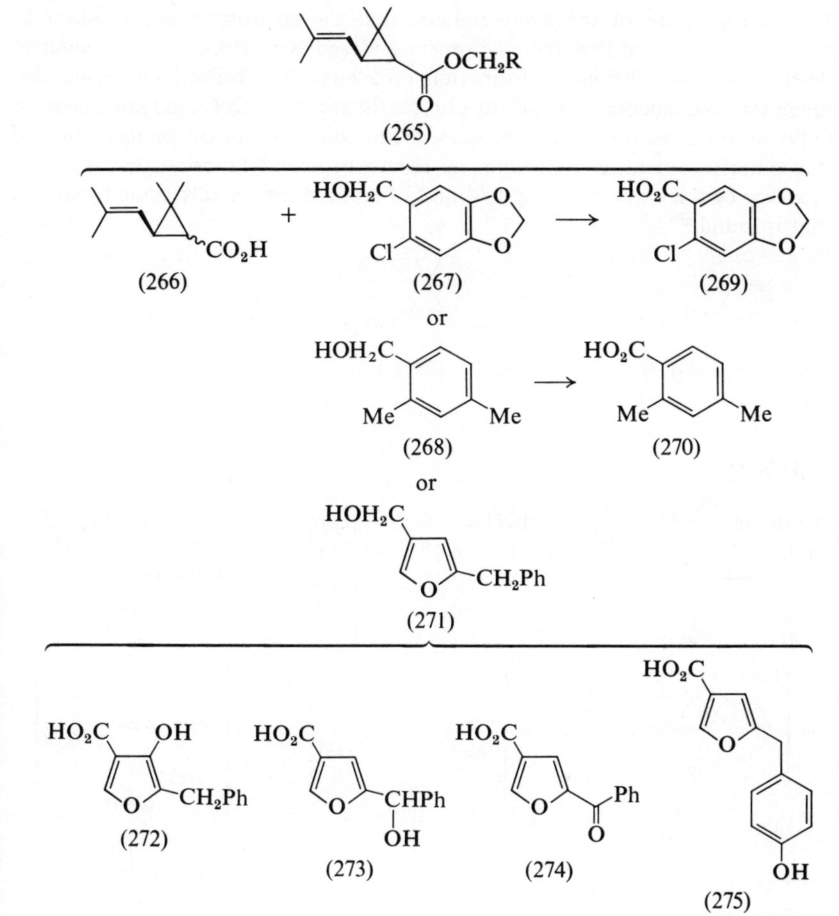

(265) (266) (267) (269) (268) (270) (271) (272) (273) (274) (275)

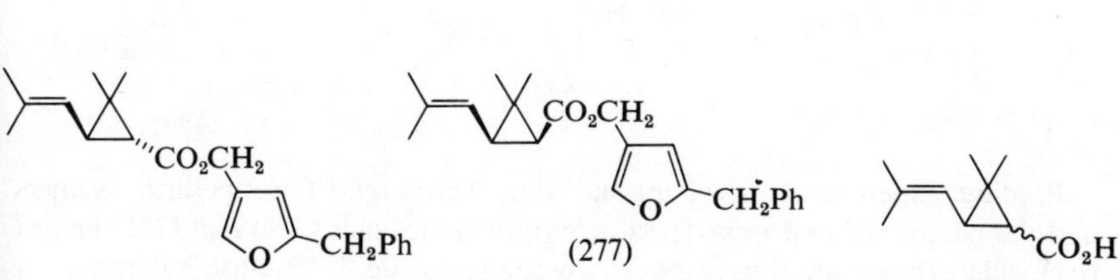

(276) (277) (266)

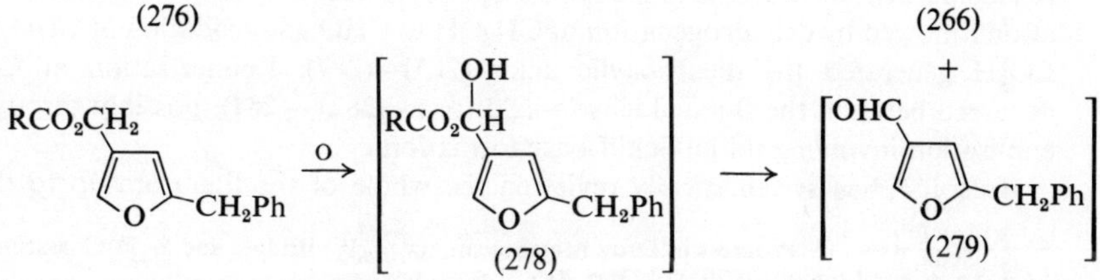

(278) (279)

biotransformation of the *trans*-isomers, that the *cis*-isomers are resistant to esteratic fission, and that the *cis*-isomers undergo NADPH-catalysed oxidative de-esterification. The initial formation of a lactol (278),[273] which would disintegrate spontaneously to afford chrysanthemic acid (266) and an aldehyde (279) would explain the latter process. Whilst direct proof of the formation of this putative aldehyde is lacking, its reactivity would be consistent with the recovery of the corresponding acid and of some microsomally bound material that is found.[273]

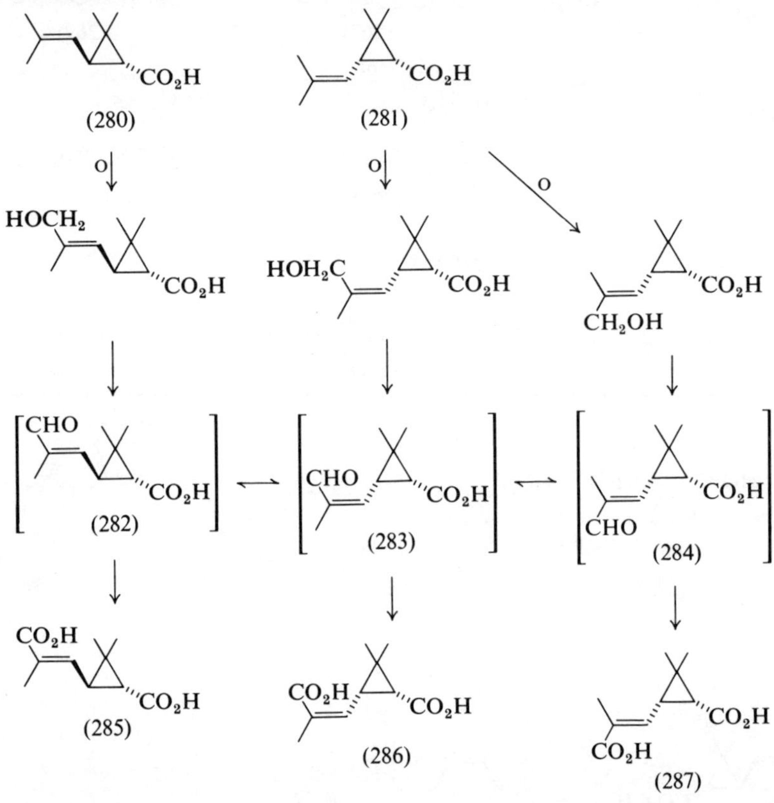

Feeding experiments involving all four [carbonyl-^{14}C]resmethrin isomers and the parent *cis*- and *trans*-[1-^{14}C]chrysanthemic acids (280) and (281) helped to elucidate the metabolism of the cyclopropane residue.[272,273] ω-Methyl hydroxylation followed by dehydrogenation of CH_2OH to CHO and oxidation of CHO to CO_2H generated the dicarboxylic acids (285)—(287). Epimerization at C-3 occurred between the three aldehydo-acid forms (282)—(284), possibly through enolisation involving initial Schiff-base formation.

Hutson[274] has systematically reviewed the whole of the literature up to the

[274] D. H. Hutson, in 'Progress in Drug Metabolism,' ed. J. W. Bridges and L. F. Chasseaud, John Wiley, London, 1979, vol. 3, p. 215.

end of 1977 on allethrin, tetramethrin, resmethrin, ethanomethrins, proparthrin, prothrin, dimethrin, barthrin, phenothrin, permethrin, cypermethrin, fenvalerate, and some miscellaneous compounds. The present account ends with brief mention of the metabolism of WL 41706 or Sumitoma S-3306 (288) and decamethrin (295).

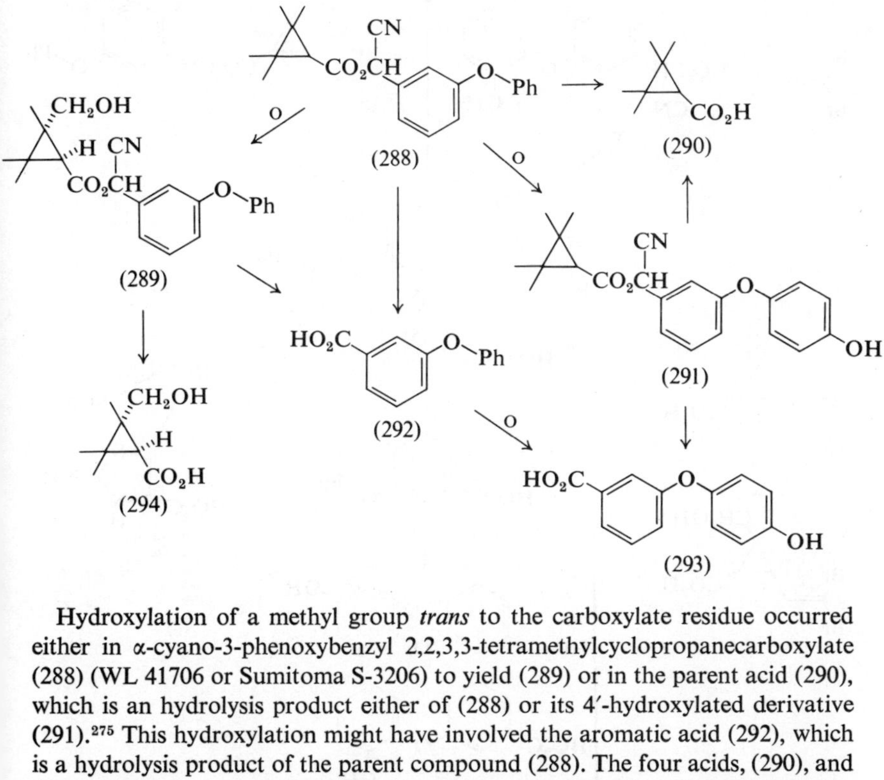

Hydroxylation of a methyl group *trans* to the carboxylate residue occurred either in α-cyano-3-phenoxybenzyl 2,2,3,3-tetramethylcyclopropanecarboxylate (288) (WL 41706 or Sumitoma S-3206) to yield (289) or in the parent acid (290), which is an hydrolysis product either of (288) or its 4′-hydroxylated derivative (291).[275] This hydroxylation might have involved the aromatic acid (292), which is a hydrolysis product of the parent compound (288). The four acids, (290), and (292)—(294) were excreted, partly as conjugates, in the urine of treated animals. Unchanged insecticide and other metabolites with an intact ester linkage were excreted faecally. Compound (289) was the major (288) metabolite in rats, in which esteratic breakdown was negligible.[275] Incidentally, 4′-hydroxylation did not take place *in vitro*.[275]

The appended Scheme 4 appears to be a fair representation of the metabolism of another synthetic pyrethroid (295) in rats and mice,[276,277] although the precise metabolic steps have not been proved experimentally. It will be seen that metabolic pathways implicate ester hydrolysis and oxidation at the 4′-position of the alcohol residue. Glucuronide, glycine, and sulphate conjugates facilitated total excretion (2—4 days) of the many metabolites from the body.

[275] M. J. Crawford and D. H. Hutson, *Pestic. Sci.*, 1977, **8**, 579.
[276] L. O. Ruzo, T. Unai, and J. E. Casida, *J. Agric. Food Chem.*, 1978, **26**, 918.
[277] L. O. Ruzo, J. L. Engel, and J. E. Casida, *J. Agric. Food Chem.*, 1979, **27**, 725.

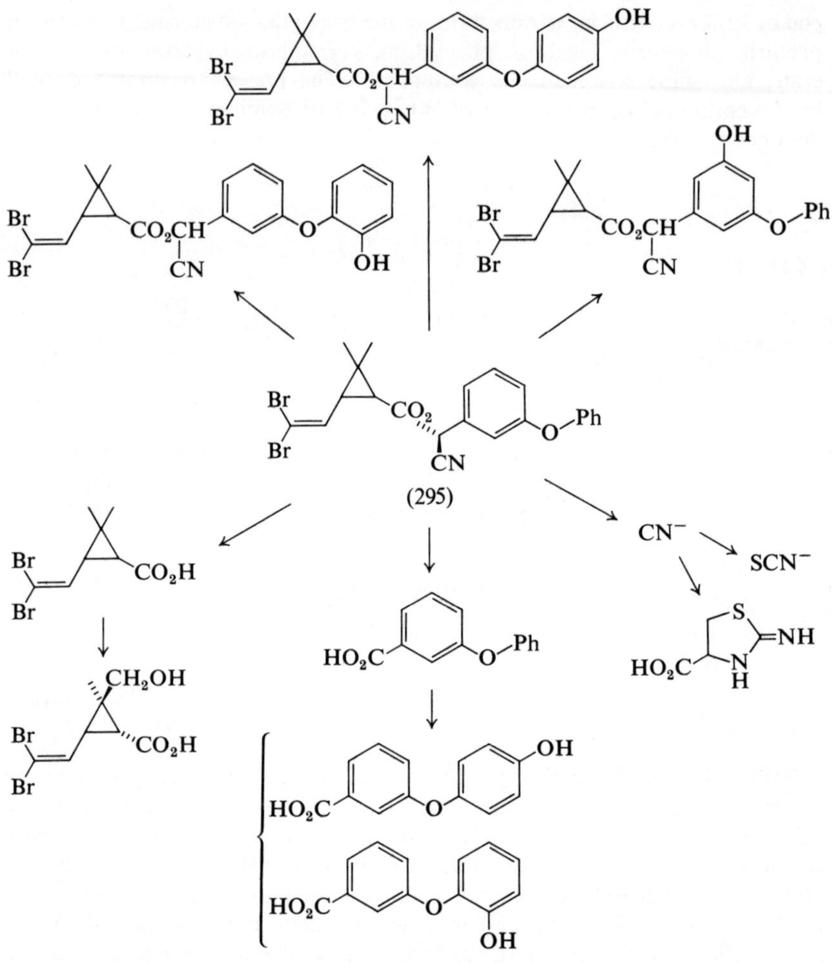

Scheme 4

5 Fungicides

Dinobuton.—By means of [*carbonyl*-^{14}C]-labelled material, dinobuton (296), the isopropyl carbonate of dinoseb (127; R = H), was found to undergo rapid hydrolysis in rats: 92% of the label was excreted as CO_2.[278] Whilst much of the dose of [*phenyl*-^{14}C]-(296) was excreted in the urine of rats and mice as very polar material, resistant to enzymic hydrolysis, small amounts of the aminophenols (297) and (298) and of the carboxylic acids (299) and (300) were identified.[278]

[278] S. K. Bandal and J. E. Casida, *J. Agric. Food Chem.*, 1972, **20**, 1235.

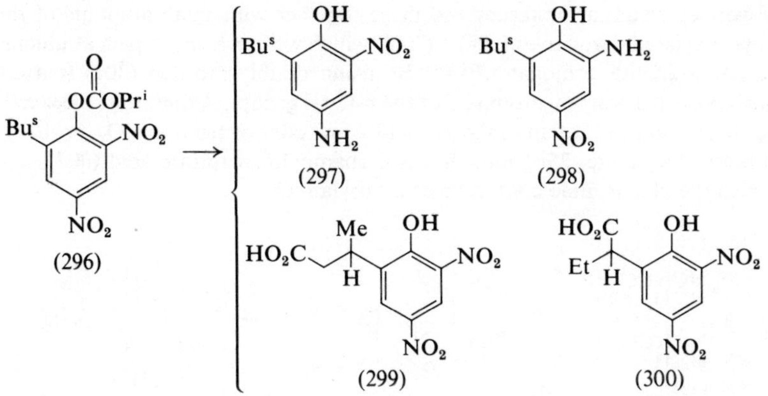

Benomyl.—In rabbits, sheep, and mice, benomyl (301) is completely metabolized:[279] the major metabolites were the simple hydrolysis products, (302) and (303), which had lost the n-butylcarbamoyl side-chain. The metabolites (302) and

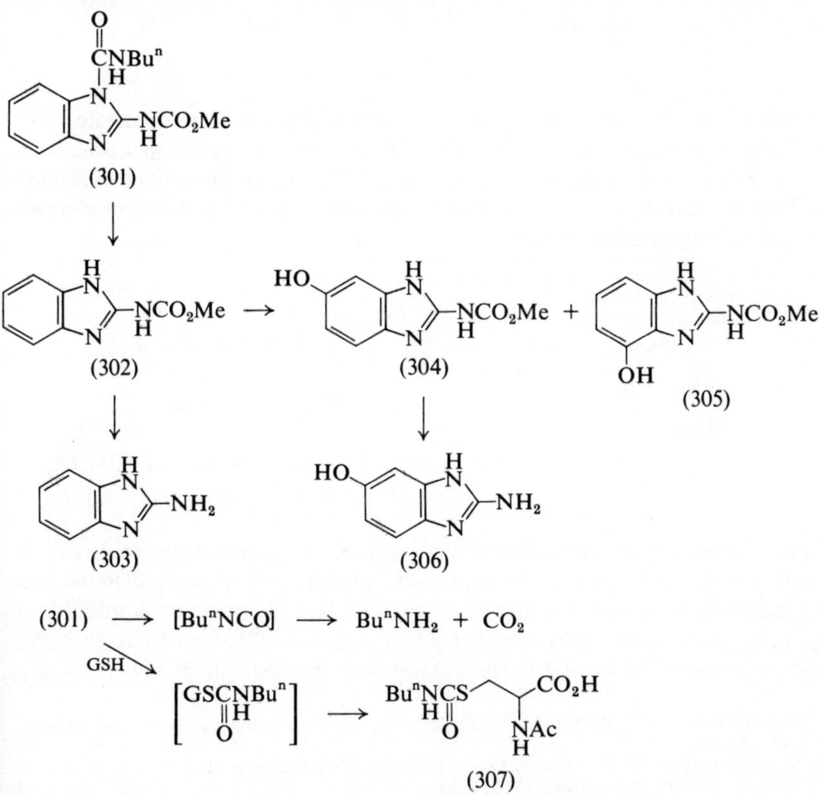

[279] P. G. C. Douch, *Xenobiotica*, 1973, **3**, 367.

(303) were excreted in the faeces and urine together with small amounts of the ring-hydroxylated derivatives (304)—(306), which were present in part as glucuronide and sulphate conjugates.[279,280] By using doubly labelled (301) (tritium was also present at carbon atom C-1 of the n-butyl group), Axness and Fleeker[281] found that in rats 40% of an oral dose of (301) was converted into CO_2, probably *via* n-butyl isocyanate, 25% into n-butylcarbamoylmercapturic acid (307), and 40% into the glucuronide conjugate of n-butylamine.

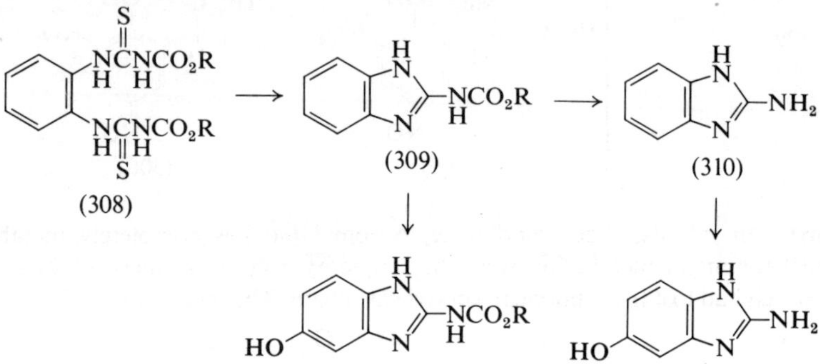

(308) (309) (310) (311) (312)

Thiophanates.—In mice and sheep,[282] major metabolites of thiophanate (308; R = Et) and thiophanate-methyl (308; R = Me) are 2-aminobenzimidazole (310) and its derivatives, (309), (311), and (312). Both carbamate hydrolysis and the aromatic hydroxylations found are predictable, and so is the mechanism of the initial cyclization process.

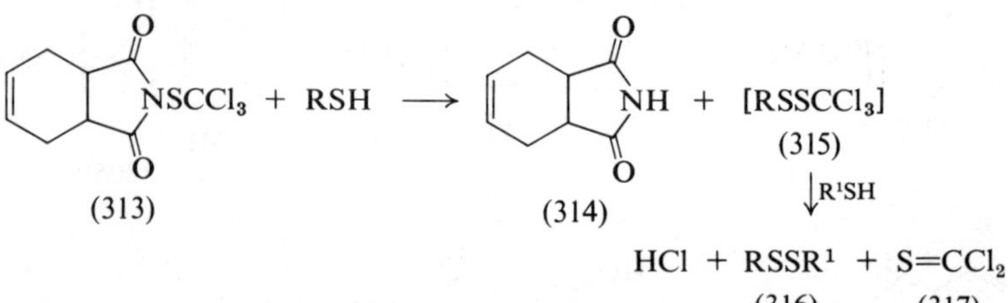

(313) (314) (315) (316) (317)

Captan.—Because of the known, high degree of spontaneous reactivity of thiols for the $SCCl_3$ group of captan-like compounds, it is predictable that the major initial biotransformation of captan (313) in mammals is thiolysis to tetrahydrophthalimide (314) and (315).[283] Compound (315) is of course highly reactive towards thiols, and in the general case reaction with R′SH would give

[280] J. A. Gardiner, J. J. Kirkland, H. L. Klopping, and H. Sherman, *J. Agric. Food Chem.*, 1974, **22**, 419.
[281] M. E. Axness and J. R. Fleeker, *Pestic. Biochem. Physiol.*, 1979, **11**, 1.
[282] P. G. C. Douch, *Xenobiotica*, 1974, **4**, 457.
[283] J. R. De Baun, J. B. Mianllis, J. Knarr, A. Mihailovski, and J. J. Menn, *Xenobiotica*, 1974, **4**, 101.

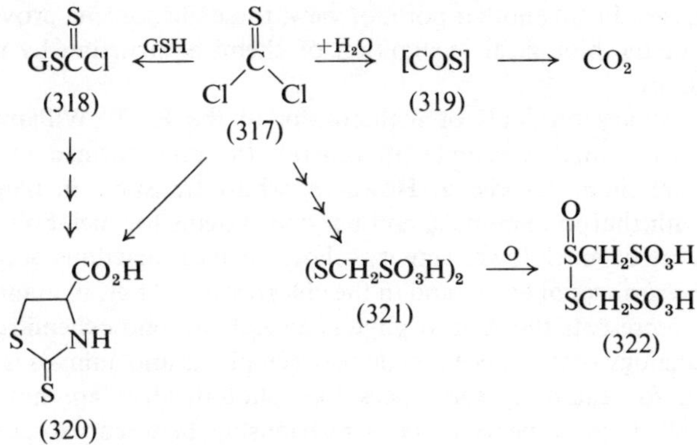

the disulphide (316), thiophosgene (317), and HCl. This sequence is suspected to occur largely spontaneously *in vivo*, involving liver glutathione. Thus, GSH is involved in each of these reactions, as follows:

$$2\ \text{GSH} + \text{captan} \longrightarrow \text{GSSG} + \text{products}$$

captan might be understood to undergo a reductive metathesis between two molecules of glutathione. By using [*trichloromethyl*-^{14}C]-(313) in rats dosed *p.o.*, DeBaun *et al.*[283] have been able to establish that a very complicated reaction sequence yields 4-carboxythiazolidine-2-thione (320), dithiobis(methanesulphonic acid) (321), and the (321) *S*-oxide, (322), as the principal urinary (313) metabolites. The acid (320) is either the product of (313)-derived thiophosgene (317) and cysteine or a breakdown product of (318), formed from (317) through initial reaction with glutathione. Endogenous sulphite is involved in the generation of (321) and (322) from (317), as ^{35}S is found to be incorporated into the isolated products (321) and (322) when rats are dosed unlabelled captan plus [^{35}S]-sulphite.[283] Further, the reaction between (317) and sulphite must occur in the gut, as compounds (321) and (322) were not produced in those cases, where the animals were injected (313) i.p.[283] A small amount of exhaled $^{14}CO_2$ in these experiments was formed probably from hepatic oxidation of COS (319), the hydrolytic product of (317).

6 Concluding Remarks

Three comments seem to be pertinent. Firstly, metabolic pathways, even of the limited number of industrial chemicals and pesticides that have been discussed, present an array of alicyclic, aliphatic, aromatic, and heterocyclic compounds and of reaction mechanisms which interlaces the whole field of synthetic organic chemistry.

Secondly, in the mammalian body, foreign compounds become enmeshed in the available physiological mechanisms. This applies to transport within the body and within cells, to biotransformations mediated by the different sub-cellular components, and to interactions between reactive metabolites and cellular macromolecules. From another point of view, these phenomena provide copious illustration of the biological recognition of chemical structure by mammalian cells and tissues.

Thirdly, primary products of metabolism, in the R. T. Williams-sense, of herbicides in mammals resemble, in general, the ones formed in plants and this is, at first sight, surprising. However, whilst transport in plants is poor compared with that in mammals, and enzyme systems for metabolizing foreign compounds are of much lower activity, photochemical reactions occur spontaneously on the surfaces of leaves and in the chloroplasts. Thus, in plants, apparent metabolism represents the sum of phytochemical and photochemical reactions. Whilst the analogy that has been made between plants and animals is not strictly correct and, for example, substances like photodieldrin are not formed in animals at all, there appears to be a relationship between oxidative reaction processes mediated by the highly developed mammalian cytochrome P-450 system and corresponding photochemical oxidations.

Chapter 7 Kinetic Considerations

1 Introduction

Ever since the beginning of this century, experiments in animals have been made to measure the blood levels of administered foreign compounds, especially ones with biological activity. The importance of these results stimulated the growth of kinetic studies *in vivo*, and this development was accelerated by (i) the growing recognition in the early 1940s that the blood level, at any particular time, represents the pharmacological status of the body better than the dose; (ii) the publication of two books in the 1950s;[1,2] and (iii) the availability in the 1960s of vastly improved techniques for the detection and measurement of the exceptionally small amounts of the substances concerned. This progress opens up the possibility of correlating blood levels with the adverse effects of food additives, industrial chemicals, and pesticides, which become apparent during long-term toxicity testing.

Whilst complicated pharmaco-kinetic calculations may now be made involving compartmentalized models, (i) in attempts to assess absorption and other physiological processes in the design of new drugs, (ii) in determining dosing regimens for therapy, and (iii) in analysing individual responses to particular drugs, on the other hand, a simple kinetic treatment provides much useful information. It is the latter approach that is developed in the present chapter. (Contributions from the writer's laboratory will be cited at various places in the narrative, and while these are not necessarily the most pertinent, they are the ones which he understood best.)

2 Blood levels

Time Courses after Different Routes of Administration.—Model curves for blood levels (plasma concentrations), after the administration of a foreign compound to a mammal by various routes, are shown in Figure 1. For i.v. injection, the curve represents the time course of distribution (metabolism) and elimination from vascular circulation, and is exponential in nature, whereas that for the i.m. injection reflects a period of increasing blood concentration whilst all of the dose disappears from the site of injection and reaches a peak blood concentration (Figure 1). Thereafter, this curve intersects the i.v. time

[1] F. H. Dost, 'Der Blutspiegel: Kinetik der Konzentrationsablaüfe in der Kreislaüfflussigkeit,' Arbeitsgemeinschaft Medizinischer Verlage (ehemals Georg Thieme), Leipzig, 1953.
[2] A. Rescigno and G. Segre, 'La cinetica dei farmaci e dei traccianti radioattivi,' Universitarie Boringhieri, Torino, 1961

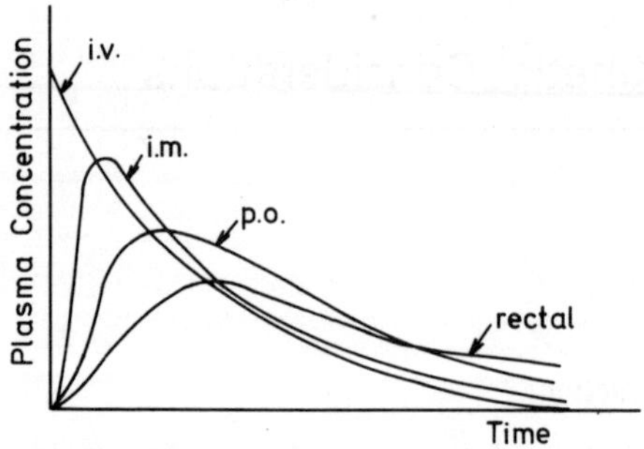

Figure 1 *Time courses of drug concentration in blood after various routes of administration*

course, and follows its decline (Figure 1). The blood-level curves for i.m. injection and oral dosing are rather similar in shape, but peak concentration is usually reached earlier by i.m. absorption than p.o. (Figure 1). In the case of ingestion, it is clear that the area under the blood level–time course represents the amount of substance which has been absorbed from the gastro-intestinal tract. Where the oral dose is completely absorbed, the corresponding time course would be similar to that for i.m. injection, and would intersect the i.v. plot (Figures 1 and 2),[3] but where absorption is incomplete, the entire curve would fall below the i.v. curve, and would be a degenerate form of that representing complete absorption. In general, peak blood levels would be attained more rapidly, and would be higher, by the i.m. than the oral route, but some cases

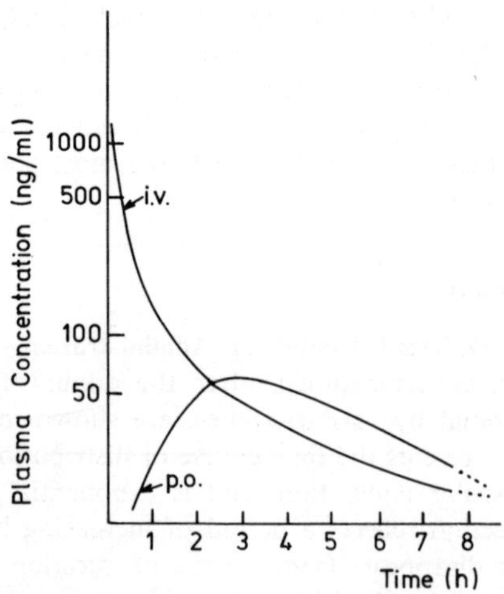

Figure 2 *Time courses for the plasma concentration of pantothenate in dogs after i.v. and p.o. administrations*

[Reproduced by permission from *Res. Vet. Sci.*, 1974, **16**, 271—275]

[3] T. Taylor, B. D. Cameron, D. E. Hathway, and H. Partington, *Res. Vet. Sci.*, 1974, **61**, 271.

are known where retention of foreign compound by the muscular tissue results in a slower absorption than that after ingestion. Phenylbutazone, which is used as an anti-inflammatory agent for aching muscles, is a case in point. Clearly, oral and rectal dosing follow a similar pattern (Figure 1), and in the latter case, peak blood levels are reached more slowly than by any other administrative route. All of the material absorbed is taken by the hepatic portal system, and the time-lag largely reflects the clearance by the liver. Rectal application is made so that the circulation, after the first liver passage, does not involve the highest rectal segments.

A typical comparison of blood-level curves after i.v. and p.o. administration in rats[4] is shown in Figure 3. The ratio of blood-level curve areas oral/i.v. is

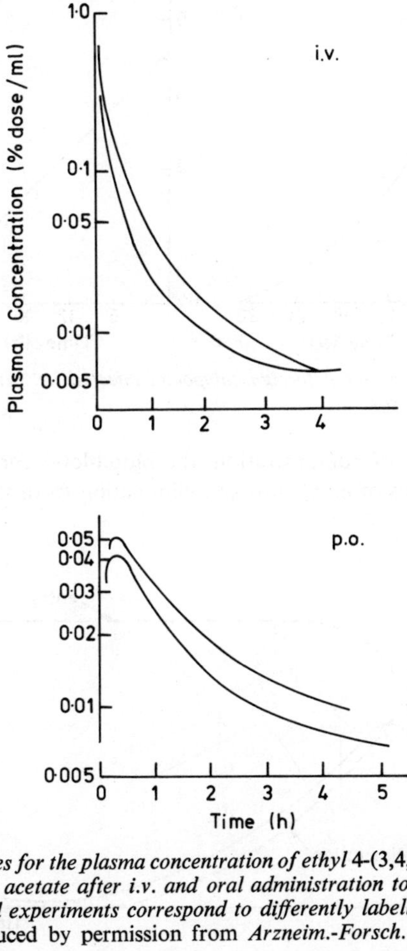

Figure 3 *Time courses for the plasma concentration of ethyl* 4-(3,4,5-*trimethoxycinnamoyl*) *piperazinyl acetate after i.v. and oral administration to rats. The two curves in the parallel experiments correspond to differently labelled forms of the drug.*
[Reproduced by permission from *Arzneim.-Forsch.*, 1972, **22**, 1726—1732]

[4] L. F. Chasseaud, D. R. Hawkins, B. J. Fry, J. D. Lewis, D. H. Moore, T. Taylor, and D. E. Hathway, *Arzneim.-Forsch.*, 1972, **22**, 1726.

approximately unity in the several animals tested, and using differently labelled forms of the drug, and the absorption rate constant was an appropriately high one.

Attention is drawn to the exponential nature of the elimination curve (Figure 4) by inclusion of the corresponding log-linear plot, which is linear (Figure 4). The so-called biological half-life $t_{0.5}$, which is the time which elapses whilst a certain plasma concentration of the test substance decreases to one-half of the original value, would be the same in both cases, but it is more easily read from the linear plot.

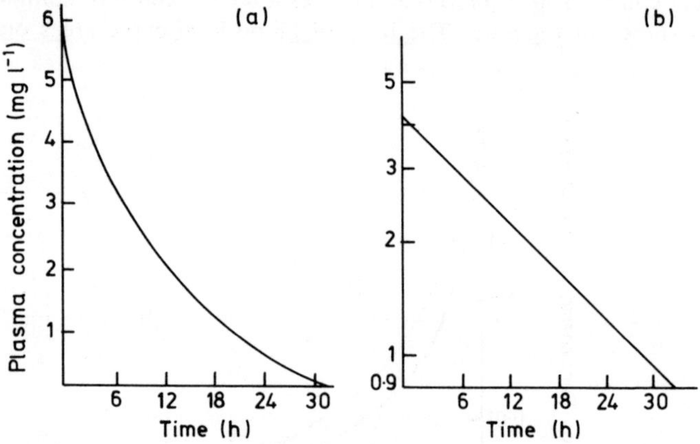

Figure 4 *Elimination curve for a foreign compound injected i.v. (a) Linear–linear axes; (b) log–linear axes*

Whatever the route of administration, the blood-level curve is the resultant of continuing processes of entry into and elimination from vascular circulation (Figure 5).

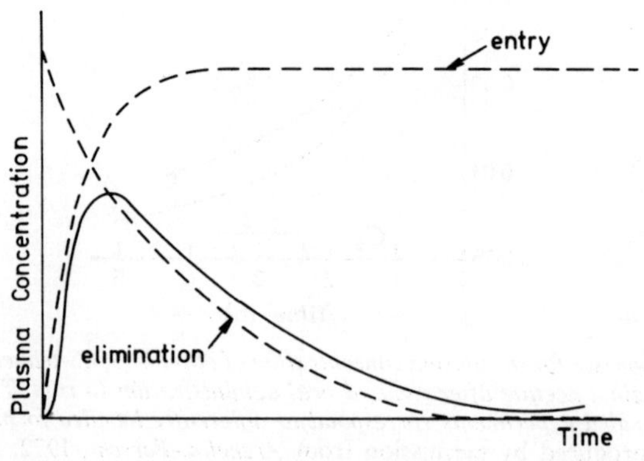

Figure 5 *The blood-level curve as a resultant of continuing entry (absorption) and elimination processes. The full line represents the blood-level curve, and the broken lines the entry (absorption) and elimination processes respectively*

Mathematically, the entry/'absorption' curve might be represented by the expression:

$$\frac{dy_1}{dt} = ak_1e^{-k_1t}$$

the elimination curve by:

$$\frac{dy_2}{dt} = -k_2y_2$$

and the interaction of the two processes by:

$$\frac{dy}{dt} = \frac{dy_1 + dy_2}{dt} = ak_1e^{-k_1t} - k_2y_2$$

and, at equilibrium, by:

$$\frac{dy}{dt} = ak_1e^{-k_1t} - k_2y \qquad (1)$$

Whence, by Lagrange's method of solution:

$$y = C_1e^{-k_2t} + C_2e^{-k_1t} \qquad (2)$$

Differentiation of this gives:

$$\frac{dy}{dt} = -\ C_1k_2e^{-k_2t} - C_2k_1e^{-k_1t} \qquad (3)$$

It follows from equations 1—3 that:

$$-\ C_1k_2e^{-k_2t} - C_2k_1e^{-k_1t} = ak_1e^{-k_1t} - C_1k_2e^{-k_2t} - C_2k_2e^{-k_1t}$$

or

$$(C_1k_2 - C_1k_2)e^{-k_2t} = (C_2k_1 + ak_1 - C_2k_2)e^{-k_1t}$$

For this expression to hold for all values of t, the bracketted expressions on each side of the equation must be zero.

For $C_2k_1 + ak_1 - C_2k_2 = 0$, it follows that:

$$C_2 = \frac{ak_1}{k_2 - k_1}$$

The general solution of equation 1 can be obtained by substituting this value of C_2 into equation 2:

$$y = C_1e^{-k_2t} + \frac{ak_1}{k_2 - k_1}e^{-k_1t} \qquad (4)$$

C_1 can now be evaluated, for, under the condition that $t = 0$, y becomes zero, and also:

$$C_1 = \frac{ak_1}{k_2 - k_1}$$

Whence:

$$y = \frac{ak_1}{k_2 - k_1}(e^{-k_1 t} - e^{-k_2 t}) \qquad (5)$$

This exponential function has a wider connotation, for example, the expression has been used to represent the genesis and decomposition of radioactive elements.[5]

Biological Half-life and Plasma Clearance.—Reference has been made already to the biological half-life $t_{0.5}$ (*v. supra*), which is the time taken for the concentration of the test substance to decrease to one-half of the initial value.

Thus, in the foregoing elimination curve $y = ae^{-k_2 t}$, where k_2 represents the elimination constant, if $y = a/2$, then:

$$t_{0.5} = \frac{1}{k_2} \ln 2 = \frac{0.6931}{k_2} \qquad (6)$$

e.g., for PAS, $k_2 = 0.68\ h^{-1}$, and $t_{0.5} = 1$ h 1 min; for Congo-red, $k_2 = 0.28\ h^{-1}$, and $t_{0.5} = 2$ h 28 min;* and for horse-serum diphtheria anti-toxin, $k_2 = 0.0055\ h^{-1}$, and $t_{0.5} = 5$ days 6 h.

* The relatively short $t_{0.5}$ value is due to the action of azo-reductase, and it contrasts with that of other amino compounds, which do not contain an azo-group.

Table 1 *Biological half-lives of some chemicals and pesticides*

	$t_{0.5}$ *Values in man*			
	(*years*)	(*days*)	(*h*)	(*min*)
p-$NH_2.C_6H_3(OH).CO_2H$			1	1
Chloroform			1	30
Ethanol			1	35
1,1,2-Trichloroethylene			2	
Congo-red			2	28
Benzylamine			2—3	
Pentachlorophenol		1	6	
Warfarin		2		
Styrene		2—4		
Hg^{2+}		{60 45*		
DDT		115		
Dieldrin	1			
HCB	2.5—3.5†			

* In lactating women. † In rhesus monkeys.

[5] Lord Rutherford, 'Radioactive substances and their relations,' Cambridge, 1913.

The Table displays some $t_{0.5}$ values for industrial chemicals and pesticides. Some of them, such as *p*-aminosalicylate, are eliminated rapidly from the body while others, such as inorganic Hg^{2+} and dieldrin, which accumulate in the body, show long periods of tissue retention.

In general, substances which are highly hydrophilic and ones which are converted rapidly into water-soluble metabolites have very short $t_{0.5}$ values. After oral and rectal administrations in particular, the absorption may extend over a considerable period of time, and during the first phase after administration, the blood-level curve represents the resultant of absorption and eliminative processes. In this context, dose-related blood levels of chloroform in man are of interest, especially as they would be expected to be of the same order of magnitude as those for the blood levels of halothane and of the chlorinated alkane and alkene solvents after comparable exposures. Peak blood concentrations of chloroform[6] after an oral dose of 0.5 g exceed 1 $\mu g\ ml^{-1}$. Breaks in the eliminative part of the time courses for chloroform concentrations in blood are consistent with the compartmentalization of chloroform in the body (Figure 6). In agreement with a previous argument (*v. supra*), the first half-life of the biphasic curves for four human subjects (Figure 6) would seem to represent the rapid unloading of the blood before the distribution equilibrium was established. The second half-life, $t_{0.5}$ = 90 min (Figure 6: 96 min for one subject, 92 min for another, and

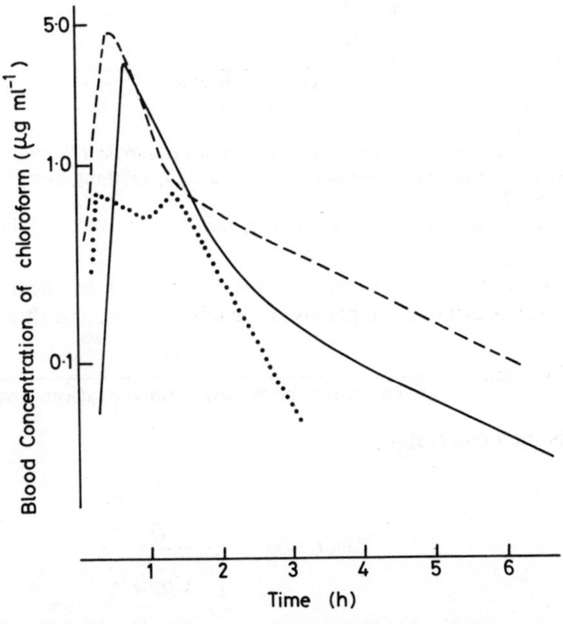

Figure 6 *Semi-log plots for the blood concentration–time relationships in human subjects after administration of a gelatin capsule containing chloroform* (500 ml) *in olive oil* (1 ml), *at zero time*

[Reproduced by permission from *Arch. Int. Pharmacodyn. Ther.*, 1972, **196**, 98—111]

86 min for the two others) represents the unloading of blood after equilibration within the total distribution volume.

After i.v. injection, a rapid decrease in blood level follows a rapid increase, as a result of redistribution. A real $t_{0.5}$ value is determined from the second phase of the curve (*v. supra*), which is found to be linear on a logarithmic scale, and in this connection, the case of the elimination of acrylonitrile (75 mg kg^{-1}, i.v.) from the blood of rabbits, pre-treated with sodium thiosulphate, might be cited.[6] In this example, the second part of the curve (Figure 7) is linear when plotted on log-linear axes: $t_{0.5} = 68.5$ min.[7]

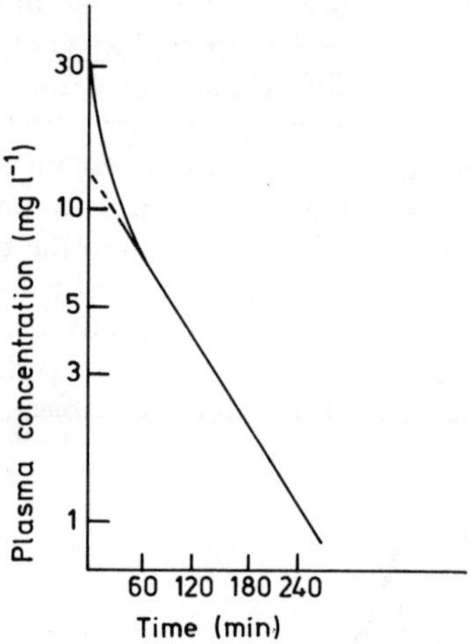

Figure 7 *Log–linear plot of the elimination of acrylonitrile* (75 mg kg^{-1} *i.v.*) *from the plasma of rabbits, pre-treated with* $Na_2S_2O_3$ (320 mg kg^{-1}, *i.v.*) *as an antidote to* HCN

[Reproduced by permission from *Ind. Health*, 1965, **3**, 30]

Plasma clearance is conceived as the proportion of the drug distribution volume which is cleared completely of drug/unit time, and thus:

$$\text{Clearance} = \frac{D}{\text{Area under the plasma concentration–time curve}} \quad (7)$$

where D is the dose employed.

Thus:

$$\text{Clearance} = \frac{D}{\int_0^\infty Cp_t \, dt}$$

Since Cp_t is the plasma concentration, the denominator involves a D/V term.

[6] B. J. Fry, T. Taylor, and D. E. Hathway, *Arch. Int. Pharmacodyn.*, 1972, **196**, 98.
[7] K. Hashimoto and R. Kanai, *Ind. Health*, 1965, **3**, 30.

The disposition of pantothenate in dogs (Figure 2)[3] accords with these concepts. Calculated values of the apparent initial distribution volumes as 2 380 and 2 310 ml and of the plasma vitamin clearances as 135 and 276 ml min^{-1} showed that the latter were in fact fractions of the distribution volumes, which approximated to those of the total extracellular fluid in the animals concerned.

Repeated and Chronic Dosings.—Three factors, *viz.* the size of the dose, the interval between consecutive dosings, and the $t_{0.5}$ value for the substance concerned, determine whether a substance will accumulate in the body. Provided that the $t_{0.5}$ value is relatively small compared with the time interval between dosings, the foreign compound would be almost entirely eliminated before the next dose, in which case, the blood level on dosing for the second time would be very little greater than that after the first dose (Figure 8). However, where

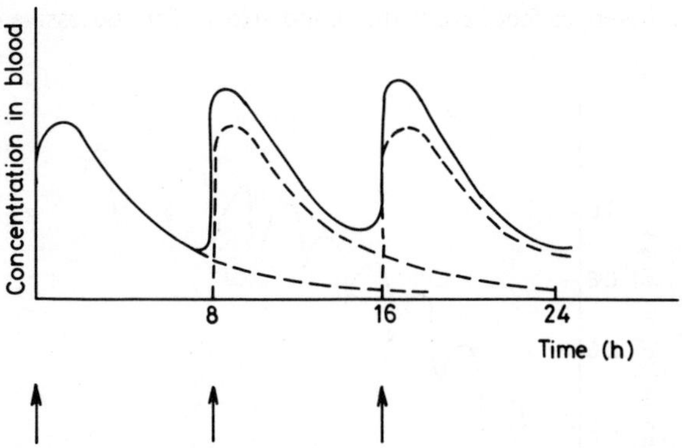

Figure 8 *Repeated dosage. Administration of the test substance* ($t_{0.5}$ = 4 h) *t.i.d.*

the $t_{0.5}$ value is of the same order of magnitude as the dose interval (Figure 9), then an appreciable amount of the substance would still be present at the end of each dose interval. The second dose gives an appreciably higher blood

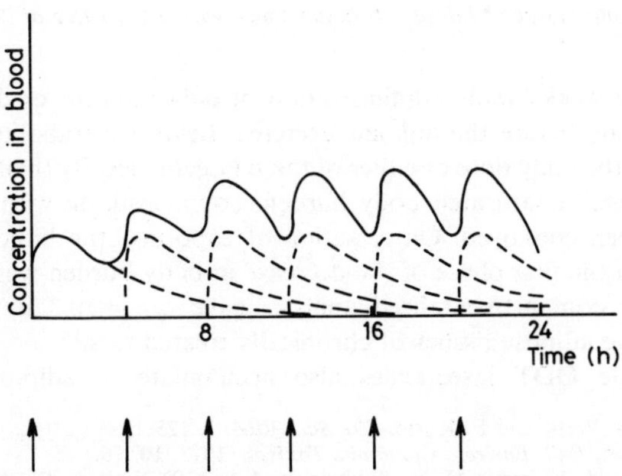

Figure 9 *Repeated dosage. Administration of the test substance* 6 times/day

level than the first one. Repeated doses would be followed by increasing blood levels and a gradually increasing rate of excretion. This process recurs until equilibration, when the rate of excretion matches the amount absorbed from the given dose, and a steady-state concentration or plateau value is reached in the blood. Figure 9 illustrates a case where equilibration is attained during 8—12 h, and shows the benefit accruing to therapy from multiple dosage.

A chronic situation might be represented by the case where the $t_{0.5}$ value greatly exceeds the dose interval (Figure 10), and equilibration would be reached only after several days' treatment. Dependent upon the dose interval, a great proportion of the first doses might remain in the body at the time of successive dosages. This is especially true for exposure to very lipophilic substances, such as the insecticides DDT, aldrin, dieldrin, and endrin, and softeners, such as the chlorinated biphenyl derivatives. However, in other instances, there is evidence of more rapid disappearance from the blood stream for successive doses.

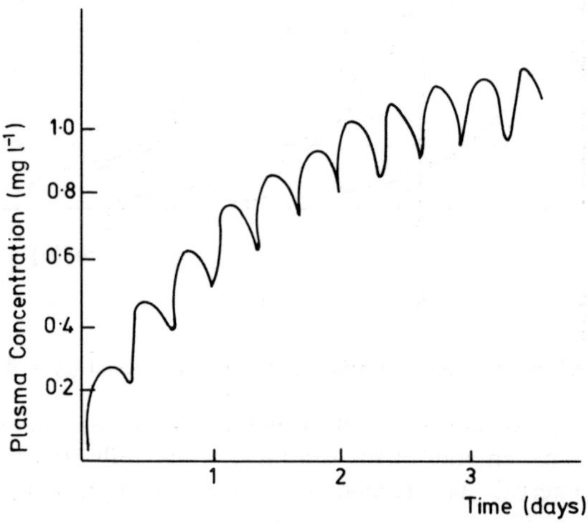

Figure 10 *Chronic dosage t.i.d. of a test substance with a* $t_{0.5}$ *value of* 24 h

Six to eight weeks' daily administration of either aldrin[8] or dieldrin[9] had to be made to rats before the animals excreted dieldrin metabolites in quantities equivalent to the daily dose of either of these insecticides. By that time, there had been established a saturated body burden, commensurate with the dose level which had been employed. On cessation of exposure, the biological $t_{0.5}$ value for dieldrin in the first phase of the decrease in body burden was 11 days,[8] and a much later compartmentalized analysis gave $t_{0.5} = 10.3$ days for dieldrin retained by the adipose tissues of chronically treated rats.[10]

Lipid-soluble DDT insecticides also accumulate in adipose tissues, and

[8] G. Ludwig, J. Weis, and F. Korte, *Life Sci.*, 1964, **3**, 123.
[9] K. L. Davison, *Bull. Environ. Contamin. Toxicol.*, 1973, **10**, 16.
[10] J. Robinson, M. Roberts, M. K. Baldwin, and A. I. T. Walker, *Food Cosmet. Toxicol.*, 1969, **7**, 317.

considerable interest is attached accordingly to such storage by human populations, and in this connection, the investigations of W. J. Hayes, jun.,[11–14] of Hunter *et al.*,[15] and of Hoffman *et al.*[16] merit attention.

Investigation of the co-administration of two substances on a chronic basis, and with the same dosage interval, showed the steady-state blood concentrations to be proportional to the $t_{0.5}$ values.[17] This result means that a substance with twice the $t_{0.5}$ value of another reaches twice the steady-state blood concentration of the latter. The same consideration applies when the $t_{0.5}$ value of a particular substance is increased, for example through injury to the liver or kidneys. In patients with liver disorders or kidney disturbances, the $t_{0.5}$ value of a drug may be considerably enhanced.

3 Kinetics of Excretion

Predictably, curves representing both the excretion of foreign compounds from the body, by the urinary, biliary, and pulmonary eliminative routes, and the elimination of substances which have accumulated in the body tissues, for example the unloading of adipose tissue retention of lipophilic substances, would be exponential in nature. In this connection, the blood level–time course is properly described by the exponential function in equation 5. This section of the chapter is a short one, as over-lavish illustration would be tedious.

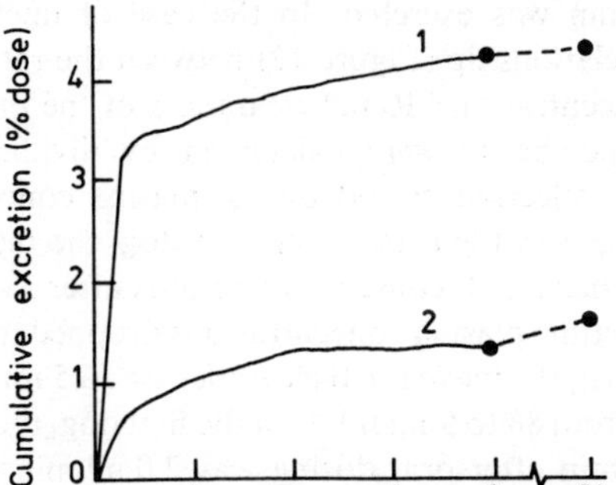

Figure 11 *Cumulative urinary excretion of unchanged pantothenate after i.v. administration* (6.68 mg) *to dogs 1 and 2*
[Reproduced by permission from *Res. Vet. Sci.*, 1974, **16**, 271—275]

Two dogs injected i.v. with sodium pantothenate (6.68 mg) excreted vitamin-related material mostly in the urine: 52.6 and 40.8% of the dose respectively in 7 days (see Figure 11) and the remainder as the β-glucuronide metabolite over

[11] G. E. Quinby, W. J. Hayes, jun., J. F. Armstrong, and W. F. Durham, *J. Am. Med. Assoc.*, 1965, **191**, 175.
[12] W. J. Hayes, jun., *Arch. Ind. Health*, 1958, **18**, 398.
[13] W. E. Dale and G. E. Quinby, *Science*, 1963, **142**, 593.
[14] W. J. Hayes, jun. and W. E. Dale, *Nature*, 1963, **199**, 1189.
[15] C. G. Hunter, J. Robinson, and A. Richardson, *Br. Med. J.*, 1963, **8**, 221.
[16] W. S. Hoffman, W. I. Fishbein, and M. B. Andelman, *J. Am. Med. Assoc.* 1964, **188**, 819.
[17] J. M. van Rossum, *J. Pharm. Sci.*, 1968, **57**, 2162.

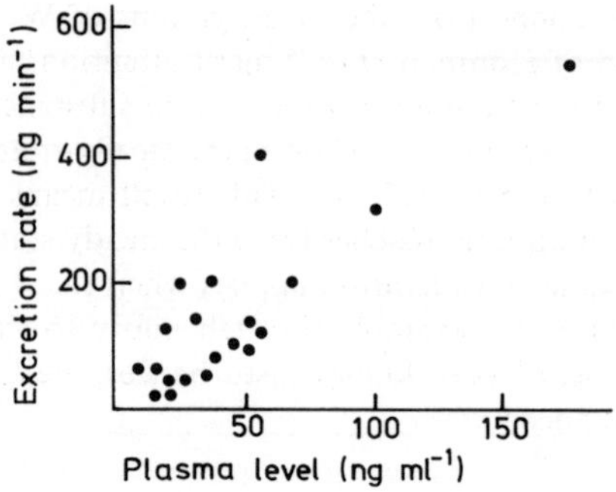

Figure 12 *Relationship of urinary excretion with plasma concentration of unchanged pantothenate after i.v. administration to dogs 1 and 2 and after oral dosing of dog 1*

[Reproduced by permission from *Res. Vet. Sci.*, 1974, **16,** 271—275]

several months.[3] During the first 2 h after injection, 1 and 4% respectively of unchanged vitamin was excreted in the urine and a further 0.6 and 0.7% during the next 22 h, but thereafter no more unchanged vitamin was excreted. Much the same pattern followed oral doses (1.67 or 6.68 mg), but a smaller proportion of unchanged vitamin was excreted. In the case of unchanged pantothenate, there was a linear relationship (Figure 12) between the rate of urinary excretion and the plasma concentration.[3] Renal clearances of the unchanged vitamin and its β-glucuronide metabolite were calculated by dividing the mean rate of excretion over any collection period by the plasma concentration at the mid-point of that period.[1,3] In the case of the first dog, the mean renal clearance of unchanged vitamin during 10 consecutive periods after i.v. injection was 2.1 ml min^{-1}, during which time plasma concentrations dropped from 500 to 15 ng ml^{-1}. For the second animal, the mean renal clearance was 6.5 ml min^{-1} and the plasma concentrations fell from 88 to 9 ng ml^{-1}. In the first dog, the mean renal clearance for unchanged vitamin after oral dosing was 2.0 ml min^{-1}. Renal clearance of the β-glucuronide metabolite was variable: 36.7 ml min^{-1} in dog 1 injected i.v. and 37.4 ml min^{-1} in dog 2, but 25.4 ml min^{-1} in dog 1, dosed p.o. Pantothenate did not bind to plasma proteins.[3]

In the case of a simple drug, for example ethyl 4-(3,4,5-trimethoxycinnamoyl) piperazinyl acetate, experiments with rats equipped with biliary fistulae showed that 35—40% of the dose of either of two differently labelled forms of the drug was secreted into the 12-h bile (Figure 13).[4] The maximum rate of secretion of drug-related material into bile occurred within a few hours of oral administration. In longer collections, up to 50% of the dose was secreted into the bile, and this together with substantial urinary excretion (*ca.* 25%) during each period shows that good absorption had occurred. Moreover, the similar rate of secretion of drug-related material into the bile after oral dosing as after i.v. injection implied that ethyl 4-(3,4,5-trimethoxycinnamoyl)piperazinyl acetate was rapidly absorbed from the gastro-intestinal tract.[4]

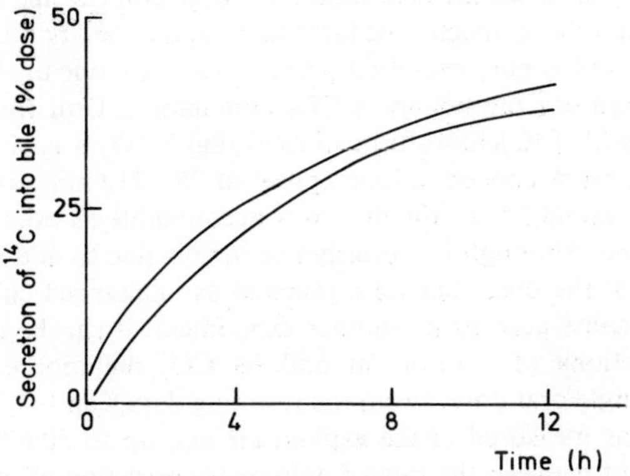

Figure 13 *Time courses for secretion into bile after the oral administration to rats of two labelled forms of ethyl* 4-(3,4,5-*trimethoxycinnamoyl*)*piperazinyl acetate*
[Reproduced by permission from *Arzneim.-Forsch.*, 1972, **22**, 1726—1732]

Pulmonary excretion after i.g. administration of chloroform and its CO_2 metabolite was thoroughly investigated in man.[6] Cumulative plots (Figure 14) for excretion of chloroform *via* the lungs showed a lag-phase before chloroform was detected in the exhaled air, and maximum pulmonary excretion occurred between 40 min and 2 h after dosage. Thereafter, the rate of pulmonary excretion diminished, and the curves became nearly parallel to the time axis (Figure 14).[6]

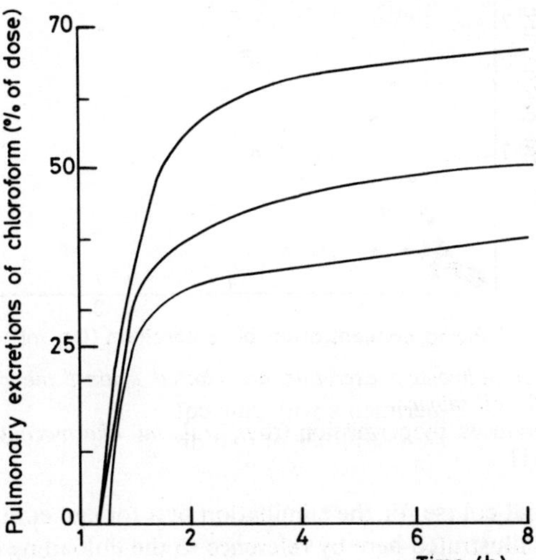

Figure 14 *Cumulative plots for the pulmonary excretions of chloroform in representative human subjects after the administration of a gelatin capsule containing chloroform* (500 mg) *in olive oil* (1 ml)
[Reproduced by permission from *Arch. Int. Pharmacodyn. Ther.*, 1972 **196**, 98—111]

Delayed excretion followed the dissolution of the gelatin capsule and absorption of chloroform from the stomach. The fact that CO_2 is a metabolite of chloroform in man makes its pulmonary excretion predictable, since one of the functions of mammalian respiratory physiology is CO_2 elimination. Oral treatment of two human subjects with [^{13}C]chloroform showed that $^{13}CO_2$ was eliminated in the expired air; maximum concentrations appeared 75—210 min after administration.[6] In the woman 48.5% of the dose was accountable as exhaled $^{13}CO_2$, and 50.6% in the man.[6] Although it is clearly not permissible to add these results to the proportions of the dose that were excreted as unchanged chloroform from the lungs of the same persons in another experiment, it can be concluded that pulmonary excretions of chloroform and its CO_2 metabolite account substantially for a single oral dose. From the resulting data,[6] up to 68.3% of a dose of chloroform was measured in the expired air and up to 50.6% as CO_2. The linear relationship[6] between the rate of pulmonary excretion of chloroform and its concentration in the blood (Figure 15) reflects the diffusion of chloroform from pulmonary arterial blood into alveolar air.

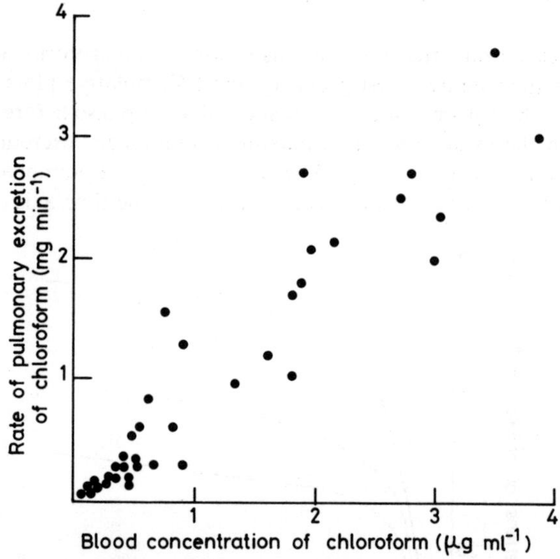

Figure 15 *Rates of pulmonary excretion are plotted against the corresponding blood levels for all subjects*
[Reproduced by permission from *Arch. Int. Pharmacodyn. Ther.*, 1972, **196**, 98—111]

The exponential course for the elimination of a foreign compound from body tissues might be illustrated here by reference to the unloading of DDT from the adipose tissues of a subject, who had been exposed to the insecticide at zero time (Figure 16).[18] DDT has $t_{0.5} = 3.7$ years in human adipose tissue.

[18] W. J. Hayes, jun., in 'Essays in Toxicology,' Academic Press, New York, 1974, vol. 5, p. 39 *et seq.*

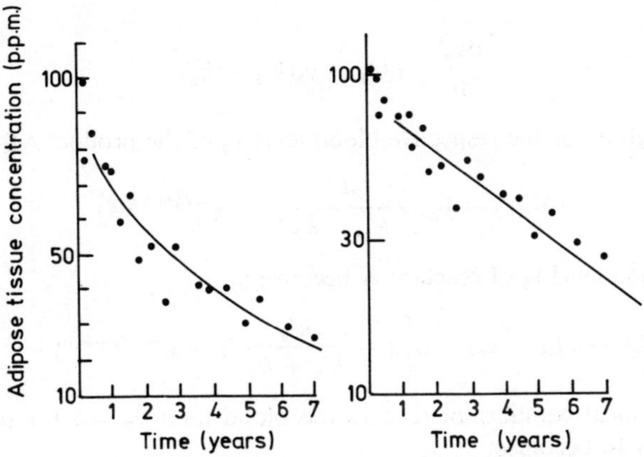

Figure 16 *Fall in the DDT level in adipose tissue of an individual, exposed to DDT at zero time. (a) Linear scale. (b) Semi-log plot. The lines represent calculated values*

4 Combined Elimination Processes

It is possible to consider a reaction:

$$A + B \underset{k_3}{\overset{k_2}{\rightleftharpoons}} AB$$

occurring *in vivo* under the conditions considered in relation to the blood-level curve for an unchanged foreign compound in the body (*v. supra*).

If a is the initial concentration of A and y_3 the concentration under consideration of AB, which takes the ($\rightharpoonup$) direction following the rate of build-up of AB:

$$\frac{dy_3}{dt} = k_2(a - y_3)(a - y_3)$$

and takes ($\leftharpoondown$) direction with regard to the rate of breakdown of AB:

$$\frac{-dy_3}{dt} = k_3y_3$$

then at equilibrium:

$$\frac{dy_3}{dt} = k_2(a - y_3)(a - y_3) - k_3y_3 \qquad (8)$$

In respect of one of the reactants, A or B, equation 8 becomes modified, so that:

$$\frac{dy_3}{dt} = k'_2(a - y_3) - k_3y_3$$

and thus

$$\frac{dy_3}{dt} = ak'_2 - y_3(k'_2 + k_3) \tag{9}$$

Integration gives for the respective blood level y_3 of the product AB:

$$F_3(t) = y_3 = \frac{ak'_2}{k'_2 + k_3}(1 - e^{-(k'_2+k_3)t}) \tag{10}$$

Thus the blood level y_2 of reactant A becomes:

$$F_2(t) = (a - y_3) = a\left[1 - \frac{k'_2}{k'_2 + k_3}(1 - e^{-(k'_2+k_3)t})\right] \tag{11}$$

When chemical equilibrium reaches the blood level $y_3 = b$ for the product AB, equation 10 becomes:

$$\underset{(\text{Lt } t = \infty)}{y_3 = b} = \frac{ak'_2}{k'_2 + k_3}$$

and

$$F_4(t) = y_4 = ae^{-k_4t} \tag{12}$$

The foregoing equations can now be brought together in respect of the reversible chemical exchange and excretion of reactant A, through the sum of the differential quotients of equations 11 and 12. Under these circumstances, all concentrations of y become equal to one another, $y_2 = y_3 = y$, thus giving equation 13:

$$\frac{dy}{dt} = -ak'_2e^{-(k'_2+k_3)t} - k_4y \tag{13}$$

Whence by Lagrange's method and with regard to unchanged initial substance A, equation 14 is obtained (see Figure 17 for this blood-level curve):

$$F_{el}(t) = F_{2,4}(t) = y$$
$$= a\left[\left(1 + \frac{k'_2}{k_4 - (k'_2 + k_3)}\right)e^{-k_4t} - \frac{k'_2}{k_4 - (k'_2 + k_3)}\,e^{-(k'_2+k_3)t}\right] \tag{14}$$

For the origin and elimination of the product AB, equation 13 becomes:

$$\frac{dy}{dt} = ak'_2e^{-(k'_2+k_3)} - k_4y$$

Integration under the stipulation that $t = 0$ gives the blood-level $y = 0$ itself, and thus:

$$F_{el}(t) = F_{3,4}(t) = \frac{ak'_2}{k_4 - (k'_2 + k_3)}[e^{-(k'_2+k_3)t} - e^{-k_4t}] \tag{15}$$

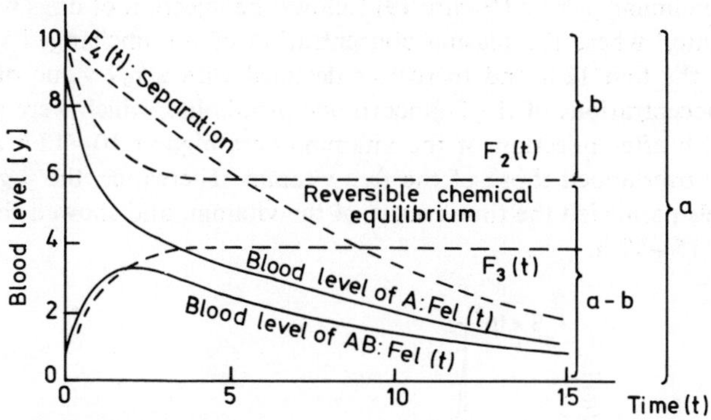

Figure 17 *Blood-level curve in respect of a substance A which has undergone a reversible chemical reaction to give a substance AB, and its blood-level curve*
[Reproduced by permission from F. H. Dost, 'Der Blutspiegel', Arbeitsgemeinschaft Medizinischer Verlage G.m.b.H, Georg Thieme, Leipzig, 1953, p.51]

The new blood-level curve for the product AB is essentially similar to the one (equation 5) that holds for a single substance which is eliminated from the blood unchanged (*v. supra*), and both functions, *viz.* equations 5 and 15, are exponential ones.

The underlying principle is a most important one, which applies both to the synthesis of conjugates and to catabolic reactions *in vivo*.

Thus, in the case of the injection of patients with Sulphapyridine,[19] the expression (equation 15) for the blood-level curve is consistent with the fact that the concentration of acetylation product reaches that of unchanged Sulphapyridine, overlaps it, and eventually parallels the time course of the free drug (Figure 18).

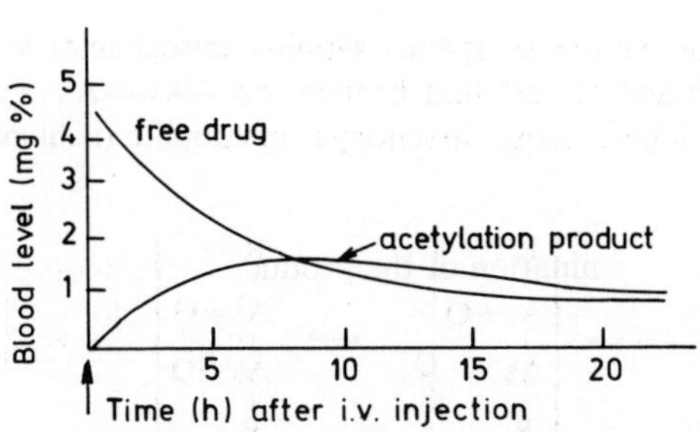

Figure 18 *Blood-level curves of free Sulphapyridine and its acetylation product after i.v. injection of* 1.841 g *in man*

[19] A. R. Frisk, Dissertation Karolinska Inst., Stockholm 1943; *Acta Med. Scand.*, 1943, supplement CXL11.

A rather similar picture (Figure 19) follows the injection of dogs with sodium pantothenate,[3] where the plasma concentration of the unchanged vitamin fell rapidly in the first 12 h and thereafter declined with a $t_{0.5}$ value of 15—17 h. Plasma concentrations of the β-glucuronide metabolite, which were measurable from *ca.* 1 h after injection of the vitamin, were highest 10—12 h afterwards, when they overlapped those of the free vitamin. Thereafter, the β-glucuronide blood levels paralleled the time course of the vitamin, and showed the same $t_{0.5}$ value, *viz.* 15—17 h.

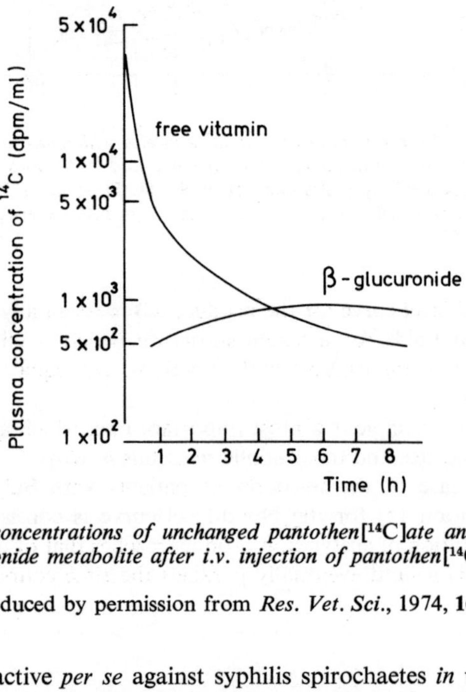

Figure 19 *Plasma concentrations of unchanged pantothen*[^{14}C]*ate and the* ^{14}*C-labelled β-glucuronide metabolite after i.v. injection of pantothen*[^{14}C]*ate* (6.68 mg) *in dogs*

[Reproduced by permission from *Res. Vet. Sci.*, 1974, **16**, 271—275]

Salvarsan is inactive *per se* against syphilis spirochaetes *in vitro*, and it was only when Ehrlich and Hata[20] had broken the —As=As— double bond that they obtained the highly active 'arsenoxyd' metabolite (Scheme).

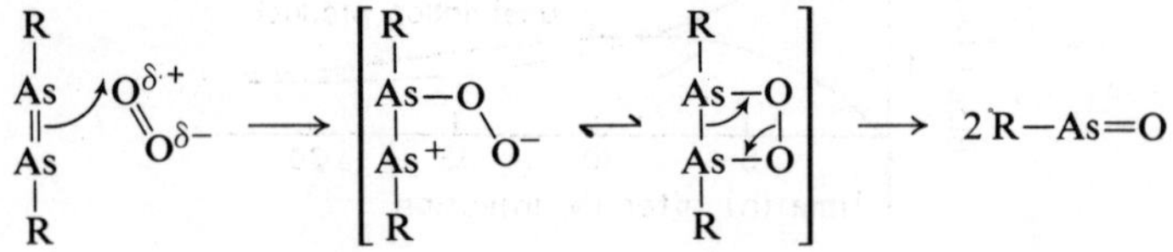

R = 3-amino-4-hydroxyphenyl

Scheme

[20] P. Ehrlich and S. Hata, 'Die experimentelle Therapie der Spirillosin,' Berlin, 1910.

The occurrence of this oxidative fission *in vivo*, by what would now be termed the electrophilic addition of oxygen, would explain the mode of action of this wonder drug, which had been discovered empirically. On this basis, as well, it is possible to reconstruct the accompanying blood-level curves for Salvarsan and its active 'arsenoxyd' metabolite (Figure 20).[21,22] A short time after the blood levels of the 'arsenoxyd' metabolite begin to build up and to overlap the ones of unchanged Salvarsan, the elimination of the drug is complete.

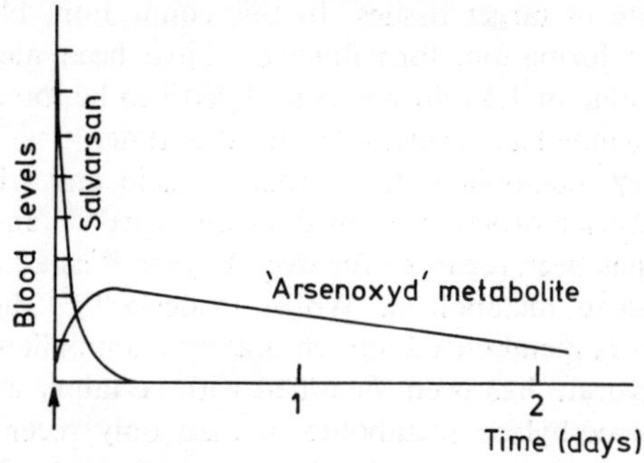

Figure 20 *Blood-level curves for Salvarsan and its active 'arsenoxyd' metabolite after the injection of man i.v. with Salvarsan at zero time*

Aspirin affords an excellent example of combined elimination. A dose of aspirin (650 mg) was given orally to human subjects, and the blood-level curves which were measured (Figure 21) represent the fraction of the dose remaining in the blood as aspirin (the lower curve) and the fraction which is hydrolysed to salicylic acid (the upper curve).[23] The experimental curves are in complete agreement with the ones that were calculated[23] from an open two-compartment model.

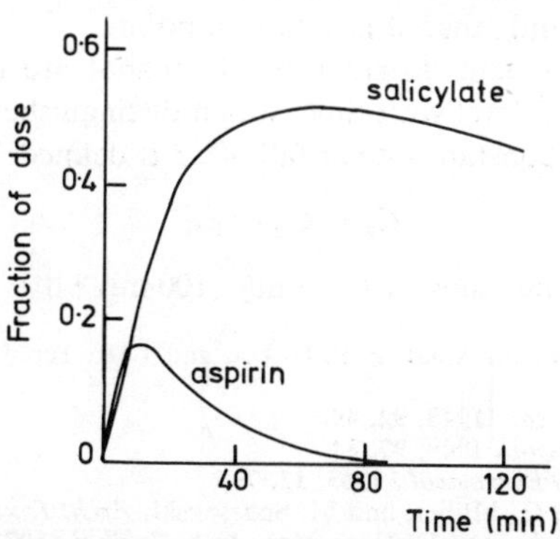

Figure 21 *Blood-level curves for the fraction of the dose as aspirin and as salicylate after oral administration to man of a solution containing* 650 mg *of aspirin*
[Reproduced by permission from *J. Pharm. Sci.*, 1972, **61**, 379]

[21] J. Danysz, *Ann. Inst. Pasteur*, 1917, **31**, 114.
[22] F. Eichhorn, 'Lehrbuch der Pharmakologie,' 5 Aufl., Berlin–Heidelberg, 1947.
[23] M. Rowland, S. Riegelman, P. A. Harris, and S. D. Sholkoff, *J. Pharm. Sci.*, 1972, **61**, 379.

It is clear that kinetic investigations of combined elimination processes mirror the network of biotransformations that characterizes the metabolism of foreign compounds. Such kinetic studies are particularly useful in revealing the formation and disappearance of key intermediates which, on account of their rapid turnover, are not excreted from the body and would escape detection by excretion–retention study.

As is explained elsewhere (chapter 8), animals, sensitive to methanol poisoning, accumulate formate in target tissues. In this connection, blood levels of the intermediate in its formation, formaldehyde, have been measured recently,[24] but its blood $t_{0.5}$ value of 1.5 min was considered[24] to be too short to modulate the effects which spanned a considerable period of time.

Since the urinary metabolites, trichloroacetic acid and trichloroethanol, of chloral[25] and 1,1,2-trichloroethylene in dogs and rats[26,27] and in man[28–30] are the same, chloral has been regarded for over 30 years[26] as a key intermediate in 1,1,2-trichloroethylene metabolism. Whilst evidence[31–33] showed that 1,1,2-trichloroethylene was metabolized into chloral by mammalian liver microsomes *in vitro*, chloral hydrate has been identified with certainty and measured as a blood 1,1,2-trichloroethylene metabolite in man only recently[34] (*cf.* ref. 35). This finding is very important as chloral is formed from 1,1,2-trichloroethylene only through rearrangement of 1,1,2-trichloroethylene oxide (*see* chapter 6), which is likely to be responsible *per se* for 1,1,2-trichloroethylene toxicity. The number of references in this paragraph seems to be justified to establish the sequence of results and the missing evidence.

5 Unusual Forms of Elimination

In the preceding sections of this chapter, consideration has been given to a variety of eliminations which have been always exponential functions, but there are some exceptions, and ethanol is a case in point.

After the absorption and distribution of ethanol are complete, there is a zero-order fall of blood level with time, which distinguishes it (Figure 22) from other substances. The constant rate of fall off, β is defined[36] by the expression

$$C_t = C_0 - \beta t,$$

where β lies within the range 10—25 mg $(100\ \text{ml})^{-1}\ \text{h}^{-1}$ for most individual

24 K. E. McMartin, G. Martin-Amat, P. E. Noker, and T. R. Tephly, *Biochem. Pharmacol.*, 1979, **28**, 645.
25 T. C. Butler, *J. Pharmacol.*, 1948, **92**, 49.
26 T. C. Butler, *J. Pharmacol.*, 1949, **97**, 84.
27 J. W. Daniel, *Biochem. Pharmacol.*, 1963, **12**, 795.
28 T. Ertle, D. Henschler, G. Müller, and M. Spassovski, *Arch. Toxikol.*, 1972, **29**, 171.
29 G. Müller, M. Spassovski, and D. Henschler, *Arch. Toxikol.*, 1972, **29**, 335.
30 J. F. Powell, *Br. J. Ind. Med.*, 1945, **2**, 142.
31 K. H. Byington and K. C. Leibman, *Mol. Pharmacol.*, 1965, **1**, 247.
32 K. C. Leibman, *Mol. Pharmacol.*, 1965, **1**, 239.
33 K. C. Leibman and W. J. McAllister, *J. Pharmacol.*, 1967, **157**, 574.
34 W. J. Cole, R. G. Mitchell, and R. F. Salamonsen, *J. Pharm. Pharmacol.*, 1975, **27**, 167.
35 G. Scansetti, G. F. Rubino, and G. Trompeo, *Med. Lav.*, 1959, **50**, 743.
36 E. M. P. Widmark, 'Die theoretischen Grundlagen und die praktische Verwertbarkeit der gerichtlich-medizinischen Alkoholbestimmung,' Berlin-Wein, 1932.

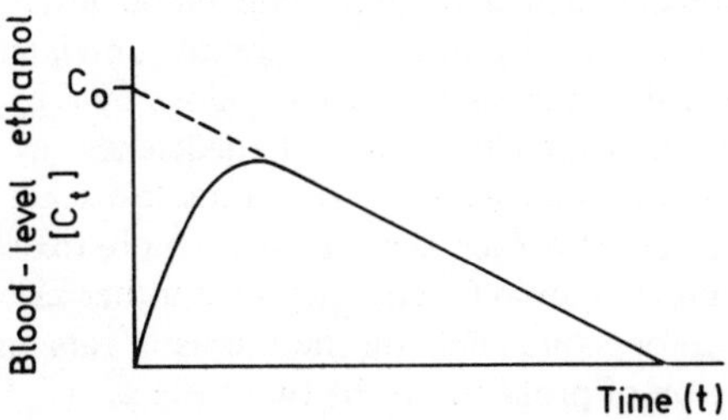

Figure 22 *Schematic representation after Widmark of the linear fall-off in blood alcohol in man*

subjects. More than 90% of exogenous alcohol is oxidized by LAD, and the resulting acetaldehyde enters the metabolic pool of C_2 compounds. Catabolism to CO_2 is negligible, and excretion of unchanged ethanol *via* the pulmonary and urinary routes accounts for less than 10% of a dose. Thus, the precise value of β would seem to depend upon the liver mass and hepatic blood flow, as there is a rapid turnover of exogenous acetaldehyde and acetate.[37] Of the many substances which have been tested, (−)-fructose alone produces a significant increase in β, to about 18—24 mg (100 ml)$^{-1}$ h^{-1}, but the mechanism involved is obscure.

6 The Contribution of the Kinetics Approach

Scope and Limitations of a Possible Relationship between Toxicity and Blood Levels.—Previous sections of this chapter stress the importance of blood levels, and the toxicity of foreign compounds has been associated with the compounds *per se* or with particular metabolites, both in the present chapter and in chapters 6 and 8. The toxicity that is produced appears to be related to the quantity and duration of the presence of the causative agent in the blood. This argument is crucial to section 4 of this chapter, where Sulphapyridine and pantothenate were the active agents *per se*, but Salvarsan was itself non-toxic to syphilis spirochaetes. Aspirin is an excellent analgesic, and both aspirin and the salicylate metabolite have anti-inflammatory properties. 1,1,2-Trichloroethylene oxide appears to be responsible for 1,1,2-trichloroethylene toxicity. The scope of the relationship between toxicity and the blood levels of foreign compounds is very general and, in the absence of differences, spans the species (*v. infra*). Nevertheless, for example, calculations of toxicity would be incorrect in those cases where the degree of absorption is disproportional to the areas under the plasma concentration–time relationships,[38] and this occurs where, as in the case of dieldrin and Telodrin, the toxicants are absorbed very rapidly and withdrawn from the blood stream just as rapidly.[39]

Some confusion occurs in the case of some drugs, where pharmacological

[37] K. J. Freundt, *Arch. Exp. Pathol. Pharmakol.*, 1968, **260**, 114.
[38] D. E. Hathway, in 'Foreign Compound Metabolism in Mammals,' ed. D. E. Hathway, Specialist Periodical Report Series, The Chemical Society, London, 1972, vol. 2, p. 3.
[39] J. A. Moss and D. E. Hathway, *Biochem. J.*, 1964, **91**, 384.

activity is undoubtedly related to prevailing blood levels, but where adverse side-effects may be caused by other, apparently unrelated factors. Thus, for example the myocardial necrosis produced in dogs by a hypolipidaemic agent[40] was considered to be related to vitamin E deficiency, as the drug was interchangeable with cod-liver oil in causing white muscle disease in lambs, susceptible to vitamin E deficiency. However, the drug is no more toxic than cod-liver oil to man, who is resistant to vitamin E deficiency. In another case, some hypothalamic tranquilizers had an opposite effect on the uterus in rats and in dogs,[41] because of the different action of prolactin in the two species.

In general, anti-inflammatory drugs (aspirin, indomethacin, phenylbutazone, *etc.*) cause gastric ulceration by preventing the healing of minor traumatic injury and, as there is great variability in susceptibility to this lesion, deaths through ulcer perforation are unpredictable and LD_{50} values in animals are erratic. A case[40] might be cited where the time-course for lethality is hyperbolic and, whilst mortality is dose- (and blood level-) related at low levels, where anti-inflammatory action is incomplete, it is very erratic at high dose levels, where the dose affording maximum anti-inflammatory action has been surpassed.

Absence of Species Differences.—The problem posed by the extension of data that were found in animals to man can be approached, where the absence of species differences in metabolism/toxicity between a representative rodent species, for example rats, and a representative non-rodent species, for example dogs or baboons, has been established with certainty. In this connection, the kinetic approach is a very versatile and sensitive tool, which takes into account the absorption, metabolism, and excretion of foreign compounds. Of the standards, therefore, that could be used for comparison in treated animals, the following might be considered:[42,43] (i) the rates of excretion from the body by a urinary, biliary, or pulmonary eliminative route, as the case may be; and (ii) plasma kinetics after the same route of administration and at comparable dose levels as in (i).

It would be wise to implement both exercises after i.v. injection and after dosing p.o. As an additional test, the array of foreign-compound metabolites in the body fluids of the species concerned ought to be investigated. Provided that the foregoing stringent tests did not reveal any marked differences between the selected species, that no adverse effects were found in toxicity, and that there was no serious accumulation of foreign compound in any of the animals, it ought to be feasible to apply them to man.

[40] S. B. de C. Baker and D. M. Foulkes, in 'Biological Effects of Drugs in Relation to their Plasma Concentration (Proceedings of a Symposium held by the British Pharmacological Society, London, 1972),' ed. D. S. Davies and B. N. C. Prichard, Macmillan, London, 1973, pp. 42—50.
[41] S. B. de C. Baker and M. J. Tucker, *Proc. Eur. Soc. Study Drug Toxic.* **IX**, Suppl. ICS 145, 113.
[42] Ref. 38, pp. 1, 2.
[43] D. E. Hathway, in 'International Aspects of Drug Evaluation and Usage (Based on an International Meeting of Medical Advisers to the Pharmaceutical Industry organized by the Association of Medical Advisers in the Pharmaceutical Industry, London, 1972),' ed. A. J. Jouhar and M. F. Grayson, Churchill Livingstone, Edinburgh and London, 1973, pp. 19—32.

Validation in Man.—Under the conditions stipulated, the foregoing tests appear to meet this objective. Three points ought to be mentioned. The first one has to do with the selection of healthy subjects with normal kidney and liver function by medical examination, from amongst volunteers. Secondly, the volunteers, who are selected, ought to remain under medical supervision throughout the experiment and to be subject to subsequent checks. For a metabolic investigation in man, a single administration should be made, and in the case of a drug, a dose level should be used which is unlikely to exceed its therapeutic dose in the event of possible clinical use. The third point concerns the use of an isotopically labelled foreign compound, which may be essential to identify the exceptionally small amounts of substances involved.[42] The very small amounts of labelled drug, which may be permitted for administration to man, make difficult the comparison of the blood levels of labelled compound in man with those in animals, and for that purpose, all of the blood levels would have to be corrected for dose level and body weight, *i.e.* the concentration of a foreign compound would have to be expressed in terms of μg of compound/unit dose level/kg body weight/ml plasma.

Selection of Animals for Long-term Toxicity Testing.—Rats and beagle hounds have come to be regarded as the animals of choice,[41–48] but their selection for toxicity testing has usually been on an empirical basis. In this connection, sub-human primates have received some attention. With a large majority of drugs, it is significant that in the past the transition from experiments in animals to those in man has been safely negotiated. Many adverse effects of established drugs in human subjects were reproducible in animals on re-testing. Comparative drug metabolism studies in animals and in man ought to be fundamental to the selection of animals for toxicological purposes, and the battery of tests discussed (*v. supra*) might serve here. Alternatively, it might be reasonable to determine the renal clearances of the foreign compound and its major metabolites after i.v. injection and oral dosing, in conjunction with liver-function tests in the animals concerned.

Useful data can be derived from experiments in a very few, carefully selected animals, such as baboons, dogs, or rhesus monkeys, and the work[3] with pantothenate in dogs is an instance of this.

[44] 'Procedures for testing of intentional food additives to establish their safety for use,' *WHO Techn. Rep. Ser.*, no. 144, Geneva, 1958.
[45] 'Procedures for investigating intentional and unintentional food additives', *WHO Techn. Rep. Ser.*, no. 348, Geneva, 1967.
[46] 'Principles and procedures for evaluating the safety of food additives,' *Nat. Acad. Sci. Nat. Res. Council Publ.*, no. 750, Washington D.C., 1960.
[47] 'Memorandum on procedure for submissions on food additives and on methods of toxicity testing,' Ministry of Agriculture, Fisheries and Food, London, 1965.
[48] 'Notification of pesticides: Scheme agreed between government and industry,' Ministry of Agriculture, Fisheries and Food, London, 1960.

Part IV
Pharmacogenetics

Chapter 8 Species Differences in Metabolism and Toxicity

1 Introduction

A knowledge of (mammalian) species variability in the metabolism of a foreign compound would appear to be a prerequisite of an understanding of its toxicity in these animals and the extension of these results to man. This chapter is concerned mainly with species differences in the metabolic fate of foreign compounds in living animals and to some extent with the appropriate enzyme activities of the liver and other organs that may be relevant, as well as with those of the gut flora. Whilst some recourse is had to model compounds, greater emphasis is given to species variability in the metabolism of important industrial chemicals, food additives and constituents, and pesticides.

Some of this information may also be found in reports on foreign compound metabolism.[1] Reference might be made also to reviews[2,3] dealing with all aspects of variability, to the position of man,[4] to a monograph[5] dedicated to the late R. T. Williams and providing a number of articles covering strain differences in metabolism and pharmacogenetics, and to a stimulating review[6] on oxidation

[1] 'Foreign Compound Metabolism in Mammals,' ed. D. E. Hathway, The Royal Society of Chemistry, London, Specialist Periodical Report series, Vol. 1 (1970)—Vol. 6 (1981).
[2] R. T. Williams, *Biochem. Soc. Trans.*, 1974, **2**, 359.
[3] A. H. Conney, C. Coutinho, B. Koechlin, R. Swarm, J. A. Cheripko, C. Impellizzeri, and H. Baruth, *Clin. Pharmacol. Therap.*, 1975, **16**, 176.
[4] 'Pharmacology and the Future of Man,' Proceedings of the 5th International Congress on Pharmacology, San Francisco, 1972, ed. G. T. O. Kita, Karger, Basel, 1973.
[5] 'Drug Metabolism: From Microbe to Man,' eds. D. V. Parke and R. L. Smith, Taylor and Francis, London, 1977.
[6] R. T. Williams, *Environ. Health Perspectives*, 1978, **22**, 133.

and conjugation pathways of metabolism. There appears to be much less information about the limiting capacities of the metabolic pathways available and about the transport mechanisms in the different species, yet such factors are indisputably pertinent to the toxicity which is apparent.

The actual genetic elements which are involved, wherever real differences in enzymic activities have been established, cannot be clearly defined, except in the case of a very few drugs that do not come within the scope of this book. In the present article, attention is given instead to species differences in mammalian metabolism and their relationship with toxicity. For convenience' sake, these differences have been subdivided as comparative catabolic reactions, as comparative differences in conjugation, as comparative differences in enzymic activities, and as comparative differences in biliary excretion and metabolism by the gut flora. Many examples of minor quantitative differences in foreign-compound metabolism between various mammals, including man, have been omitted purposely in order to make evident more pronounced variability. Finally, the sections devoted to enzymes and species differences in metabolism are not meant as definitive reviews but rather to provide the various metabolic pathways, which have been described in chapter 6, with a biochemical basis and some biological relevance.

2 Comparative Catabolic Reactions

Ethylene Glycol.—In mammals, ω or (ω — 1) oxidation of ethylene glycol affords (i) CO_2 by a major metabolic pathway, which involves glycolic aldehyde, glycolic acid, and glyoxylic acid,[7] and (ii) oxalic acid by a minor one, which is likely to proceed *via* glyoxal.[8] Two enzyme systems seem to be implicated, one of which distinguishes between the two terminal groups and the other which does not. Severe acidosis, which large acute doses of ethylene glycol produce in dogs and monkeys, is due entirely to accumulation of glycolic acid.[9] However, formation of oxalic acid is species dependent,[8] the order of species dependence rabbits $<$ rats $<$ cats being also that of increasing chronic toxicity of ethylene glycol. Thus, ethylene glycol chronic toxicity is attributable at any rate in part to oxalic acid and local deposition of calcium oxalate in the bladder and renal tubules, for example, of rabbits and rats. On the other hand glyoxal, which belongs to the same metabolic pathway as oxalic acid, has been incriminated also as a causative agent of chronic toxicity, particularly in cats which suffer from pancreatic necrosis. Both ethylene glycol and alloxan generate glyoxal *in vivo*, which acts on the pancreas, as all the other mammalian tissues contain glyoxalase.[10]

[7] S. Weinhouse and B. Friedmann, *J. Biol. Chem.*, 1951, **191**, 707.
[8] P. K. Gessner, D. V. Parke, and R. T. Williams, *Biochem. J.*, 1961, **79**, 482.
[9] K. L. Clay and R. C. Murphy, *Toxicol. Appl. Pharmacol.*, 1977, **39**, 39.
[10] W. Doerr, *Sitzungsber. Heidelb. Akad. Wiss. Math. Naturwiss. Kl.*, 1949, **7**, 112.

Biphenyl.—2-Hydroxylation of biphenyl is species dependent.[11,12] A high proportion of the 2-hydroxy derivative is formed in the liver of mice, but not in those of guinea-pigs, rabbits, and rats.

***trans*-Stilbene.**—Similarly, *trans*-stilbene (1) has been found to be metabolized differently by mice than by guinea-pigs and rabbits.[13] In guinea-pigs and rabbits, biotransformation into 4-hydroxy- (2), 4,4′-dihydroxy- (3), 4-hydroxy-3-methoxy- (4), and 3-hydroxy-4-methoxy-stilbenes (5) occurs, whereas in mice, only limited conversion into (3) takes place.

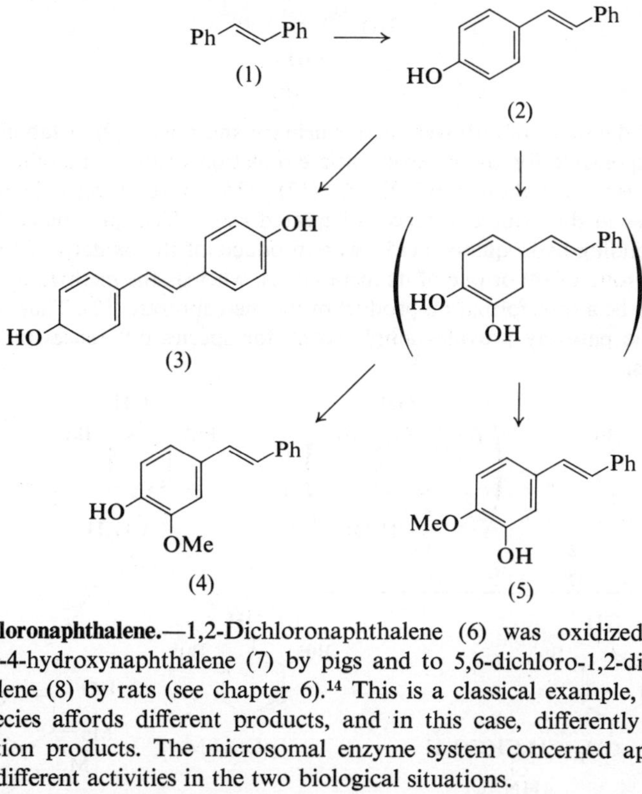

1,2-Dichloronaphthalene.—1,2-Dichloronaphthalene (6) was oxidized to 1,2-dichloro-4-hydroxynaphthalene (7) by pigs and to 5,6-dichloro-1,2-dihydroxy-naphthalene (8) by rats (see chapter 6).[14] This is a classical example, in which each species affords different products, and in this case, differently oriented substitution products. The microsomal enzyme system concerned appears to express different activities in the two biological situations.

Hydroxy-3,5-di-t-butyltoluene (BHT).—In man,[15] urinary BHT (9) metabolites were the dihydrobenzofuran (11) (21% of the dose), BHT-acid (10) (trace amount), and *N*-acetyl-*S*-(4-hydroxy-3,5-di-t-butylbenzyl)cysteine (12) (trace amount), whereas in rats[16,17] the mercapturate (12) and the ester glucuronide

[11] P. J. Creaven, D. V. Parke, and R. T. Williams, *Biochem. J.*, 1965, **96**, 390.
[12] P. J. Creaven, D. V. Parke, and R. T. Williams, *Biochem. J.*, 1965, **96**, 879.
[13] J. E. Sinsheimer and R. V. Smith, *Biochem. J.*, 1969, **111**, 35.
[14] L. O. Ruzo, D. Jones, S. Safe, and O. Hutzinger, *J. Agric. Food Chem.*, 1976, **24**, 581.
[15] L. I. Wiebe, J. R. Mercer, and A. J. Ryan, *Drug Metab. Dispos.*, 1978, **6**, 296.
[16] J. W. Daniel, J. C. Gage, and D. I. Jones, *Biochem. J.*, 1968, **106**, 783.
[17] J. W. Daniel and J. C. Gage, *Food Cosmet. Toxicol.*, 1965, **3**, 405.

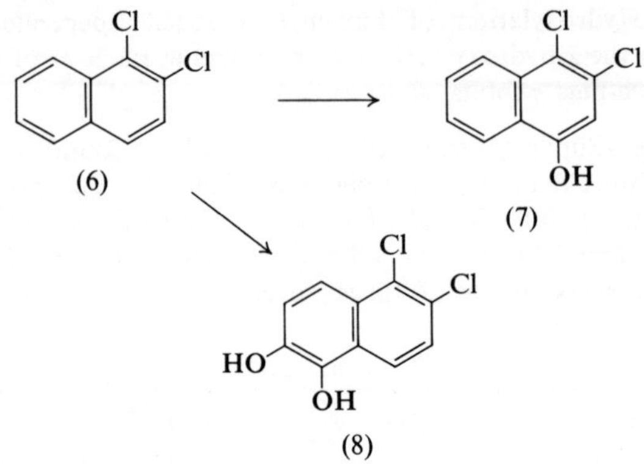

(15% of the dose) of (10) were major urinary and biliary (9) metabolites, which were responsible for the enterohepatic circulation of (9) metabolites in rats.[17] Three further metabolites of (9), *viz.* (13)—(15), were excreted in very small quantities in the urine and faeces of treated rats.[18] The quinone (14), and the corresponding hydroquinone (15), were products of the oxidative fission of the methyl group of (9) or one of its metabolites, whereas the methylthio derivative (13) may be a transformation product of the mercapturate (12). Thus, a complex metabolic pathway provides ample scope for species differences in metabolic reactions.

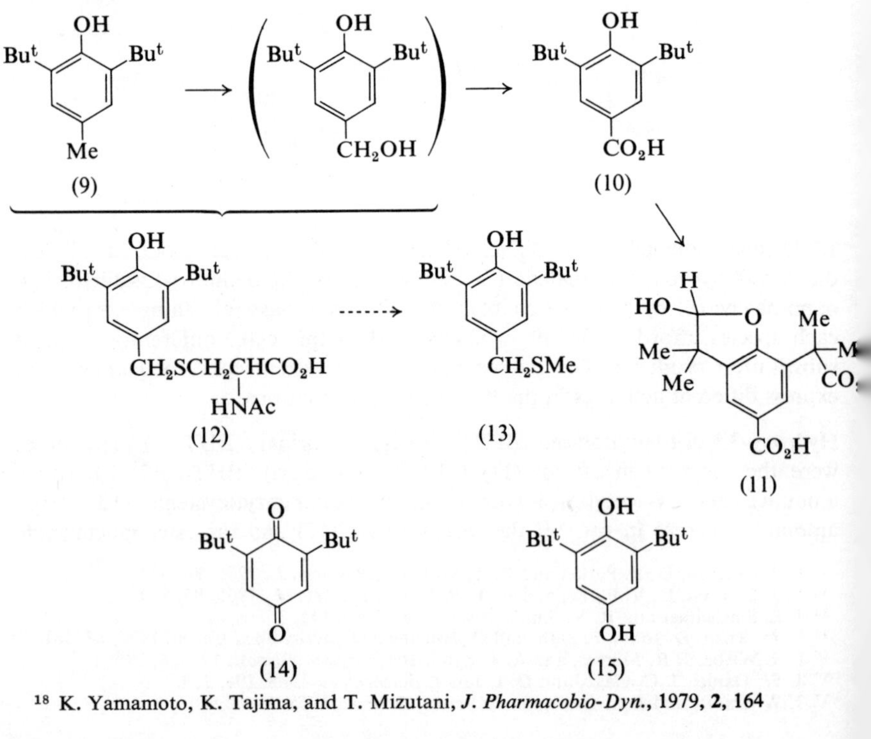

[18] K. Yamamoto, K. Tajima, and T. Mizutani, *J. Pharmacobio-Dyn.*, 1979, **2**, 164

Chlorfenvinphos [2-Chloro-1-(2,4-dichlorophenyl)vinyl Diethyl Phosphate].—It is worthwhile recording here that a species difference between dogs and rats in the rate of *O*-de-ethylation, (17) and (18), of the insecticide, chlorfenvinphos (16), resulting in a difference in rate of excretion *via* the kidneys of different proportions of the (16) metabolites,[19] does not account for the very pronounced difference in acute oral toxicity shown by those animals towards (16),[20]

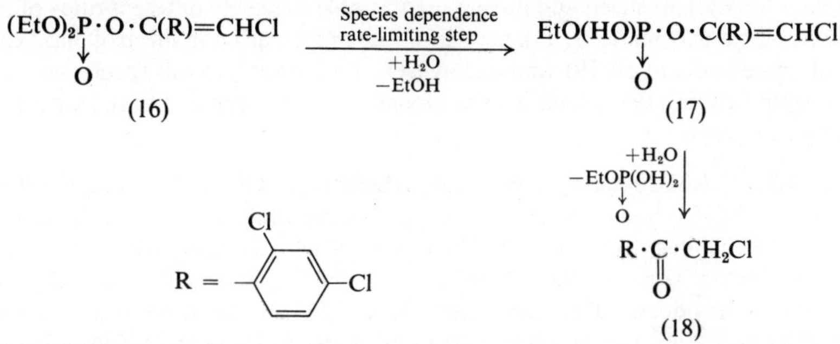

Diazinon [*O*,*O*-Diethyl *O*-(2-Isopropyl-4-methylpyrimidin-6-yl) Thiophosphate].—In sheep, (20) and (21) were urinary diazinon (19) metabolites (see chapter 6),

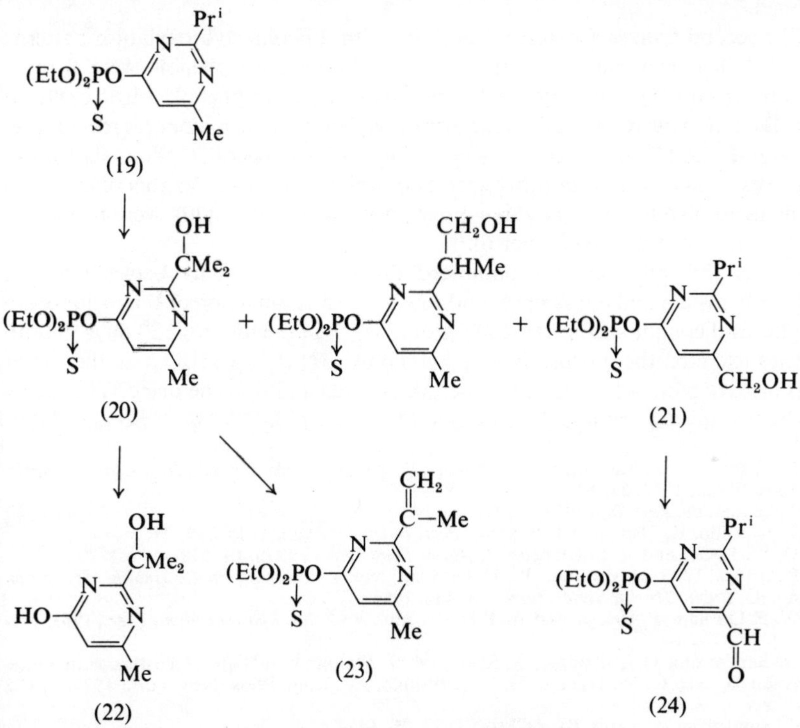

[19] D. H. Hutson, D. A. A. Akintonwa, and D. E. Hathway, *Biochem. J.*, 1967, **102**, 133.
[20] D. H. Hutson and D. E. Hathway, *Biochem. Pharmacol.*, 1967, **16**, 949.

and the alkene (23) was isolated from adipose tissues,[21] whereas in mice, (20)–(24) were all excreted (19) metabolites.[22] It might be recalled that the further metabolism of (20) *in vitro* gave the corresponding oxon, diethyl phosphorothionate, and diethyl phosphate,[23] together with the hydroxylated pyrimidine (22) and its structural isomer derived from (21),[23] both of them known (19) metabolites in rats.[24] Formation of the vastly different proportions of (19) metabolites, (20)–(24), in sheep and mice is attributable to widely different rates of the various biotransformations. The very slow rate of formation in sheep of diazoxon, the ultimate toxicant of (19), and its low LD_{50} (> 1 g kg^{-1}) in this species account for the toxicity of (19), which is exceptionally low in sheep compared with that in other animals.

DDT [1,1,1-Trichloro-2,2-bis(*p*-chlorophenyl)ethane].—Of various species differences in DDT (25) metabolism (see chapter 6) three which belong to this section, are considered here. Firstly, rats, in common with several other species of mammal including man, when dosed chronically (25) accumulate the dehydrochlorination product, DDE (26); male rats, 22% of the dose, and females, 29%.[25] In fact, (26) may be formed from unchanged (25) in the adipose tissues. On the other hand, monkeys do not convert any (25) into (26), but they have the capacity for tissue retention of this substance (26), if it is given to them preformed.[26]

The second species difference has to do with different hydroxylation patterns (see 1,2-dichloronaphthalene, this section). In pigs, no phenols were formed directly from (25), but very small amounts of a single phenol, 3-hydroxylated *p,p′*-DDE (27), were excreted in the urine together with the major (25) metabolite, *viz. p,p′*-DDA (31; R = H and R = $C_6H_9O_6$).[27] In general, (25) metabolism in pigs was similar to that in other species of animal but, whereas this phenol (27) is the major product in rats, three other phenols, *viz.* (28)—(30), were formed as well in that species (see chapter 6).[28]

Lastly, (25) afforded a pronounced difference in toxicity between Syrian golden hamsters and Swiss mice, and this led to a comparison of the metabolism of (25) in these animals, given 250 μg of (25) g^{-1} in the diet for 120 days.[29] Both species excreted the glucuronide of *p,p′*-DDA (31; R = $C_6H_9O_6$) as the major (25) urinary metabolite, but only the mice excreted (26) in the urine. The faeces of the two species contained unchanged (25) and *p,p′*-DDD (32).[30] Because DDE

[21] N. F. Janes, A. F. Machin, M. P. Quick, H. Rogers, D. E. Mundy, and A. J. Cross, *J. Agric. Food Chem.*, 1973, **21**, 121.
[22] B. Sekine, *Jpn. Pest. Inf.*, 1972, **10**, 77.
[23] T. Shishido, K. Usui, and J. Fukami, *Pest. Biochem. Physiol.*, 1972, **2**, 27.
[24] G. W. Lucier and R. E. Mentzer, *J. Agric. Food Chem.*, 1970, **18**, 698.
[25] P. Ortega, W. J. Hayes, jun., W. F. Durham, and A. Mattson, *Public Health Monograph* no. 43, *Public Health Series*, publ. no. 484, 1956.
[26] W. F. Durham, P. Ortega, and W. J. Hayes, jun., *Arch. Int. Pharmacodyn., Ther.*, 1963, **141**, 111.
[27] G. Sundström, O. Hutzinger, S. Safe, and N. Platonow in 'Fate of Pesticides in Large Animals,' eds. G. W. Ivie and H. W. Dorough, Academic Press, New York, 1977, p. 175 *et seq.*
[28] G. Sundström, *J. Agric. Food Chem.*, 1977, **25**, 18.
[29] R. Gingell and L. Wallcave, *Toxicol. Appl. Pharmacol.*, 1974, **28**, 385.
[30] L. Wallcave, S. Bronczyk, and R. Gingell, *J. Agric. Food Chem.*, 1974, **22**, 904.

$(p\text{-}ClC_6H_4)_2CH{-}CCl_3$

(25)

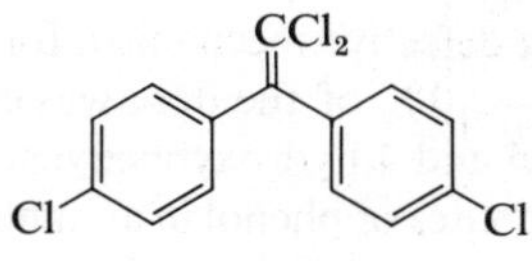

(26)

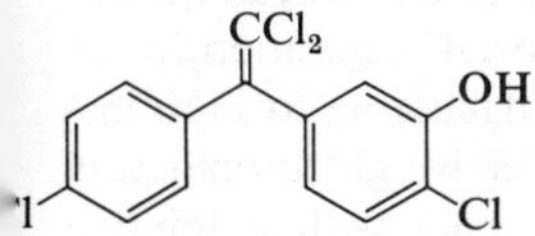

(27)

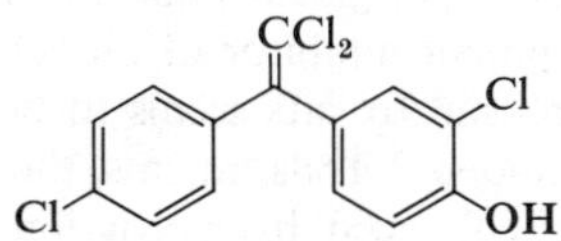

(28)

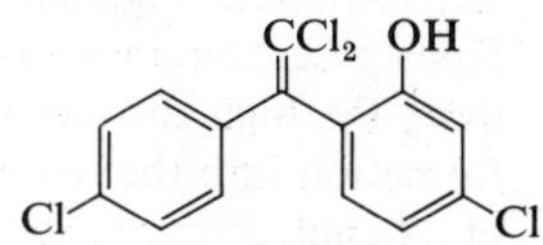

(29)

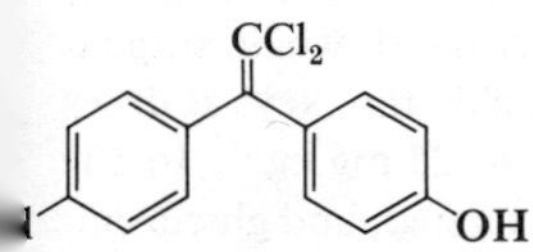

(30)

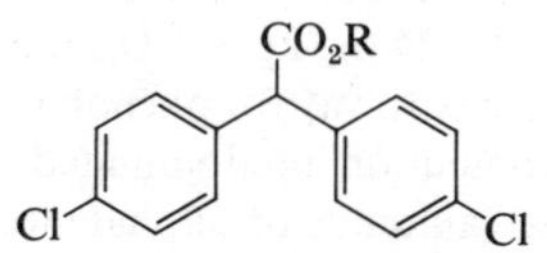

(31)

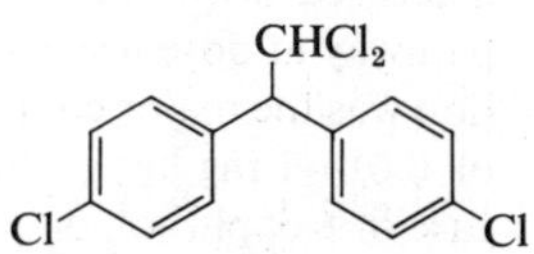

(32)

(26) was absent from the excretory products of hamsters, in which it was produced in only trace amounts in the liver,[29] there is a strong supposition that this metabolite is the ultimate liver carcinogen in mice,[31] and this is substantiated by the fact that (26) is carcinogenic to mice.[32] The parallel between the alkene (26) and vinylidene chloride, which is known now to be also characteristically carcinogenic to mice (chapter 11), although this had not been discovered at that time,[32] is now apparent.

3 Comparative Differences in Conjugation

Phenol.—Rats and sheep excreted 80—90% of an oral dose of phenol in the 24-h urine, and pigs *ca.* 50% in that period: phenyl glucuronide and phenyl sulphate were major urinary metabolites.[33] Pigs have a defective mechanism for sulphate conjugation,[33,34] and in sheep, pigs, and rats the sulphate accounted for 32, 1, and 55% of the dose and the glucuronide for 49, 83, and 42%. The defective mechanism for sulphation by pigs contributed to the slower rate of excretion[33] in that species (*v. supra*).

Phenyl phosphate accounted for 12% of the urinary metabolites in sheep, but it was not formed in pigs and rats.[33]

The authors[33] observe that differences in rates of distribution and excretion are as important to the elimination of conjugates as the rate of synthesis, and this stresses the importance of the point that was made in the Introduction to chapter 8 (*v. supra*) about transport mechanisms in different species.

[31] R. Gingell, *Xenobiotica*, 1976, **6**, 15.
[32] L. Tomatis, V. Turosov, R. T. Charles, and M. Boicchi, *J. Nat. Cancer Inst.*, 1974, **52**, 883.
[33] J. Kas, J. W. Bridges, and J. K. Faulkner, *Xenobiotica*, 1979, **9**, 141.
[34] I. D. Capel, M. R. French, P. Millburn, R. L. Smith, and R. T. Williams, *Xenobiotica*, 1972, **2**, 25.

Cats have a defective mechanism for glucuronide conjugation (see chapter 6), and only 0.1—2.0% of the dose was excreted as glucuronide by that species.[34] In fact, phenyl and 4-hydroxyphenyl sulphates accounted for 80 and 20% of the urinary metabolites of phenol in animals dosed 20 mg kg^{-1}, and at twice that dose level, a similar ratio of the two sulphates was excreted as well as 2% of free phenol and 4% of quinol.[35] When quinol was dosed to cats, 87% of the dose was excreted as its sulphate, together with 3% of glucuronide and 10% of unchanged quinol. Since *p*-benzoquinone is a potent inhibitor of mitochondrial respiration in cat liver, the high toxicity of phenol to cats seems to be attributable to biotransformation into the toxic quinone.[35] Thus, in cats, the defective glucuronidation of phenol is paralleled by enhanced hydroxylation coupled with a limiting capacity for quinol conjugation.

In cynomolgus and rhesus monkeys, sulphation both of phenol and 1-naphthol decreased with increasing dose, but sulphation was the major conjugative pathway at dose levels of 0.01—24 mg kg^{-1}.[36] On the other hand, whilst sulphation was the major conjugative pathway for phenol in capuchin monkeys at doses of 0.01—1 mg kg^{-1}, glucuronidation predominated at 10—25 mg kg^{-1}. In the case of 1-naphthol, only small amounts of sulphate were excreted, and glucuronidation was the major metabolic pathway at all four dose levels.[36]

Aniline.—Different species of animal eliminated the various metabolites of aniline at different rates. In rats and sheep, 80—100% of an acute oral dose was excreted in the 24-h urine, but in pigs, only 56% was recovered in that time, and in all three species, faecal excretion amounted to 2% of the dose. In pigs, sheep, and rats, *N*-acetylation products accounted respectively for 85, 82, and 76% of the urinary metabolites. *p*-Acetylaminophenyl glucuronide and *p*-acetyl aminophenyl sulphate were the major metabolites of aniline. The former accounted for 66% of the dose in pigs and 60% in sheep, and the latter for 56% in rats [37] (*cf.* ref. 38). Minor urinary aniline metabolites in these species included *O*-conjugates of *o*- and *p*-aminophenol (*ca.* 20%), acetanilide (*ca.* 3%), and *p*-acetylaminophenol (*ca.* 10%). The proportion of the dose excreted as sulphate conjugates was significantly less in pigs than in the other species, and this incapacity to effect sulphation is reflected in the slower rate of excretion in pigs, compared with that in rats and sheep (*v. supra*).[37]

An unidentified sulphur-containing metabolite of aniline, which was considered[37] to be a mercapturic acid derivative, was found in pigs, but not in rats and sheep.

Saccharin Impurities.—Toluene-2-sulphonamide (33), an impurity in commercial saccharin (34), afforded 2-sulphamoylbenzyl alcohol, its sulphate and glucuronide conjugates (80% of the dose in rats; 35% in man), and (34) (3% in rats; 35% in man).[39] Other urinary metabolites were 2-sulphamoylbenzoic acid (2% in

35 J. J. Miller, G. M. Powell, A. H. Olavesen, and C. G. Curtis, *Biochem. Soc. Trans.*, 1973, **1**, 1163.
36 R. Mehta, P. C. Hirom, and P. Millburn, *Xenobiotica*, 1978, **8**, 445.
37 J. Kao, J. Faulkner, and J. W. Bridges, *Drug Metab. Dispos.*, 1978, **6**, 549.
38 D. V. Parke, *Biochem. J.*, 1960, **77**, 493.
39 A. G. Renwick, L. M. Ball, D. L. Corina, and R. T. Williams, *Xenobiotica*, 1978, **8**, 525.

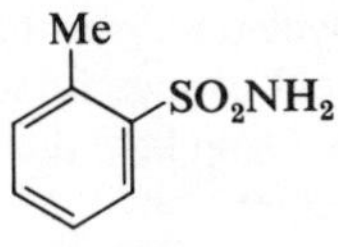

(33)

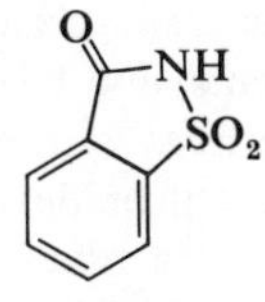

(34)

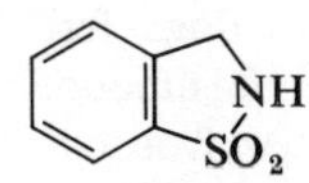

(35)

rats; 4% in man), *N*-acetyltoluene-2-sulphonamide (6% in rats; 2% in man), and unchanged (33) (5% in rats; 3% in man).

Another impurity, BIT (2,3-dihydrobenz[*d*]isothiazole 1,1-dioxide) (35), yielded 2-sulphamoylbenzoic acid, (34), 2-sulphamoylbenzyl alcohol, and polar metabolites as urinary metabolites in rats and man.[40] In addition, rats excreted a labile conjugate of (35) itself (12% of the dose), but none was formed in man. Renwick[41] has argued that, since labile conjugates of aromatic amines play a role in environmental bladder cancer, and at high dose levels commercial saccharin is supposed to cause bladder cancer in rats, this polar metabolite of the saccharin impurity (35) might merit detailed investigation (see chapter 6).

Phenylacetic Acid.—The glutamine conjugate of phenylacetic acid was excreted in the urine of old-World monkeys (rhesus, cynomologus, green, drill, white collared mangabey, and baboon) and of man, but a mixture of glutamine and glycine conjugates was excreted in that of new-World monkeys (capuchin and squirrel).[42] Non-primate mammals, dogs, cats, ferrets, rabbits, guinea-pigs, rats, hamsters, mice, and vampire bats, as well as the slow lorris and bush baby excreted only glycine conjugates.[42]

Similarly, indole-3-acetic acid was converted into the glutamine conjugate by old-World, and into a mixture of glutamine and glycine conjugates by new-World monkeys, and into the glycine conjugate by non-primates.[43]

Homoanisic acid (*p*-methoxyphenylacetic acid) was conjugated with glutamine by man and with glycine by guinea-pigs, as well as affording other metabolites, notably *O*-demethylated compounds and glucuronides.[44]

Naphthylacetic Acids.—The foregoing evidence suggests that amino-acid conjugation of arylacetic acids by non-primate mammals is confined to one particular amino acid, and since 2-naphthylacetic acid differs (*v. infra*) from the usual pattern of metabolism by undergoing simultaneous synthesis with glutamine, glycine, and taurine, it might be useful for testing the conjugating capacity of various species. In fact, 2-naphthylacetic acid was conjugated by ferrets, rabbits, and rats with glutamine, glycine, and taurine as well as with glucuronic acid.[45] Amino-acid conjugation of 2-naphthylacetic acid was more important than its glucuronic-acid conjugation in the species in question, whereas the isomeric 1-naphthylacetic acid was conjugated almost entirely with glucuronic acid; amino-acid conjugation was minimal.[45]

[40] A. G. Renwick and R. T. Williams, *Xenobiotica*, 1978, **8**, 475.
[41] A. G. Renwick, *Xenobiotica*, 1978, **8**, 487.
[42] M. James, R. L. Smith, and R. T. Williams, *Biochem. J.*, 1971, **124**, 15P.
[43] R. T. Williams, *Ann. N. Y. Acad. Sci.*, 1971, **179**, 141.
[44] S. E. Oakley and J. W. T. Seakins, *Biochem. J.*, 1971, **121**, 17*P*.
[45] T. S. Emudianughe, J. Caldwell, P. A. F. Dixon, and R. L. Smith, *Xenobiotica*, 1978, **8**, 525.

Benzoic Acid.—Benzoic acid was conjugated by cats, dogs, ferrets, hedgehogs, monkeys, pigs, rabbits, and rodents, and by man with glycine to yield hippuric acid; by dogs, ferrets, and hedgehogs with glucuronic acid to give in addition substantial amounts of benzoyl glucuronide (*ca.* 20% of a 50 mg kg^{-1} dose); and by Indian fruit bats with glucuronic acid almost exclusively.[46]

4 Comparative Differences in Enzymic Activities

Fate of Methanol.—Methanol (see chapter 6) is quite toxic to monkeys and to man, but it is practically innocuous to guinea-pigs, mice, and rats. Clearly, methanol would be expected to be oxidized to formaldehyde and formic acid, and infusion experiments in monkeys showed that formaldehyde had too short a $t_{0.5}$ value (1.5 min) in blood[47] to be connected with the effects observed. Whereas blood concentrations of formate and bicarbonate were raised in monkeys after an acute dose of methanol, rats did not accumulate formate even after very large doses.[48] This is due to the ready biotransformation of formate into CO_2 by folate-dependent enzymes in rats.[48] In agreement with this supposition, rats maintained on a folate-deficient diet were susceptible to methanol poisoning.[49] Formate retention by target tissues is associated with methanol poisoning in susceptible species.

Fate of Vinylidene Chloride (DCE).—The rate of DCE metabolism in mice was faster than in rats: a greater proportion of an oral dose was excreted as metabolites in the murine urine.[50] Increased metabolism in mice was balanced by increased formation of a single DCE metabolite, *viz.* the *N*-acetyl-*S*-cysteinylacetyl derivative in mice, compared with rats.[50] In terms of enzyme activities, the efficiency of DCE metabolism parallels the greater activity of cytochrome P-450 in the drug-metabolizing organs, kidneys, liver, and lungs, of mice than of rats, and this evidence is entirely consistent with the metabolic pathway for DCE (see chapter 6), involving initial DCE epoxidation. (Real exposure of mice, apparently exposed identically with rats, is greater than that of rats, and this ranking concurs with the order of the LD_{50} values: DCE is considerably more toxic to mice than to rats, and this toxicity is associated with the DCE reactive metabolites, 1,1-dichloroethylene oxide and chloroacetyl chloride.) The relative proportions of the *N*-acetyl-*S*-cysteinylacetyl derivative formed in mice and rats parallel the activities of liver glutathione *S*-epoxide transferase in these species. It follows that the greater production of this excretory product of DCE in mice than rats is due (i) to the higher cytochrome P-450 activity in the drug-metabolizing organs of mice, (ii) to a saturable chloroacetic acid metabolism, and (iii) to correspondingly higher activity of glutathione *S*-epoxide transferase for the more available murine 1,1-dichloroethylene oxide.

[46] J. W. Bridges, M. R. French, R. L. Smith, and R. T. Williams, *Biochem. J.*, 1970, **118**, 47.
[47] K. E. McMartin, G. Martin-Amat, P. E. Noker, and T. R. Tephly, *Biochem. Pharmacol.*, 1979, **28**, 645.
[48] T. R. Tephly, *Fed. Proc., Fed. Am. Soc. Exp. Biol.*, 1977, **36**, 1627.
[49] A. B. Makar and T. R. Tephly, *J. Toxicol. Environ. Health*, 1976, **2**, 1201.
[50] B. K. Jones and D. E. Hathway, *Br. J. Cancer*, 1978, **37**, 411.

Moreover, the fact that DCE is weakly positive in *S. typhimurium* TA1535 strain mediated by the S-9 mix from normal mice, but strongly positive with that from induced animals, in comparison with the mediation by rat tissue, where only liver S-9 mix from induced animals afforded a significant response, agrees with the greater availability of the reactive DCE metabolites in mice than rats, and with DCE carcinogenicity in mice but not in rats.[51]

It might be noted that the foregoing evidence is an acceptable proof of a genetic mechanism for DCE carcinogenicity.

Fate of 1,1,2-Trichloroethylene (TCE).—The evidence on DCE (*v. supra*) and TCE metabolism (see chapter 6) shows that similar mutagenic and carcinogenic properties in mice may be ascribed to rearrangement of the two halogenoalkene-derived epoxides, respectively, into chloroacetyl chloride and dichloroacetyl chloride. However, on the other hand, the innocuous nature of TCE in rats and in man is due to the alternative rearrangement of TCE-oxide into chloral and the further products of its metabolism, as is well-known. Recent identification in mice[52] of the new TCE metabolite, *viz.* dichloroacetic acid, in addition to trichloroacetic acid, strongly supports the foregoing supposition. In fact, the small proportion of dichloroacetic acid relative to the large one of trichloroacetic acid in the urine of TCE-treated mice agrees with a spill-over model, proposed for TCE metabolism in mice.[52]

Enzymically, greater cytochrome P-450 activity in murine liver and kidneys favours faster epoxidation than in rats, and there would be a matching tendency in mice for TCE-oxide rearrangement into chloral to become saturated, as well as for the lower activity of the cytosol enzymes responsible for chloral disposition in mice (compared with rats) to become rate-limiting. It is under these conditions, and in an excess of substrate to enzyme situation, in mouse-liver cells *in vivo* that some of the TCE-oxide, which is continuing to be formed, would be expected to be transformed into dichloroacetyl chloride at the cytosol surface of the vesicles (see ref. 52).

A small proportion of the dichloroacetyl chloride, which is formed in mice, would be expected to react with DNA nucleoside to give cyclized products. By analogy with DCE carcinogenicity, the biochemical lesion proposed for TCE would seem to account for TCE tumourogenicity, reported in mice but not in rats.

Benzene Metabolism.—A comparative study of benzene metabolism *in vitro* has shown[53] that the rate of hydroxylation to afford phenol is greater by mouse-liver microsomal enzymes than by rabbit- and rat-liver microsomal systems.

Coumarin Metabolism.—The hepatic enzyme system, coumarin-7-hydroxylase, is responsible for much of the hydroxylation of coumarin (36) by cats, guinea-pigs, hamsters, and rabbits[54] and by man,[55] but it is absent from the livers of ferrets,

[51] B. K. Jones and D. E. Hathway, *Cancer Lett.*, 1978, **5**, 1.
[52] D. E. Hathway, *Cancer Lett.*, 1980, **8**, 263.
[53] I. M. Gonasun, C. Witmer, J. J. Kocsis, and R. Snyder, *Toxicol. Appl. Pharmacol.*, 1973, **26**, 398.
[54] M. Keighen and R. T. Williams, *J. Med. Chem.*, 1961, **3**, 25.
[55] W. H. Shilling, R. F. Crampton, and R. C. Longland, *Nature*, 1969, **221**, 664.

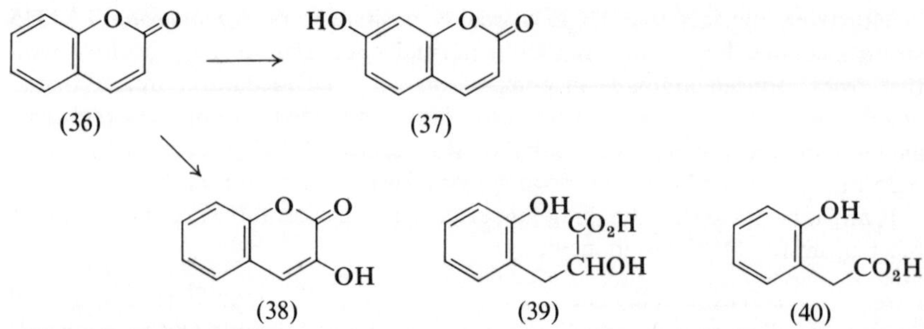

(36) (37) (38) (39) (40)

mice, and rats.[56] In fact, rat liver contains an enzyme inhibitor. In man, 7-hydroxycoumarin (37) is the major metabolite (68—92% of the dose), but in rabbits and rats, 3-hydroxycoumarin (38) and its degradation products, (39) and (40), predominate (39—49%). Of all the (36) metabolites, only *o*-hydroxyphenylacetic acid (40) causes liver enlargement and affects glucose-6-phosphatase activity.

Cytochrome P-450 and P-448.—Different forms of these enzymes are known to exist, which show marked inter- and intra-species variability.[57] This may provide a basis for the marked species differences in activity that have been expressed by this highly developed mammalian enzyme system towards a common substrate (*v. supra*). In consequence, there has been extensive enzymological investigation, but the outcome of work involving the various *in vitro* systems and cell cultures is not clear-cut, and, for example, Nebert *et al.*[58] have warned against the extension of cell-culture data to the *in vivo* situation. The following results illustrate some of the difficulties occasioned. Thus, a cytochrome P-448 partially purified from rabbits, when treated with 3-methylcholanthrene, showed 10% of the activity of an essentially similar rat cytochrome P-448 in catalysing the hydroxylation of benzo[*a*]pyrene in a reconstituted mixed-function oxidase system. 7,8-Benzoflavone and SKF 525-A inhibited the rabbit cytochrome P-448 more completely than the rat enzyme.[59,60] These results suggest an inverse hydroxylation capacity for rabbits/rats to those of Gram *et al.*,[61,62] which showed that the rabbit had enhanced mixed-function oxidase activity compared with rats. The results of Nebert *et al.*[58] *in vitro* differed from those of their studies of benz[*a*]pyrene hydroxylase activity in living animals. Species differences in the induction of the mixed-function oxidase system by polychlorinated biphenyl have been studied.[63] In rabbits, compared with rats, no induction of microsomal aminopyrene and *p*-nitroaniline *N*-demethylation or of aniline and *p*-chlorobiphenyl hydroxylation was found. In both species, *p*-chlorobiphenyl pretreatment raised the activity of cytochrome P-450.[63] Organ variability is also

[56] P. J. Creaven, D. V. Parke, and R. T. Williams, *Biochem. J.*, 1965, **96**, 390.
[57] D. A. Haughen, T. A. van der Hoeven, and M. J. Coon, *J. Biol. Chem.*, 1975, **250**, 3567.
[58] I. S. Owens and D. W. Nebert, *Mol. Pharmacol.*, 1975, **11**, 94.
[59] J. C. Kawalek and A. Y. U. Lu, *Mol. Pharmacol.*, 1975, **11**, 201.
[60] R. M. Philpot and J. R. Bend, *Life Sci.*, 1975, **16**, 985.
[61] C. L. Litterst, E. G. Mimnaugh, R. L. Reagan, and T. E. Gram, *Drug Metab. Dispos.*, 1975, **3**, 259.
[62] T. E. Gram, C. L. Litterst, and E. G. Mimnaugh, *Drug Metab. Dispos.*, 1974, **2**, 254.
[63] T. Wolff and S. Hesse, *Biochem. Pharmacol.*, 1977, **26**, 783.

significant. It follows that interpretation of data concerning enzyme activity, which have been obtained *in vitro*, is often exceptionally difficult. Even with carefully controlled parallel measurements, and using animals of the same identifiable strain, great differences in enzyme activity have been encountered.

This sub-section ends with an investigation,[64] which illustrates some features relating to the present enzymological situation, and which involves the *in vitro* effects of α-naphthoflavone on aromatic hydrocarbon hydroxylase, 2-acetylaminofluorene *N*-hydroxylase and biphenyl 2- and 4-hydroxylases before and after methylcholanthrene pre-treatment of guinea-pigs, hamsters, C75BL/6N and DBA/2N mice, rabbits, and rats. The electrophoretic pattern of cytochrome P-450 sub-units and reduced CO-haemoprotein difference spectra of the microsomal fractions were also examined. α-Naphthoflavone inhibited selectively all four mono-oxygenase activities of methylcholanthrene pre-treated C57 BL/6N mice, rats, and hamsters, 2-acetylaminofluorene *N*-hydroxylase and biphenyl 4-hydroxylase activities of rabbits, and aromatic hydrocarbon hydroxylase, 2-acetylaminofluorene *N*-hydroxylase, and biphenyl 4-hydroxylase activities of guinea-pigs. α-Naphthoflavone raised the activities of aromatic hydrocarbon hydroxylase and biphenyl 2-hydroxylase in liver microsomes from control and methylcholanthrene pre-treated rabbits, biphenyl 2-hydroxylase of guinea-pigs, and 2-acetylaminofluorene *N*-hydroxylase in control and methylcholanthrene pre-treated DBA/2N mice, as well as in control C57 BL/6N mice. These results showed that liver cytochrome P-448 is made up of multiple cytochromes, showing species differences, and each of them catalysing different mono-oxygenase activities.

Alcohol Dehydrogenase (LAD).—The activity of this enzyme system is 5—10-fold greater in horse liver than in guinea-pig, mouse, rat, sheep, and human liver, and much greater than in cat, dog, ferret, shrew, and bovine liver.[65] Thus, LAD may play a physiological role in the detoxification of ethanol produced by the gut flora of the various species.

Rhodanese.—The activity of the liver mitochondrial enzyme rhodanese,[66] which converts cyanide ion into the 200 times less toxic thiocyanate ion (detoxification) [equation (1)],[67] is greater in rabbit, sheep, and bovine (herbivore) liver

$$^{-}C{\equiv}N \xrightarrow{+S} {}^{-}S{-}C{\equiv}N \qquad (1)$$

than in human (omnivore) liver, and it is least in dog (carnivore) liver. This reaction protects herbivores from a normal intake of cyanogenetic glycosides in the natural herbage. However, the amount of cyanide ion that can be detoxified depends ultimately on the availability of sulphur substrate, and the physiological metabolite, thiosulphate, behaves as a source of sulphur to rhodanese, which

[64] S. S. Thorgeirsson, S. A. Atlas, A. R. Boobis, and J. S. Felton, *Biochem. Pharmacol.*, 1979, **28**, 217.
[65] H. A. Krebs and J. R. Parkin, *Biochem. J.*, 1970, **118**, 635.
[66] K. Lang, *Biochem. Z.*, 1933, **259**, 243.
[67] S. Lang, *Arch. Exp. Path. Pharmakol.*, 1894, **34**, 247.

may possess a disulphide linkage, capable of reacting with cyanide and thio-sulphate ions [equation (2)]. Cobalamin derivatives afford effective protection

$$^{-}CN + S_2O_3{}^{2-} \longrightarrow {}^{-}SCN + SO_3{}^{2-} \qquad (2)$$

against large concentrations of cyanide by formation of cyanocobalamin and depletion of the cyanide-ion pool.

Catalase, Hydrogen Peroxide: Hydrogen Peroxide Oxidoreductase.—The bulk of the liver catalase activity in all ten species of mammal which have been investigated,[68] except mice, is associated with the cytosol. Guinea-pigs, pigs, sheep, and human beings provided the richest sources of supernatant liver catalase, and mouse, pig, and rat liver yielded peroxisomal catalase of the highest activity.

UDP-glucuronyltransferase.—By means of labelled *p*-nitrophenol and UDP-glucuronic acid, UDP-glucuronyltransferase activity has been identified in the microsomal fractions of guinea-pig and rat lung.[69] The activity of the lung enzyme was between 30 and 60% of that of the liver one, and the activity of guinea-pig was twice that of the rat enzyme. Separate forms of UDP-glucuronyltransferase were involved in the synthesis of *p*-nitrophenyl glucuronide and *o*-aminophenyl glucuronide by guinea-pigs.[70] Different forms of this enzyme were considered to effect glucuronidation of bilirubin and *p*-nitrophenol by Gunn and Wistar rats and by cats,[71] because Gunn rats either with or without pre-treatment with phenobarbitone had no bilirubin glucuronidating activity, but their capacity to make *p*-nitrophenyl glucuronide was greatly enhanced through phenobarbitone pre-treatment. Phenobarbitone pre-treatment of cats induced bilirubin glucuronidation, but was irrelevant to that of *p*-nitrophenol. Similarly, separate forms of UDP-glucuronyltransferases have been shown to be involved in the synthesis of morphine glucuronide and *p*-nitrophenyl glucuronide by rat-liver microsomes.[72] *p*-Nitrophenyl glucuronide competitively inhibited glucuronidation of *p*-nitrophenol, but not of morphine, and pre-treatment of the animals with different inducing agents affected the two metabolic pathways differently. In work with rabbit-liver microsomes, two bands, each with different enzymic activities towards morphine and *p*-nitrophenol, were separated chromatographically, and the results obtained[73] agreed with those from the experiments with rat-liver microsomes.[72] In further work,[74] where kidney and liver bilirubin glucuronyltransferase activities in Gunn rats were about one-tenth of those in Wistars, both enzyme activities in Gunn, Wistar, and heterozygous Gunn–Wistar rats were unaffected by pre-treatment of the animals with 2,3,7,8-tetrachlorodibenzo[1,4]dioxin (TCDD) or with diethylnitrosamine (DEN). Pre-treatment

[68] R. S. Holmes and C. J. Masters, *Arch. Biochem. Biophys.*, 1972, **148**, 217.
[69] A. Aitio, *Xenobiotica*, 1973, **3**, 13.
[70] D. Zakim, J. Goldenberg, and D. A. Vessey, *Biochim. Biophys. Acta*, 1973, **309**, 67.
[71] P. L. M. Jansen and P. Th. Henderson, *Biochem. Pharmacol.*, 1972, **21**, 2457.
[72] E. Sanchez and T. R. Tephly, *Drug. Metab. Dispos.*, 1974, **2**, 247.
[73] E. del Villar, E. Sanchez, and T. R. Tephly, *Drug Metab. Dispos.*, 1977, **5**, 273.
[74] A. Aitio, M. G. Parkki, and J. Marniemi, *Toxicol. Appl. Pharmacol.*, 1979, **47**, 55.

of Wistars with TCDD induced liver glucuronyltransferase activity towards 4-methylumbelliferone almost eight-fold and the kidney enzyme nearly two-fold but there was no induction of corresponding activities in the two organs of Gunn rats. Similarly, TCDD raised the glucuronyltransferase activity towards *o*-aminophenol, seven- to nine-fold in Wistar and heterozygous animal livers and two-fold in the kidneys of those strains, but not in the corresponding organs of Gunn rats. In Gunn, Wistar, and heterozygous Gunn–Wistar rats, DEN provoked, respectively, an 8-, 2-, or 3-fold increase in hepatic glucuronyltransferase activity.

N-Acetyltransferase.—The highest *N*-acetyltransferase activity was shown to be present in the liver cytosol of hamsters, followed by that successively of guinea-pigs, mice, and rats, where 2-naphthylamine, 4-aminobiphenyl, and 2-aminofluorene were used as substrates.[75] Dog-liver cytosol did not effect *N*-acetylation of the three aromatic amines,[75] and dogs had been found previously to be incapable of acetylating aromatic amines *in vivo*.[76] This finding may be important, as it has been known for several decades that dogs and human subjects inadvertently exposed either to 2-naphthylamine or to 4-aminobiphenyl suffer from bladder cancer, which cannot be induced in rodents. Later experiments,[77] in which toluene-2,4-diamine was incubated with liver cytosol and acetyl-CoA, confirmed those results.[75] The 4-amino group was acetylated. Hamster-liver cytosol had the highest *N*-acetyltransferase activity, followed by that from hamster kidneys, intestinal mucosa, and lungs.[77] Only a trace of *N*-acetyl derivative was synthesized by human-liver cytosol, and none by dog-liver cytosol.[77]

Epoxide Hydratase.—The order of epoxide hydratase activities in rats is liver > testes > kidneys > lungs > intestine ≃ skin, and in mice, testes > liver, lungs > skin > kidneys > intestine.[78] The mouse-testis enzyme activity is more than twice that of the liver.[78,79] In both species, lungs and skin enzyme activities were about the same, but murine liver- and kidney-enzyme activities were 7—10 times lower than those of rats.[78] There is a higher activity of skin epoxide hydratase in human beings than in mice, which have a higher level than rats: there was considerable intra-species variability on the part of the human subjects who were monitored.[80] *trans*-Stilbene oxide has been found to be a potent inducer of epoxide hydratase activity in rat (males and females) liver: the enhanced enzyme activity is 300—400% of that in control, untreated animals.[79] The induction of liver epoxide hydratase activities, expressed in terms of percentage of controls, was respectively 350:180:140 for rats, mice, and hamsters. Induction of epoxide hydratase in rat and hamster livers was selective, but in mouse liver, benzo[*a*]-pyrene mono-oxygenase activity was induced to approximately the same extent

[75] G. M. Lower and G. T. Bryan, *Biochem. Pharmacol.*, 1973, **22**, 1581.
[76] L. A. Poirier, J. A. Miller, and E. C. Miller, *Cancer Res.*, 1963, **23**, 790.
[77] T. Glinsukon, T. Benjamin, P. H. Grantham, E. K. Weisburger, and P. P. Roller, *Xenobiotica*, 1975, **5**, 475.
[78] F. Oesch, H. Glatt, and H. Schmassmann, *Biochem. Pharmacol.*, 1977, **26**, 603.
[79] F. Oesch and H. Schmassmann, *Biochem. Pharmacol.*, 1979, **28**, 171.

as epoxide hydratase. The only other organs where *trans*-stilbene oxide increased epoxide hydratase activity were the kidneys of the rat.[79] On the other hand, s.c. and topical treatment of the skin of living rats with *trans*-stilbene oxide diminished the activity of rat-skin epoxide hydratase to about 70% of that in the skin of control, untreated animals. Thus *trans*-stilbene oxide emerges from these investigations as a selective inducer of rat-liver epoxide hydratase activity.

Response of Liver Glutathione to Paracetamol Injury.—Interestingly, the severity of hepatic injury caused by paracetamol, *p*-HOC_6H_4NHAc, in guinea-pigs, hamsters, mice, rabbits, and rats was matched by depletion of the liver pool of glutathione.[81] A reactive arylating paracetamol metabolite, derived probably by *N*-hydroxylation, is suspected to be the causative agent. Hamsters and mice were the most vulnerable species and their hepatic glutathione was reduced by 80% within 90 min of treatment, whereas in guinea-pigs and rats which were resistant to injury even at doses over the LD_{50}, hepatic glutathione was decreased respectively by only 30 and 10%.[81]

In this connection, the exposure of mice to vinylidene chloride might be expected to deplete liver-glutathione pools, as its metabolism is singularly dependent on glutathione and on GSH *S*-epoxide transferase plus GSH *S*-acyltransferase and, if operative, this might be a contributing factor to vinylidene chloride cancer in mice, but not in rats and other creatures.

It is worthwhile mentioning that the mammalian body pools of glutathione would be expected to be maintained, as far and as soon as possible, by the normal physiological mechanisms.

GSH *S*-Transferases.—Not many species differences in GSH *S*-transferase activities seem to have been found, but the investigation of hepatic GSH *S*-transferase activities towards four substrates, 1,2-dichloro-4-nitrobenzene, diethyl maleate, cyclohex-2-en-1-one, and *trans*-benzylideneacetone, is of some interest.[82] Thus, DDT pre-treatment induced the enzyme activity in Sprague–Dawley rats, but not in baboons and rhesus monkeys. Phenobarbitone pre-treatment induced significantly rat-liver GSH *S*-transferase activity towards two of the four substrates, *viz.* 1,2-dichloro-4-nitrobenzene and cyclohex-2-en-1-one, but there was no induction of enzyme activity by similar pre-treatment of the non-human primates, except in activity towards 1,2-dichloro-4-nitrobenzene. Thus, the inducibility of GSH *S*-transferases is much less significant in non-human primates than in rodents.

Age is a contributing factor in the development of GSH *S*-transferase γ-glutamyltranspeptidase and *S*-substituted *N*-acetyltransferase in the livers and kidneys of neonatal (*versus* adult) rats,[83] and this parameter must be considered in experiments involving drug-metabolizing enzymes.

[80] F. Oesch, H. Schmassmann, and P. Bentley, *Biochem. Pharmacol.*, 1978, **27**, 17.
[81] D. C. Davis, W. Z. Potter, D. J. Jollow, and J. R. Mitchell, *Life Sci.*, 1974, **14**, 2099.
[82] W. H. Down and L. P. Chasseaud, *Biochem. Pharmacol.*, 1979, **28**, 3525.
[83] S. P. James and A. E. Pheasant, *Xenobiotica*, 1978, **8**, 207.

5 Biliary Excretion and Metabolism by Intestinal Flora

Topanol (4-Hydroxy-3,5-di-t-butylanisole).—There was considerable variability in the elimination of a single oral dose of topanol (41). In rats and dogs and in man, major urinary and biliary (41) metabolites are glucuronide and/or sulphate conjugates of the phenols, 2,6-di-t-butylhydroquinone (42), (2-hydroxy-1,1-dimethylethyl)-2-t-butylhydroquinone (43), 5-hydroxy-3,3-dimethyl-7-t-butylcoumaran (44), and 2,5-dihydroxy-3,3-dimethyl-7-t-butylcoumaran (45).[84] The metabolic profile of (41) in all three species was qualitatively similar and, since in rats major urinary metabolites of 2,6-di-t-butyl-*p*-benzoquinone (46), the main autoxidation product of (41), are metabolites (42)—(44) in the form of glucuronide and/or sulphate conjugates and the major biliary metabolite of (46) is the glucuronide of (42), it is unlikely that the ingestion of small amounts of (46) in large doses of (41) would modify the metabolic pattern of excretion of (41).[84] However, whilst in man the main eliminative route was urinary, in rats one-half of the dose was excreted in the bile (and the other part in the urine), and in dogs 80% of the dose was excreted in the bile.[84]

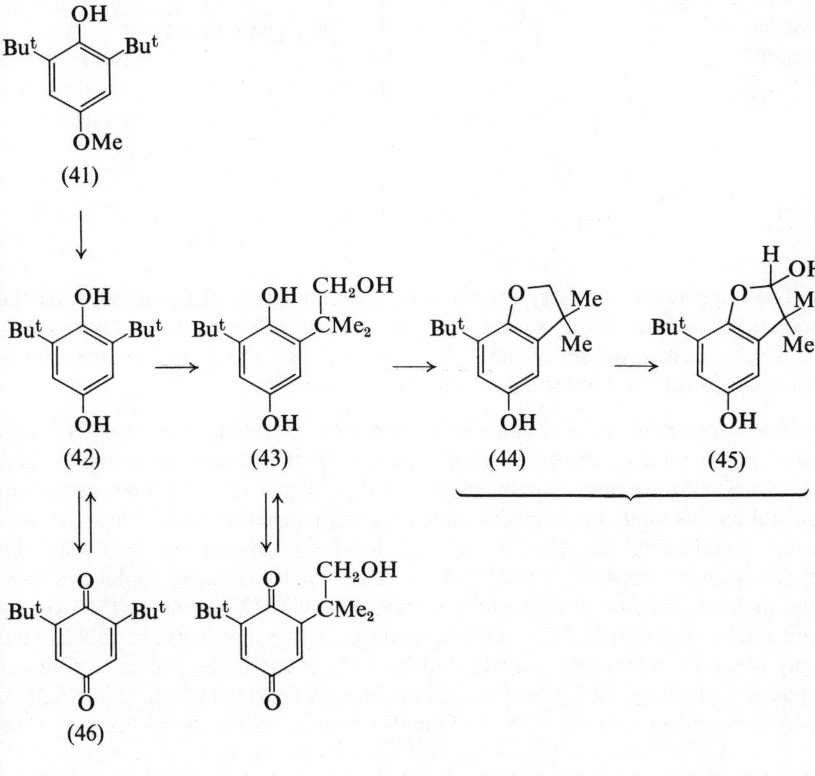

[84] J. W. Daniel, T. Green, and P. J. Phillips, *Food Cosmet. Toxicol.*, 1973, **11**, 781.

(+)-Catechin.—Species variability in the mammalian metabolism of (+)-catechin (47) has been reported.[85a] When (+)-(47) was given to rats, guinea-pigs, rabbits, monkeys, and human beings, major metabolites were δ-(3-hydroxyphenyl)-γ-valerolactone (48) (4.3% of the dose) and *m*-hydroxyphenylhydracrylic acid (49) (7.6%). These metabolites were excreted in free and conjugated forms. Gut flora play a role in (47) metabolism, and this has been shown especially in rats and guinea-pigs.[86,87] The two species together with rabbits, monkeys (*Macaca iris*), and human subjects on treatment with (+)-(47) excreted various valerolactone derivatives, but there were species variations in respect of the excretion of phenolic derivatives of (47).[85a] Monkeys produced *m*-hydroxyphenylpropionic acid, *m*-hydroxyphenylhydracrylic acid, *m*-hydroxyhippuric acid, and *m*-hydroxybenzoic acid, whereas guinea-pigs produced only the corresponding benzoic acid and hippuric acid derivatives. Different proportions of the various (47) metabolites were excreted by the biliary and urinary eliminative routes in the mammalian species investigated.[85a]

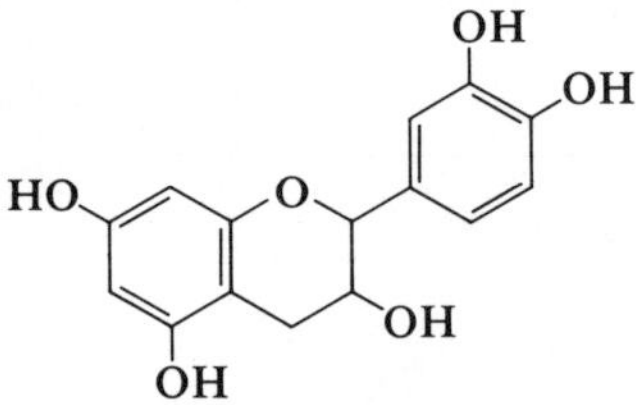

(47)

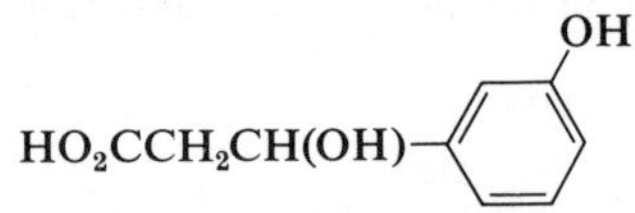

(49)

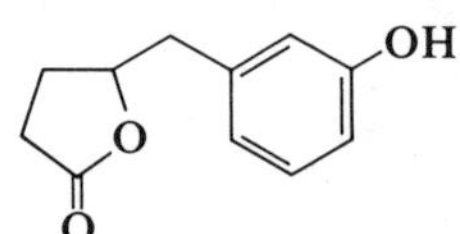

(48)

The importance of biliary excretion to the elimination of flavanoids, and the species differences arising (*v. supra*), applies also to the elimination of flavonoids, of which the metabolism of the 3′,4′, 7-tri-, 4′,7-di-, and 7-*O*-(2-hydroxyethyl)-rutosides in rats and other mammals[85b] is noteworthy.

Endrin.—Whereas male rabbits and male rats excreted respectively 65 and 68.5% of a dose of endrin (50) (see chapter 6), the urinary excretion by rats (2.5%) was lower than that by rabbits (16%). Much of the urinary excretion of rabbits was made up of glucuronide plus sulphate conjugates of the hydroxylated metabolites of (50), of which *anti*-12-hydroxyendrin (52) was the major (urinary) metabolite (7.5% of the dose). However, these conjugates were absent from male-rat urine, where highly lipophilic 12-oxoendrin (51) (0.8%) and unchanged (50) (1.4%) were the main excretory products. In rabbits, the only faecal excretory product was endrin (49% of the dose), but in rats, faecal excretory products (66%) consisted of unchanged endrin (16.6%), (52) (26.2%), 3-hydroxyendrin (53) (23.7%), and small amounts of the *trans*-diol (54). The

[85] (*a*) N. P. Das, *Drug Metab. Dispos.*, 1974, **2**, 209; (*b*) A. Barrow and L. A. Griffiths, *Xenobiotica*, 1974, **4**, 1.
[86] L. A. Griffiths, *Biochem. J.*, 1964, **92**, 173.
[87] N. P. Das and L. A. Griffiths, *Biochem. J.*, 1968, **110**, 449.

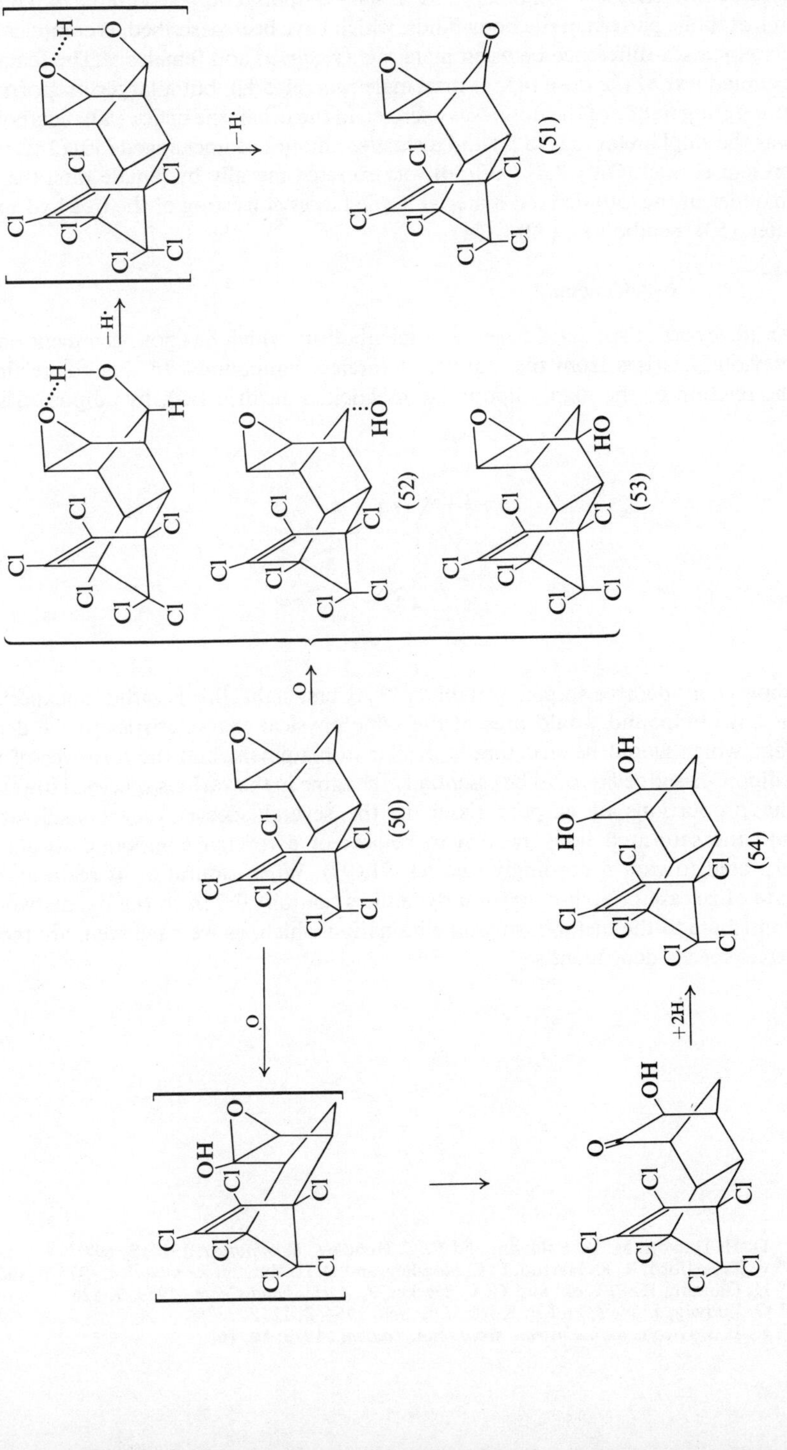

(50)
(51)
(52)
(53)
(54)
−H·
+2H

species differences[88,89] on biliary and urinary outputs, coupled with the difference in metabolic pattern in the body fluids, which have been described, is complicated also by a sex difference between male rats (*v. supra*) and females.[88] The females excreted less of the dose (45%) than male rats (68.5%), but a larger proportion, amounting to 8% of the dose, was excreted in the urine: the major (50) metabolite was the sulphate of (52) (5%) and a smaller amount of unchanged (50) (2%) was present as well. Only 2.2% of (50) was excreted faecally by female rats, the remainder of the (50)-derived material in the faeces consisting of the free hydroxylated (50) metabolites, (52)—(54).

6 Addendum

Another sort of species difference in metabolism, which has not been mentioned previously, arises from the storage of foreign compounds. In this connection, the retetion of the highly lipophilic insecticide, dieldrin (55), by adipose tissue

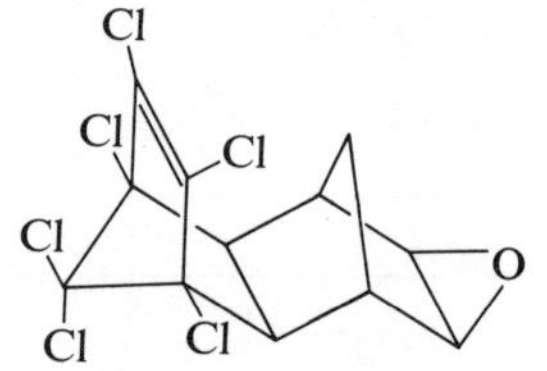

(55)

shows considerable species variability.[90] At first sight, this is rather unexpected, as any compound would present the same physical characteristics to the depot fats, which would be structurally similar in mammals, and the turnover of the adipose-tissue cells would be essentially the same in the various species. However, the proportions of adipose tissue in the several species vary considerably, and the saturated body burden in respect of a foreign compound would be expected to vary accordingly (see ref. 91, 92). When saturation is realized, the rate of release or spill-over (in a dynamic situation[91,92]) from the depots would contribute to the metabolism and elimination which, as we have seen, are themselves species dependent.

[88] D. H. Hutson, M. K. Baldwin, and E. C. Hoadley, *Xenobiotica*, 1975, **5**, 697.
[89] C. T. Bedford, R. K. Harrod, E. C. Hoadley, and D. H. Hutson, *Xenobiotica*, 1975, **5**, 485.
[90] N. Gannon, R. P. Link, and G. C. Decker, *J. Agric. Food Chem.*, 1959, **7**, 826.
[91] G. Ludwig, J. Weis, and F. Korte, *Life Sci.*, 1964, **3**, 123.
[92] K. L. Davison, *Bull. Environ. Contamin. Toxicol.*, 1973, **10**, 16.

Part V

Biochemical Lesions

Chapter 9 Mode of Action Studies

1 Introduction

The mode of action of several acute mammalian toxicities has been incompletely defined in molecular terms. Thus, for perceptible effects there must be physiological dysfunction following a disturbance in intermediary metabolism which is brought about through the binding of a particular industrial chemical or pesticide, or of a reactive metabolite, with a receptor site or tissue protein. Where interaction is irreversible, in the case for example of the organophosphorus insecticides, such binding is covalent, and where it is of a more temporary nature and reversible, as for example in that of acute carbon monoxide poisoning, weaker physicochemical forces apply. Investigation of the resulting symptomatology need not necessarily account for the 'biochemical lesion' in question, and the study of receptor and tissue binding may not explain *per se* the complex sequence of biological events which takes place. Nevertheless, a considerable body of evidence has accumulated on the mode of action of notable pesticides and industrial chemicals, and this might be amplified somewhat from the contemporary background of biochemical, pharmacological, and physiological experience.

However, the foregoing arguments are inapplicable to those intoxications where the effects seem to be unrelated to metabolic inhibition. Irritational toxicity exemplifies this, and the case might be cited where the metabolism of conjugated dienes and polyols affords oxalic acid, calcium oxalate deposits in the renal tubules, and an accompanying haematuria. In addition, the anaesthesia provoked by inhalation of volatile chloroalkanes and chloroalkenes has been mentioned already (chapter 5) in this context.

Accordingly, the present chapter attempts to sift the evidence and information on biochemical mechanisms of toxicity involved with metabolic inhibition and with the modulation of biological events, independent of receptor interaction.

2 Mechanisms Involving Metabolic Inhibition

Carbon Monoxide.—CO combines reversibly with haemoglobin, the O_2-transport carrier. It follows that: (i) a number of O_2-binding sites become occupied (by CO) thereby diminishing the transport capacity of blood for O_2; and (ii) that the binding of 1 or more moles of CO to 1 mole of haemoglobin, with its four prosthetic haem groups, increases the affinity of the three remaining haem groups for O_2.

Allosteric modification of the globin protein brings about effect (ii), and accounts for the sigmoid O_2-saturation curve for haemoglobin, whereby the binding of 1 mole of O_2 to one haem group increases the affinity of successive molecules of O_2 for the three remaining haem groups. This is a complex phenomenon,[1] as *X*-ray analysis shows that the haem groups in the haemoglobin macromolecule are spaced too far apart for interaction to occur. However, it seems to be explicable in terms of a simple model whereby haemoglobin dissociates reversibly into half-molecules, each with an α- and a β-chain.[2]
Thus, where 1 mole of O_2 [marked by an asterisk (*), *v. infra*] combines with an α-haem belonging to an αβ half-molecule, it causes the α-polypeptide, designated ○, to undergo a conformational change into the form designated □. Whence:

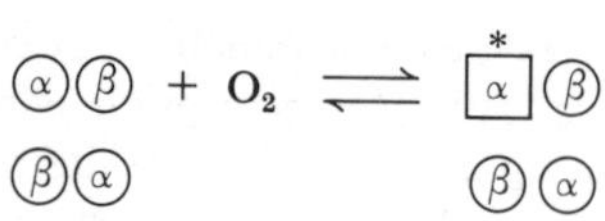

This conformational change is transmitted in the half-molecule to the tightly bound β-chain, which also undergoes a conformational change.

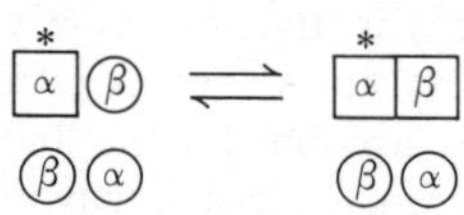

Since the affinity of $\boxed{\beta}$ > Ⓑ for O_2, the β haem also becomes oxygenated.

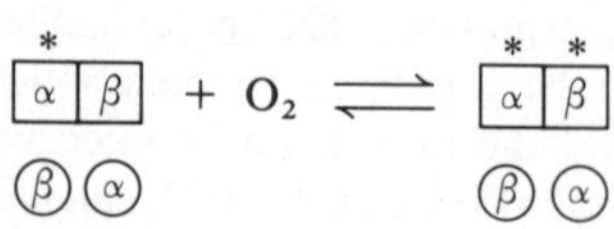

[1] J. Wyman, *Adv. Protein Chem.*, 1964, **19**, 223.
[2] A. L. Lehninger, in 'Biochemistry,' Worth Publishers, New York, 1970, p. 183 *et. seq.*

Thus, the binding of 1 mole of O_2 enhances that of another mole of O_2. Complete oxygenation of the first αβ functional subunit and its conformational change produces new internal stresses among the subunits of the haemoglobin molecule; these stresses cause the other αβ functional subunit to change from (α)(β) configuration with a low affinity for O_2 into the [α|β] form with a relatively high affinity for O_2. Hence:

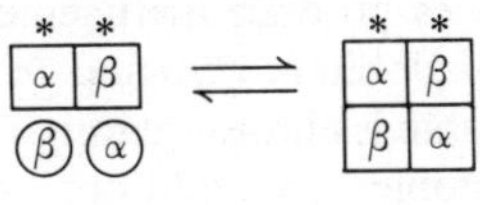

Reaction with further oxygen then gives the fully oxygenated oxyhaemoglobin.

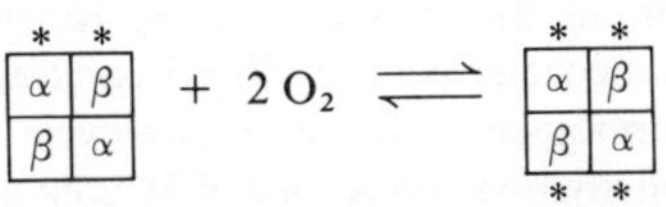

Actually, allosteric modification, which can be followed by high resolution X-ray crystallography, seems to be even more complicated than this, and it involves the removal of an α-amino acid unit from the α-helix and the modification of the transitional molecular species by diphosphoglycerate co-factor.[3]

Thus, interference with the oxyhaemoglobin dissociation by CO, *i.e.* the shifting of Roughton and Darling's[4] oxyhaemoglobin dissociation curve to the left, is accompanied by a much greater degree of tissue anoxia than is consistent with loss in O_2-transport capacity. Where dogs were poisoned with CO until 75% of the haemoglobin was converted into carboxyhaemoglobin, the animals collapsed, and the ones that survived suffered severe injury from tissue anoxia. On the other hand, in animals where 75% of the blood was replaced with CO-saturated blood, there was no serious consequence.[5]

As has already been said (chapter 5), the affinity of human haemoglobin for CO is about 210 times greater than for O_2, which means that a 50% carboxyhaemoglobin level in blood would be reached when the concentration of CO in the inspired air is 1/210 that of O_2, or 0.095%. The kinetic implications have been discussed (chapter 5). CO behaves as a high solubility agent in blood, and an active person with a high respiratory exchange will absorb CO more rapidly, and be poisoned faster, than one at rest.

CO shows all the properties of an antagonist/inhibitor of the interaction of O_2 with the haem-group receptors of haemoglobin. In the sense that the lung behaves as a separate compartment from the rest of the body, and intermediary metabolism is involved minimally, CO might be regarded as a physiological inhibitor; in this case, its description (*v. supra*) ought to be couched in physiological terms. As an O_2-antimetabolite, CO mitigates against aerobiasis.

3 J. Monod, J. Wyman, and J. P. Changeux, *J. Mol. Biol.*, 1965, **12**, 88.
4 F. J. Roughton and R. C. Darling, *Am. J. Physiol.*, 1944, **141**, 17.
5 D. L. Drabkin, F. H. Lewey, S. Bellet, and W. H. Ehrich, *Am. J. Med. Sci.*, 1943, **205**, 755.

Agents which Cause Methaemoglobinaemia.—The oxidized form of haemoglobin is a chocolate coloured pigment, known as methaemoglobin. Erythrocytes contain small amounts of methaemoglobin, presumably formed by spontaneous oxidation of haemoglobin, and representing a steady-state level. Two erythrocyte enzymes are concerned with the reduction of methaemoglobin to haemoglobin, *viz.* diaphorase I (methaemoglobin diaphorase) which uses NADH as co-enzyme, and diaphorase II (methaemoglobin reductase) which employs NADPH. A number of chemical substances produce methaemoglobin.[6] For example NO_2^- will react directly with haemoglobin *in vitro* and *in vivo*. Where pO_2 is high, the conversion into methaemoglobin is almost quantitative. ClO_3^- and quinones also react directly with haemoglobin. In addition, compounds such as aniline, acetanilide, nitrobenzene, and *p*-nitrophenol cause the formation of methaemoglobin indirectly. Thus, in the case of aniline, the phenylhydroxylamine metabolite reacts with haemoglobin in the presence of O_2 to yield nitrosobenzene and methaemoglobin, nitrosobenzene being reduced back again to phenylhydroxylamine by erythrocyte diaphorase II. In this way, a cyclic oxidation is established, and 1 mol equiv. of phenylhydroxylamine will convert many equivalents of haemoglobin into methaemoglobin.[7–11] By contrast, stoicheiometric proportions are involved in the case of NO_2^-. However, NO_2^- is the most common cause of methaemoglobinaemia, and a case of mass poisoning by this source might be mentioned.[12]

Methaemoglobin does not transport O_2, and the allosteric phenomenon with regard to haemoglobin (*v. supra*) applies in this context as well. Where one or more of the Fe atoms in the haemoglobin macromolecule is oxidized to the Fe^{3+} state, then the affinity of the other haem sites for O_2 is increased. The oxyhaemoglobin dissociation curve is shifted to the left, as in the case of carboxyhaemoglobin (*v. supra*), with the result that the delivery of O_2 to the tissues is impaired.[13] Animal experiments establish that methaemoglobin is less toxic than an equivalent amount of carboxyhaemoglobin;[14] but, even so, patients with methaemoglobinaemia are more anoxic than they would be had they suffered an equivalent loss of haemoglobin by haemorrhage, and early symptoms of anoxia are seen below 50% of methaemoglobin.[15]

The use of Methylene Blue (1) as an antidote for methaemoglobinaemia (chapter 5) illustrates therefore the repair of the receptor for O_2-transport. Irrespective of how it was produced, methaemoglobin (MHb) (Scheme 1) is reduced to haemoglobin (Hb) through the agency of (1). Methylene Blue (a) acts as an electron acceptor between NADPH and MHb, and undergoes a cyclic reduction itself to give *leuco*-Methylene Blue (2). Diaphorase II catalyses

[6] O. Bodansky, *Pharmacol. Rev.*, 1951, **3**, 144.
[7] M. Kiese, D. Reinwein, and H. D. Waller, *Arch. exp. Pathol. Pharmakol.*, 1950, **210**, 393.
[8] M. Kiese and D. Reinwein, *Arch. exp. Pathol. Pharmakol.*, 1950, **211**, 392.
[9] H. Dannenberg and M. Kiese, *Arch. exp. Pathol. Pharmakol.*, 1950, **211**, 410.
[10] M. Kiese, *Arch. exp. Pathol. Pharmakol.*, 1959, **235**, 360.
[11] J. Haan, M. Kiese, and A. Werner, *Arch. exp. Pathol. Pharmakol.*, 1959, **235**, 365.
[12] B. Roeché, in 'Eleven Blue Men,' Berkeley Publishing, New York, 1953, pp. 78—89.
[13] R. C. Darling and F. J. W. Roughton, *Am. J. Physiol.*, 1942, **137**, 56.
[14] O. Lester and L. A. Greenberg, *J. Pharmacol.*, 1944, **81**, 182.
[15] O. Bodansky and H. Gutmann, *J. Pharmacol.*, 1947, **90**, 46.

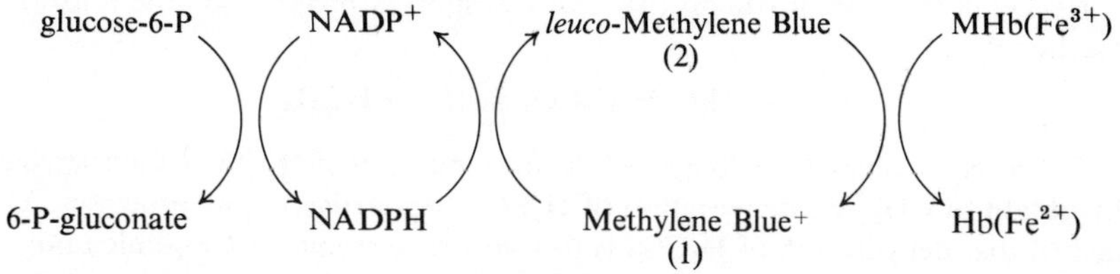

Scheme 1

the reaction between NADPH and MHb, which in turn is accelerated by the presence of (1).[16] The electron-transport sequence[17] is shown in Scheme 1, and, in the absence of MHb, O_2 would serve as terminal electron acceptor, oxidizing (2) to (1) and thus stimulating glucose oxidation.

Enough has been said to show that methaemoglobin, produced by industrial chemicals *in vivo*, behaves both as an antagonist/inhibitor *versus* the interaction of O_2 with the haem-group receptors of haemoglobin and as an O_2-antimetabolite. This situation is redressed by appropriate therapy with Methylene Blue, which acts as an antidote to methaemoglobinaemia in dogs[15] and in man.[18] O_2-Administration is indicated as well to augment the concentration of O_2 that is carried to the tissues by solution in the plasma.

Carbon Dioxide Transport.—On account of the industrial production of CO_2 and the inhibition of carbonic anhydrase (*v. infra*) by many compounds[19] including sulphonamides, some consideration might be given to CO_2-transport.

Thus, much of the carbonic acid (H_2CO_3) formed by reaction with water, is buffered within the erythrocytes by reaction with haemoglobin.

(i) Oxyhaemoglobin is a stronger acid than reduced haemoglobin, and when a solution containing HbO_2^- is reduced, it affords base and becomes more alkaline. Therefore, in the tissues H_2CO_3 reacts with the base produced by reduction of haemoglobin, without change in pH.

$$H_2CO_3 + HbO_2^- \rightleftharpoons HCO_3^- + HHbO_2$$

(ii) On the other hand, H_2CO_3 reacts with haemoglobin to give HCO_3^- and a more acid haemoglobin, and such buffering involves a small change in pH.

$$H_2CO_3 + Hb^- \rightleftharpoons HCO_3^- + HHb$$

(iii) Again, CO_2 reacts directly with haemoglobin amino groups to give carbaminohaemoglobin, without formation of H_2CO_3.

$$RNH_2 + CO_2 \rightleftharpoons RNH.CO_2 \rightleftharpoons RNH.CO_2^- + H^+$$

[16] F. M. Huennekens, R. W. Caffrey, R. E. Basford, and B. W. Gabrio, *J. Biol. Chem.*, 1957, **227**, 261.
[17] E. Beutler and M. C. Baluda, *Blood*, 1963, **22**, 323.
[18] A. F. Mangelsdorff, *Arch. Ind. Health*, 1956, **14**, 148.
[19] H. Keller, *Z. Vitam. Hormon. Fermentforsch.*, 1959, **9**, 297.

Hence, in the case of (i) and (ii), CO_2-transport is preceded by the following reactions:

$$CO_2 + H_2O \rightleftharpoons H_2CO_3 \rightleftharpoons H^+ + HCO_3^-$$

The reverse occurs in the lungs. Whilst the ionization of H_2CO_3 is spontaneous, hydration of CO_2 and dehydration of H_2CO_3 are relatively slow processes. The fact (i) that dehydration of H_2CO_3 is too slow to account for CO_2-unloading in the lungs and (ii) that the exchange of CO_2 with a gas phase is much more rapid in whole blood than in plasma, led to the recognition and eventual isolation of carbonic anhydrase[20] (*v. supra*). It should be noted that CO_2 and not HCO_3^- is the immediate product of enzyme interaction.[21]

Apparent lack of effect of the inhibition of carbonic anhydrase in human subjects treated with, for example, sulphonamides might be attributed to the fact that (i) human erythrocytes contain *ca.* 7 500 times as much enzyme as would be necessary to deal with normal CO_2-transport in man,[22] and (ii) compensatory changes in respiration permit normal CO_2-transport, even where a marked carbonic anhydrase inhibition has occurred.

In experiments where dogs were injected i.v. with acetazolamide to effect $> 97\%$ inhibition of carbonic anhydrase,[23] the total ventilation rose from 2.7 l min^{-1} to 5.0 l min^{-1} and the CO_2-output remained unchanged; the corresponding figures for O_2 were 84 and 82 ml min^{-1}. However, increased total ventilation resulted in a fall in alveolar pCO_2 from 37 to 19 mmHg and an increase in pO_2 from 103 to 123 mmHg. This means that the ensuing respiratory changes maintained a normal CO_2-output with a tissue CO_2-tension just sufficient to maintain the stimulus to the respiratory centre. In man, the largest doses of sulphanilamide administered by Roughton *et al.*[22] were well-tolerated at rest, but gave rise to choking when severe exercise was attempted, owing to the retention of CO_2 by the tissues. In practice, the principal action of carbonic anhydrase inhibitors derives more from the kidneys than from the erythrocytes.

Thus, many substances, such as the sulphonamides, behave as chemical inhibitors of CO_2-transport, and although their effect may not be evident *prima facie*, they cause stress through tissue retention of CO_2 in the subjects concerned.

Cyanide and Hydrosulphide Poisonings.—As has been stated previously (chapter 5), the dangerous toxicities of CN^- and HS^- result through terminal inhibition of the mitochondrial respiratory chain:[24] the nature of the cytochrome $a + a_3$ system[25,26] has been discussed (chapter 5).[27]

20 F. R. W. Roughton, *Physiol. Rev.*, 1935, **15**, 241.
21 H. A. Krebs and F. J. W. Roughton, *Biochem. J.*, 1948, **43**, 550.
22 F. J. W. Roughton, A. B. Dill, R. C. Darling, A. Graybiel, C. A. Knehr, and J. H. Talbott, *Am. J. Physiol.*, 1941, **135**, 77.
23 E. T. Carter and R. T. Clark, *J. Appl. Physiol.*, 1958, **13**, 42.
24 W. S. Caughley, W. J. Wallace, J. A. Volpe, and S. Yoshikawa, 'The Enzymes,' ed. P. D. Boyer, Academic Press, New York, 3rd edn., 1976, vol. 13, p. 300.
25 B. G. Malmström, *Q. Rev. Biophys.*, 1974, **6**, 389.
26 R. Lemberg and J. Barrett, 'Cytochromes,' Academic Press, New York, 1973, p. 4 *et seq.*
27 Q. H. Gibson, C. Greenwood, D. C. Wharton, and G. Palmer, 'Oxidases and Related Redox Systems,' ed. T. E. King, H. S. Mason, and M. Morrison, John Wiley and Sons, New York, 1965, vol. 2, pp. 595, 596.

Antidotal action by complexation and removal of the toxic agent is illustrated by the treatment of CN^- poisoning by i.v. injection of sodium nitrite.[28]

$$Hb(Fe^{2+}).O_2 \longrightarrow MHb(Fe^{3+}) + e^- + O_2$$

$$Hb(Fe^{2+}).O_2 \longrightarrow MHb(Fe^{3+}) + e^- + [O] + [O]$$

$$NO_2^- + [O] \longrightarrow NO_3^-$$

$$H^+ + [O] + 2\,e^- \longrightarrow OH^-$$
$$OH^- = OH^-$$

Whence, the overall reaction:

$$NO_2^- + 2\,Hb(Fe^{2+}).O_2 + H_2O \text{ —— } NO_3^- + 2\,MHb(Fe^{3+}).OH^- + O_2$$

In practice, two different methods of combating CN^- are used, *viz.* treatment with NO_2^- to yield methaemoglobin which will complex with CN^- in the manner described, and treatment with $S_2O_3^{2-}$ to accelerate the metabolic conversion of CN^- into harmless SCN^- (chapter 8). Additionally, increased plasma O_2-tension might help to replenish tissue-O_2 deprived by CN^- blockade.

The use of NO_2^- and $S_2O_3^{2-}$ as antidotes for CN^- poisoning illustrates the repair of the receptor concerned with terminal respiration.

Methanol Poisoning.—The serious effects of methanol poisoning, *viz.* acidosis and retinal-cell injury leading to blindness, which occur only in primates, are due respectively to the methanol metabolites, formate and formaldehyde (chapter 6). Since ethanol has a greater affinity for both LAD and catalase than for methanol, it can be used to inhibit methanol oxidation by acting as a competitive substrate for the two enzyme systems[29–32] until all the methanol has been eliminated from the body. In this case, the antidote, ethanol, blockades the enzyme receptors responsible for methanol metabolism.

O_2-Toxicity.—To recapitulate (chapter 5), the 'super oxide theory' of O_2-toxicity assumes: (i) that O_2^- is formed in biological systems; (ii) that O_2^- is extremely toxic to cellular constituents; and (iii) that superoxide dismutases destroy O_2^-, and are vital to aerobiasis.

$$2\,O_2^- + 2\,H^+ \longrightarrow H_2O_2 + O_2$$

However, chapter 5 indicates[33] that, whilst there is considerable experimental

[28] K. Betke, I. Greinacher, and O. Tietze, *Arch. exp. Pathol. Pharmakol.*, 1956, **229**, 220.
[29] J. R. Cooper and M. M. Kini, *Biochem. Pharmacol.*, 1962, **11**, 405.
[30] M. M. Kini and J. R. Cooper, *Biochem. Pharmacol.*, 1961, **10**, 207.
[31] M. M. Kini and J. R. Cooper, *Biochem. J.*, 1962, **82**, 164.
[32] T. R. Tephly, R. E. Parks, and G. T. Mannering, *J. Pharmacol.*, 1964, **143**, 292.
[33] J. A. Fee, in 'Oxygen and Life: Second BOC Priestly Conference,' Special Publication, no. 39, The Royal Society of Chemistry, London, 1981, pp. 77—97.

evidence for premise (i), propositions (ii) and (iii) are less credible. Thus, (ii) no reaction of O_2^- has proved to be toxic to a cell. Hence, it is not responsible for the degradative reactions attributed to it, where O_2^- is undoubtedly present, but where superoxide dismutase protects the substrates concerned. With regard to (iii), the amounts of dismutase in various anaerobes cannot be correlated easily with their capacity to withstand O_2, and the presence of this enzyme conflicts with the cellular economy for organisms which do not encounter O_2. In addition, the fact that some aerobic organisms consume O_2 and form O_2^-, but lack dismutase, contradicts the idea of the requirement of dismutases for aerobiasis. Thus, O_2-toxicity seems to depend on the rival 'sensitive enzyme theory' (chapter 5).

These ideas have repercussions in respect of paraquat toxicity and CCl_4-induced lipid peroxidation.

Paraquat Toxicity.—Paraquat (3) is accumulated selectively in the lungs[34] by an active process[35] which is inhibited by various endogenous and exogenous substances. This pulmonary-uptake is dissimilar from that for 5-hydroxytryptamine,[36] suggesting that accumulation involves different epithelial cell types. In mammalian lung, it is envisaged that paraquat undergoes a so-called cyclic redox process with formation of O_2^- since it can be reduced in the absence of O_2 to form a stable free radical,[38] which is rapidly reoxidized by O_2 to the cation with simultaneous production of O_2^-.[39] Rose *et al.*[37] considered that radical formation may lead directly or indirectly to lipid peroxidation and cell death but, as in the case of CCl_4-induced lipid peroxidation (*v. infra*), this has not been established and on account of the reappraisal of O_2-toxicity (*v. supra*) might prove to be unlikely. In this connection, the mortality of rats dosed with (3) was unaffected by their pre-treatment with superoxide dismutase.[37,40] However, (3) stimulates the pentose-phosphate pathway[41] and both reduces the level of NADPH and inhibits lung fatty acid synthesis. Since the lung cells undergo minimal structural damage, it appeared[37] that the primary biochemical lesion might be 'the extreme oxidation of NADPH which inhibits vital physiological processes and renders the cells vulnerable to (possible) attack by lipid hydroperoxides'. Extreme oxidation of NADPH leads also to diminished respiration. In this connection, the energy-dependent mitochondrial process for paraquat-uptake into the lungs is also pertinent.

Accordingly, the cyclic reactions (*v. supra*) might be illustrated (Scheme 2). It is relevant that the reduction of $NADP^+$ to NADPH is a two-electron process, whereas paraquat (PQ^{2+}) (Scheme 2) reduction is a single-electron process; for

34 M. S. Rose, A. E. Lock, L. L. Smith, and I. Wyatt, *Biochem. Pharmacol.*, 1976, **25**, 419.
35 M. S. Rose, L. L. Smith, and I. Wyatt, *Nature*, 1974, **252**, 314.
36 L. L. Smith, E. A. Lock, and M. S. Rose, *Biochem. Pharmacol.*, 1976, **25**, 2485.
37 L. L. Smith, M. S. Rose, and I. Wyatt, in 'Oxygen Free Radicals and Tissue Damage,' CIBA Foundation Series 65 (new series), Elsevier/Excerpta Medica/North-Holland, Amsterdam, 1979.
38 L. Michaelis and E. S. Hill, *J. Am. Chem. Soc.*, 1933, **55**, 1481.
39 J. A. Farrington, M. Ebert, E. J. Land, and K. Fletcher, *Biochim. Biophys. Acta*, 1973, **314**, 372.
40 A. P. Autor, *Life Sci.*, 1974, **14**, 1309.
41 M. S. Rose, L. L. Smith, and I. Wyatt, *Biochem. Pharmacol.*, 1976, **25**, 1763.

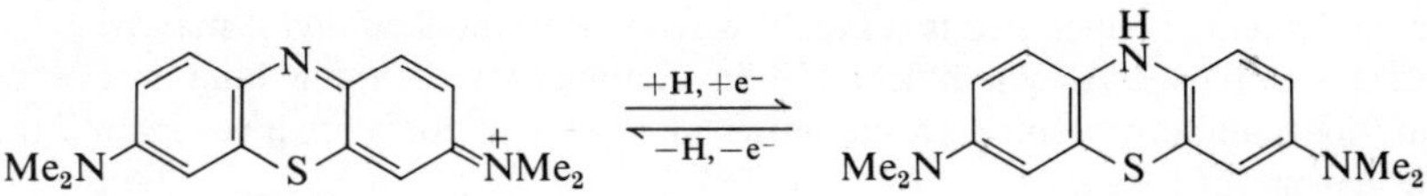

(1) (2)

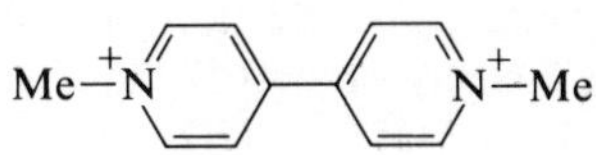

(3)

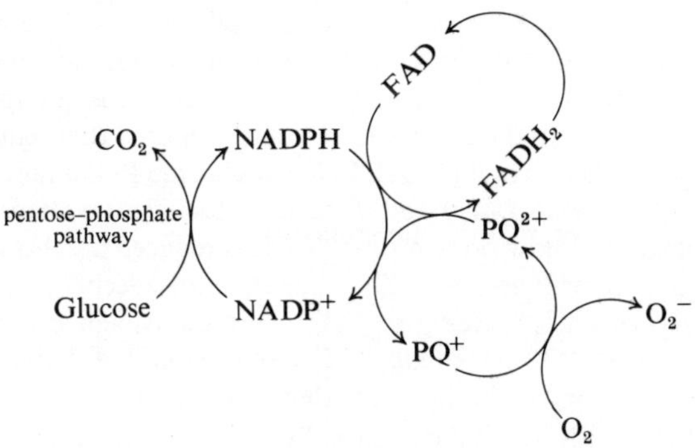

Scheme 2

this reason, a flavoprotein or iron–sulphur enzyme would be implicated. The FAD–$FADH_2$ process seems to be favoured,[42] the two-electron donor NADPH providing equivalents for the reduction of FAD and therefore a single-electron addition to paraquat.

Evidence about the link between O_2^- production and the pathological lesion of paraquat is missing, and from what has been said already, it does not look as though O_2^- is implicated directly. There is a parallel in this case with $^{\cdot}CCl_3$ production and CCl_4-induced lipid peroxidation; the latter used to be considered to be a simple linear relationship, but this no longer seems to be correct (*v. infra*). In this case, whilst formation of $^{\cdot}CCl_3$ radicals has now been proved beyond all reasonable doubt, it appears that trace amounts of $^{\cdot}CCl_3$ may react with O_2 to yield CCl_3—O—O$^{\cdot}$, and it is this molecular species which might degrade to give phosgene, and which might abstract a proton and so initiate a lipid peroxidation sequence. It follows that in the case of paraquat, where again radical formation has been established,[39] trace amounts of O_2^- might form hydroperoxide or peroxide and initiate some lipid peroxidation sequence.

In conclusion, paraquat inhibits mammalian intermediary metabolism in a way which is inconsistent with normal mitochondrial functioning, but the

[42] J. C. Gage, *Biochem. J.*, 1968, **109**, 757.

precise receptor concerned is difficult to recognize. Incidentally, it may be possible to employ analogue-blockade[43] in conjunction with the lung-uptake of paraquat, and any resulting antagonists may serve as tools for investigating the mechanism of toxicity.

Carbon Tetrachloride Induced Fatty Liver Infiltration.—It is generally recognized that the $^{\cdot}CCl_3$ radical, formed by single-electron reduction of CCl_4,[44] is the reactive intermediate in the toxicity process.[45–48]

$$CCl_4 + e^- \longrightarrow {}^{\cdot}CCl_3 + Cl^-$$

However, it remains uncertain whether cellular necrosis follows from the covalent binding of the radical to microsomal lipids and proteins or from radical induced peroxidation of the membrane unsaturated lipids,[45,46,49] and this uncertainty continues to stimulate research. In the event, Slater [45] has proposed that reduction of CCl_4 is mediated by the flavoprotein, NADPH–cytochrome P-450 reductase, despite the fact that cytochrome P-450 *per se* reduces halogenomethanes.[50,51] Accordingly it is important to know precisely how CCl_4 is reduced and how CCl_4 metabolism initiates hepatocyte necrosis. *En passant*, until recently, indirect evidence has been taken of CCl_4 metabolism, such as the covalent binding of $^{14}CCl_4$ to macromolecules[45,46,48,50,52,53] or signs of peroxidation,[45,46,48] and at the present stage in the elucidation of the problem this is too vague.

Recent results, obtained with purified enzymes,[54] show that cytochrome P-450 catalyses the single-electron and two-electron reductions of CCl_4.

$$CCl_4 + e^- \xrightarrow{-Cl^-} {}^{\cdot}CCl_3 \xrightarrow{RH} CHCl_3$$

$$^{\cdot}CCl_3 + e^- \xrightarrow{-Cl^-} :CCl_2 \xrightarrow{H_2O} CO$$

[43] J. H. Gaddum, Khan A. Hameed, D. E. Hathway, and F. F. Stephens, *Q. J. Exp. Physiol.*, 1955, **40**(1), 49.
[44] D. E. Hathway, *Arzneim. Forsch.*, 1974, **24**, 173.
[45] T. F. Slater, in 'Free Radical Mechanisms in Tissue Injury,' Pion Press, London, 1972, pp. 85—170.
[46] R. O. Recknagel, E. A. Glende, and A. M. Hruskewycz, in 'Free Radicals in Biology,' ed. W. A. Pryor, Academic Press, New York, 1977, vol. III, pp. 97—132.
[47] R. P. Mason, in 'Reviews in Biochemical Toxicology,' ed. E. Hodgson, J. R. Bend, and R. M. Philpot, Elsevier/North Holland, Amsterdam, 1979, vol. 1, pp. 151—200.
[48] E. S. Reynolds and M. T. Moslem, in 'Free Radicals in Biology,' ed. W. A. Pryor, Academic Press, New York, 1980, vol. IV, pp. 44—49.
[49] J. A. Castro, E. V. Cignoli, C. R. de Castro, and O. M. de Fenos, *Biochem. Pharmacol.*, 1972, **21**, 49.
[50] H. Uehleke, K. H. Hellmer, and S. Tabarelli-Peplawski, *Xenobiotica*, 1973, **3**, 1.
[51] C. R. Wolf, D. Mansuy, W. Nastainczyk, G. Deutschmann, and V. Ullrich, *Mol. Pharmacol.*, 1977, **13**, 698.
[52] D. Grodis, *J. Clin. Invest.*, 1969, **48**, 203.
[53] G. I. Sipes, G. Krishna, and J. R. Gillette, *Life Sci.*, 1977, **20**, 1541.
[54] C. R. Wolf, W. G. Harrelson, W. M. Nastainczyk, R. M. Philpot, B. Kalydnaraman, and R. P. Mason, *Mol. Pharmacol.*, 1980, **18**, 553.

This is important because: (i) since cytochrome P-450 is necessary for CCl_4 reduction, cytochrome P-450 reductase is not of itself responsible for the reaction; and (ii) $CHCl_3$ production under anaerobic microsomal conditions is completely inhibited by CO. There is therefore a strong supposition that NADPH–cytochrome P-450 reductase does not reduce CCl_4.

It is pertinent that, whilst CCl_4 metabolism can be detected only under anaerobic conditions,[54] the presence of CCl_4 increased significantly microsomal rates of lipid peroxidation and the corresponding utilization of co-factor in aerobic incubations. Hence, the relationship between these separate reaction processes seems to be very complicated. This result contrasts with the proposed initiation of CCl_4-induced lipid peroxidation through proton abstraction from unsaturated lipid to give $CHCl_3$ plus lipid radical(s),[45,46,48] and the supposed linear relationship (correlation coefficient, 0.82) between the rate of peroxidation and (CCl_4 concn.)$^{\frac{1}{2}}$.[55] Wolf *et al.*[54] suggest that Slater and Sawyer's argument[55] is weakened by theoretical considerations which preclude the differentiation of a square root function from equilibrium kinetics where the substrate range is limited. Thus, data from a hypothetical double reciprocal plot which are plotted as a square root function are linear (correlation coefficient, 0.91). Data from the effect of CCl_4 concn. on malonaldehyde production becomes linear in double reciprocal (correlation coefficient, 0.96) and square root plots (correlation coefficient, 0.90). In any event, the fact that air and CO do not inhibit lipid peroxidation, but completely inhibit $CHCl_3$ formation[54] (*v. supra*) strongly infers that CCl_4 induced lipid peroxidation is not initiated through proton abstraction by $^{\cdot}CCl_3$. Formation of $^{\cdot}CCl_3$ has been established by the use of $^{13}CCl_4$ and electron-spin trapping methods.[56] Thus, it is feasible that trace quantities of $^{\cdot}CCl_3$, formed anaerobically, react with O_2 to give CCl_3—O—O; which would either be degraded to phosgene[57] or which might abstract a proton to initiate lipid peroxidation. Use of the extreme co-factor, NADPH may render the hepatocytes more vulnerable to attack by radicals (see sub-section on paraquat). On the other hand, if the enzymological data of Wolf *et al.*[54] are followed *in vivo*, the CCl_4 induced lipid-peroxidation hypothesis[45] becomes superfluous. Since, $^{\cdot}CCl_3$ production has been authenticated,[54,56] it appears that the covalent binding of trichloromethyl radicals to microsomal lipids and proteins becomes the initiating circumstance in CCl_4 toxicity.

Liver Toxicity Relating to Carbon Disulphide and Phosphorothionates.—The fact that the metabolism of variously labelled forms of carbon disulphide in mammals affords CO_2 and inorganic SO_4^{2-} as end-products[58,59] does not provide any clues about the well-known toxicity of this solvent. However, rats injected i.v. with $^{14}CS_2$ eliminated $^{14}CO_2$ in quantities proportional both to the liver cytochrome P-450 activity and to the severity of the toxic changes in the liver.[59]

[55] T. F. Slater and B. C. Sawyer, *Biochem. J.*, 1971, **123**, 805.
[56] P. B. McCay, J. L. Poyer, T. Noguchi, E. K. Lai, K.-L. Fong, S. S. Alexander, and L. Olson, *Fed. Proc.*, 1980, **39**, 1949.
[57] H. Shah, S. P. Hartman, and W. Weinhouse, *Cancer Res.*, 1979, **39**, 3942.
[58] C. F. Strittmatter, T. Peters, and R. W. McKee, *Arch. Ind. Hyg. Occup. Med.*, 1950, **1**, 54.
[59] F. de Matteis and A. A. Seawright, *Chem.-Biol. Interact.*, 1973, **7**, 375.

Hence, these data[59] stress the dependence of hepatotoxicity on the metabolism of CS_2. Further work with rat-liver microsomes *in vitro*[60,61] showed carbonyl sulphide to be an intermediate in CO_2 production.

$$CS_2 + [O] \longrightarrow COS + [S]$$

$$COS + [O] \longrightarrow CO_2 + [S]$$

Both steps were mediated by cytochrome P-450–NADPH-dependent reactions, and gave atomic sulphur as a common by-product. Neal *et al.*[60,61] considered that it was this sulphur that was involved with the inhibition of cytochrome P-450 by CS_2 and COS. All this evidence suggests the probable intermediacy of singlet sulphur [S] atoms which, as they are isoelectronic with carbenes, nitrenes and oxene, are powerful electrophiles *per se*. In this connection, 50% of the sulphur that was bound covalently to rat-liver microsomes, which had been incubated with $C^{35}S_2$, was liberated on treatment with CN^- as $^{35}SCN^-$,[62] and this provides evidence for the binding of part of the sulphur, as hydrodisulphide, RS—^{35}SH. The similar results obtained in parallel experiments, where the P=S containing insecticide, [^{35}S]parathion, was incubated with rat-liver microsomes,[63] link the >C=S and ⟩P=S linkages with hepatotoxicity.[64] Finally, ^{14}COS, in addition to $^{14}CO_2$, has now been detected[65] in the exhaled air of living rats exposed to $^{14}CS_2$ by inhalation. The fact that phenobarbitone pre-treatment of the animals led to greater expiration of CO_2 at the expense of COS[65] might explain in part the delay in the making of this discovery.

Thus, singlet sulphur [S] electrophiles react with hepatocyte macromolecules, and this seems to account not only for the loss in normal cytochrome P-450 functioning, but also for the centrilobular hydropic degeneration which is seen *in vivo* following exposure to CS_2[66] and phosphorothionates.[67] As in the case of CN^- poisoning (*v. supra*), it is feasible that [S] would react also with other enzyme prosthetic groups, but the availability of those belonging to cytochrome P-450 *etc.* and the immediacy of the onset of the liver toxicity does not permit the expression of such effects.

Fluoroacetate and Lethal Synthesis.—The close structural relationship of fluoroacetate and acetate suggested that, for example, the fluoroacetate poisoning of rodents might well implicate the tricarboxylic acid cycle, and evidence for this was sought from incubations of fluoroacetate with guinea-pig kidney homogenates in which the decrease in O_2-uptake was paralleled by the accumulation of citrate, but not of acetate (chapter 5). It follows that the asymmetrical

[60] R. R. Dalvi, R. E. Poore, and R. A. Neal, *Life Sci.*, 1974, **14**, 1785.
[61] R. R. Dalvi, A. L. Hunter, and R. A. Neal, *Chem.-Biol. Interact.*, 1975, **10**, 349.
[62] G. L. Catignani and R. A. Neal, *Biochem. Biophys. Res. Commun.*, 1975, **65**, 629.
[63] F. De Mattheis, *Mol. Pharmacol.*, 1974, **10**, 849.
[64] F. De Mattheis, in 'Biological Reactive Intermediates,' ed. D. J. Jollow, J. J. Kocsis, R. Snyder, and H. Vainio, Plenum Press, New York, 1977, p. 314 *et seq.*
[65] R. R. Dalvi and R. A. Neal, *Biochem. Pharmacol.*, 1978, **27**, 1608.
[66] E. J. Bond, W. H. Butler, F. De Matteis, and J. M. Barnes, *Br. J. Ind. Med.*, 1969, **26**, 335.
[67] A. A. Seawright, J. Hrdlicka, and F. De Matteis, *Br. J. Exp. Pathol.*, 1976, **57**, 16.

fluorocitrate which is synthesized[68] inhibits the aconitase receptor,[69–71] but not isocitrate dehydrogenase,[72] and thereby blocks the normal cycling of citrate and the terminal respiration in these animals.

Whilst the fluorocitrate antagonism/inhibition of aconitase accounts completely for the mortality of rodents, there seems to have been some conjecture[73] about whether the cerebral effects in pigeons might be attributed to the same causal mechanism. However, it now seems to be pretty clear that inhibition of the cycling of cerebral citrate would diminish the supply of α-oxoglutarate available for glutamic acid and glutamine synthesis, which constitutes the principal binding mechanism for ammonia (*v. infra*) that has been liberated in the brain before the onset of convulsions and throughout their course (Scheme 3). Later in the seizure pattern, this mechanism is overwhelmed, free ammonia accumulates in the brain, and the birds die.

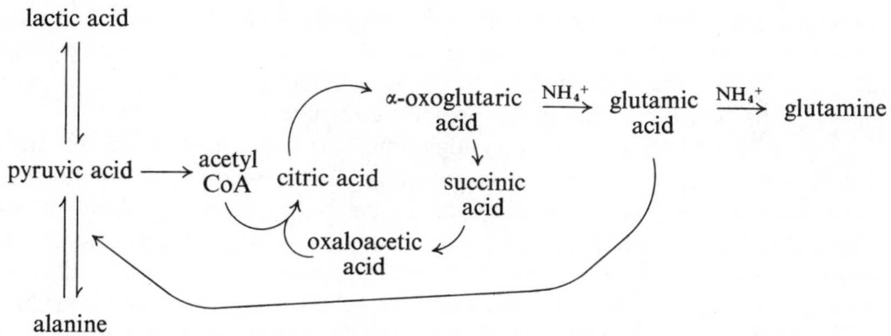

Scheme 3 *Utilization of ammonia in the brain*

Organochlorine Insecticides and Convulsive States.—Study of the endogenous cerebral metabolites illustrates the problem of disentangling changes belonging to an apparent mechanism for dieldrin (4) and Telodrin (5) convulsions from ones related purely to brain hyperactivity. Thus, the relatively large increase in cerebral lactate concentration which occurred after the onset of seizures[74] is characteristic of the convulsive state,[75] and the fact that the cerebral pyruvate concentration attained peak values after convulsions had started and fell after the tonic extensor seizure[74] was also consistent with brain hyperactivity (Scheme 3).

On the other hand, in both acute (4) and (5) intoxications the cerebral alanine concentration increased very significantly pre-convulsively, and the increased variability of values thereafter compared with the ones before strongly suggested

68 A. G. Ogston, *Nature*, 1948, **162**, 963.
69 J. F. Morrison and R. A. Peters, *Biochem. J.*, 1954, **56**, xxxvi
70 J. F. Morrison and R. A. Peters, *Biochem. J.*, 1954, **58**, 473.
71 R. A. Peters, *Biochem. J.*, 1961, **79**, 261.
72 W. D. Lopspeich, R. A. Peters, and T. H. Wilson, *Biochem. J.*, 1952, **51**, 20.
73 R. A. Peters, in 'Biochemical Lesions and Lethal Synthesis,' Pergamon, Oxford, 1963, pp. 88—130.
74 D. E. Hathway, A. Mallinson, and D. A. A. Akintonwa, *Biochem. J.*, 1965, **94**, 676.
75 H. McIlwain, in 'Biochemistry and the Central Nervous System,' 2nd edn., J. and A. Churchill, London, 1959, p. 37.

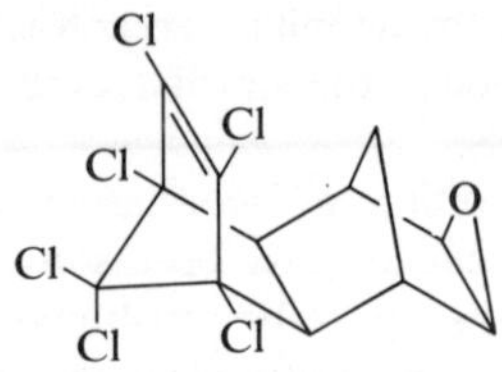

(4)

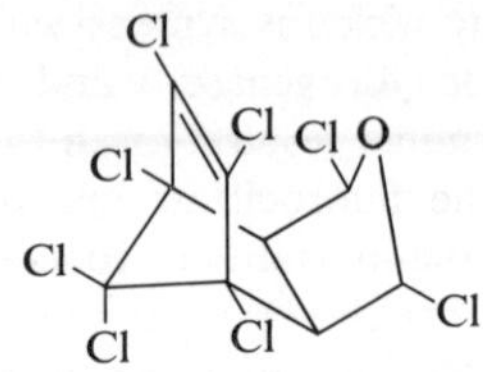

(5)

that, after convulsions hyperactivity complicated the significant change in concentration of this metabolite which occurred before them. Acute (5) intoxication was paralleled by a significant increase in glutamine concentration and a corresponding decrease in that of glutamic acid. (i) The fact that cerebral glutamine reached maximum concentration in the pre-convulsive period, (ii) the shape of the cerebral glutamine time-course, and (iii) electro-encephalographic evidence for pre-convulsive activity in the intoxicated rat brain, strongly suggested that the pre-convulsive changes in cerebral glutamine concentration relate to the causal mechanism for Telodrin convulsions.

Late in (4) and (5) seizures, very high ammonia concentrations in the brain are commensurate with ammonia poisoning. In (4) seizures, fluctuations in brain ammonia were out of phase with the periods of intense cerebral activity which alternate with periods of quiescence. The fluctuations in cerebral ammonia concentration, -8.34 μmol/100 g ($P < 0.025$), increased with time after dosage; the changes were significantly different from values from the second and third convulsions. It is reasonably certain that the fluctuating increases in cerebral ammonia concentration contribute to the seizures in question.

That glutamine synthesis (Scheme 3) represents a significant proportion of the total cerebral metabolism in acute (5) intoxication is shown by comparing the maximum rate of glutamine synthesis, 0.2 μmol/g of brain tissue min^{-1}, with the normal rate of glucose utilization, 0.4 μmol g^{-1} min^{-1}, calculated from an arteriovenous glucose difference of 13.2 mg/100 ml[76] and a flow rate of 0.6 ml g^{-1} min^{-1} for cerebral blood. The availability of pyruvate would be approximately 0.8 μmol/g of brain tissue min^{-1}, *i.e.* only four times the rate of glutamine synthesis. The latter was about the same in a dozen experiments in which the final glutamine concentration ranged from 0.6—0.8 μmol/g. Thus, this mechanism seems to have been operating at its maximum capacity, and the NH_4^+ concentration is not rate-limiting in this range.[77] These findings and the fact that the tricarboxylic acid cycle would have to proceed at 0.7 μmol g^{-1} min^{-1} to account for respiration from glucose *in vitro* at 2.0 μmol of O_2 g^{-1} [78] min^{-1} are commensurate with the later deceleration of glutamine that has been found.[79] The decrease in glutamic acid was significant[79] whereas that of α-oxoglutarate was, if anything, increased; it is uncertain whether the supply of α-oxoglutarate was in fact rate-limiting.

76 R. Rodnight, H. McIlwain, and M. A. Tresize, *J. Neurochem.*, 1959, **3**, 209.
77 J. K. Tews, S. H. Carter, P. D. Roa, and W. E. Stone, *J. Neurochem.*, 1963, **10**, 641.
78 A. Beloff-Chain, R. Catanzaro, E. B. Chain, I. Masi, and F. Pocchiari, *Proc. Roy. Soc.*, 1955, **B144**, 22.
79 D. E. Hathway and A. Mallinson, *Biochem. J.*, 1964, **90**, 51.

Transamination involving pyruvate is clearly another method for ammonia utilization in the brain, and there is high activity of the relevant transaminase in cerebral tissues.[80] In this connection, both dieldrin and Telodrin brought about a significant change in cerebral alanine concentration.[74]

There is clear evidence: (i) that the action of Telodrin caused liberation of ammonia in the brain before the onset of seizures and throughout their course; (ii) that α-oxoglutarate, glutamate, and glutamine were utilized in a principal ammonia-binding mechanism; (iii) that α-oxoglutarate, glutamate, pyruvate, and alanine were utilized in a subsidiary mechanism for ammonia disposal; and (iv) that later in the seizure pattern, these mechanisms were overwhelmed and free ammonia accumulated in the cerebral tissues.

Futhermore, the fact that parenteral administration of glutamine (50 mg kg^{-1}) which presumably penetrates the brain, causes an increase of glutamate of 230 μmol/100 g wet weight of brain, and that the equivalent amount of ammonia released is utilized in alanine formation, and not in glutamine synthesis, provides an explanation for the recovery of one-half of the animals which received a lethal dose of Telodrin after administration of 50 mg of glutamine kg^{-1}. An additional supply of glutamate thus became available for normal brain metabolism at the time when the maximum rate of glutamate synthesis, due to Telodrin, had begun to deplete the cerebral glutamate pool (and this supply was not diminished by combination with extra ammonia from injected glutamine, as this ammonia had already been incorporated into alanine). Thus, animals killed 30 min after glutamine injection and 16 min after injection of Telodrin have a cerebral alanine concentration which approximates to the sum of the separate concentrations of alanine resulting from administrations of glutamine and Telodrin respectively, a normal concentration of cerebral glutamate, and a concentration of cerebral glutamine commensurate with Telodrin intoxication. It can be argued accordingly (chapter 2) that Telodrin behaves as an antagonist/inhibitor, in which case the extra supply of glutamate that is made available cerebrally might be said to repair the damage done to the receptor, or to by-pass the 'biochemical lesion'.

In the case of dieldrin convulsions, the fluctuating release of cerebral ammonia suggests that the brain can deal effectively with changes produced in cerebral NH_4^+ ion concentration. The decreased concentration of cerebral ammonia associated with a convulsion might be related to the increased rate of circulation and of O_2-consumption by the brain which accompanies drug-induced seizures. Thus, the action of dieldrin leads to the liberation of ammonia before the onset of convulsions and throughout their course, and whilst α-oxoglutarate, glutamate, pyruvate, and alanine are utilized in an ammonia-binding mechanism, this mechanism is overwhelmed later in the seizure pattern, when free ammonia accumulates in cerebral tissues. Dieldrin seems to inhibit glutamine synthesis (*cf.* the case of Telodrin, *v. supra*).

The changes in the biochemistry of rat brain during acute insecticide intoxication imply disturbances in brain-cell economy. Work with rat-brain mito-

[80] J. Awapara and B. Seale, *J. Biol. Chem.*, 1952, **194**, 497.

chondria *in vivo*[81] and liver mitochondria *in vitro*[82] provides some evidence for mitochondrial changes. Enzymes concerned with, for example, the biotransformation of glutamate are mitochondrial enzymes, and the present evidence[74,79] implies that dieldrin and Telodrin intoxications occasion disturbances in mitochondrial function in the brain.

Mustard Gas Poisoning.—Mustard gas, bis(2-chloroethyl) sulphide (6) (Scheme 4) is an alkylating reagent, which ionizes and reacts with (cellular) nucleophiles, for example water, through the intermediacy of the epi-sulphonium ion (7),[83,84]

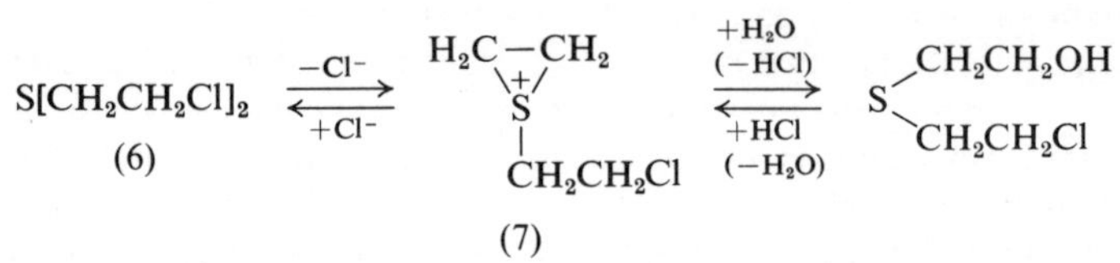

Scheme 4

and in this respect it behaves like a cysteine metabolite of vinyl chloride (chapter 6). An S_N2 reagent (see chapter 11), (6) reacts more exclusively at *N*–7 of the guanine residues of DNA than, for example, the alkyl—N_2^+ generating *N*-ethyl-*N*-nitrosourea (ENU) and *N,N*-diethylnitrosamine (DEN). The exact mechanism by which (6) produces the injury in skin leading to vesication and erythema is not as clear as its reactivity.[85] In this connection, as little as 6 μg/cm² causes vesication in 50% of the white subjects, and 1 μg/cm² causes permanent corneal injury in rats. From the evidence available,[85–87] it would appear likely that some phosphate group, presumably in a phospholipid or possibly in nucleoside (guanosine) residues of RNA, near to the surface of the cell becomes esterified. This might even take place in one of the internal surfaces where ribosomes are attached to the endoplasmic reticulum. Whilst work with alkylating agents focuses on DNA (chapter 11), and this may have a bearing in the present case, it seems unlikely that sulphur mustard does not attack some other cellular constituent besides the nuclear DNA. In this connection, there is evidence[85,88] that sulphur mustard was selectively toxic to the pyruvate oxidase system. The toxic action was exerted not only upon pyruvic dehydrogenase but on some other factor in the pyruvate oxidase system, and this might well be upon the co-enzyme A or lipoate needed for citric acid cycling both at the pyruvate and the α-oxoglutarate stage.[89]

[81] E. A. Hosein and P. Proulx, *J. Agric. Food Chem.*, 1960, **8**, 428.
[82] V. H. Parker, *Biochem. J.*, 1960, **77**, 74.
[83] A. G. Ogston, E. Holiday, J. St. L. Philpot, and L. A. Stocken, *Trans. Faraday Soc.*, 1948, **44**, 45.
[84] A. G. Ogston, *Biochem. Soc. Symp.*, 1948, No. 2, 2.
[85] R. A. Peters, *Nature*, 1947, **159**, 149.
[86] R. M. Herriott, *J. Gen. Physiol.*, 1948, **32**, 221.
[87] H. B. Fell and C. B. Allsopp, *Cancer Res.*, 1948, **8**, 145.
[88] R. A. Peters and R. W. Wakelin, *Biochem. J.*, 1947, **41**, 555.
[89] Ref. 73, pp. 58—87.

Lewisite Toxicity.—Peters found[90] that very small concentrations of arsenic blocked the vitamin stimulated respiration of pyruvate in pigeon-brain preparations in the same way that vesicants (*v. supra*) attacked selectively the pyruvate oxidase system.[91] In fact, the action of lewisite (8) (Scheme 5) increased markedly

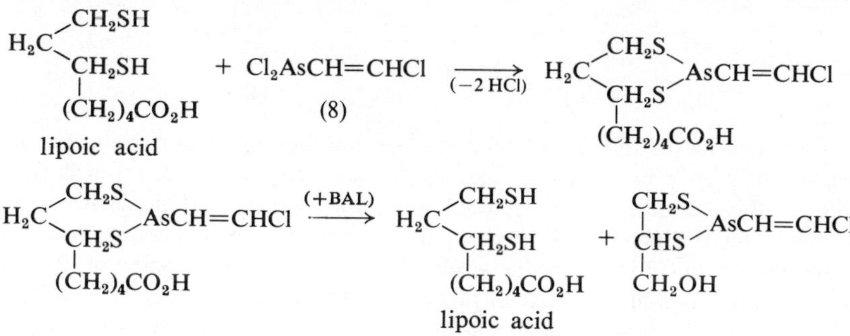

Scheme 5

blood pyruvate in the living mammal in the same way that thiamine deficiency does. A clue as to how this occurred was afforded by the discovery that BAL might act as an antidote to lewisite poisoning (Scheme 5) where it was initially considered that the SH groups *per se* belonged to a protein/enzyme. BAL does in fact reduce the blistering when applied to the skin after the beginning of erythema caused by lewisite. In addition, lewisite injected into the brain of pigeons overwhelms the cerebral pyruvate oxidase system and produces convulsions.[92] [BAL = 2,3-dimercaptopropanol]

Thus BAL overcame the biochemical lesion caused by (8). It is now clear[93,94] that the α,γ-thiol groups of lipoic acid, belonging to the pyruvate oxidase system, react with lewisite to form a six-membered ring (Scheme 5), whereas BAL chelates more effectively than this with the lewisite As atom. In other words, BAL repairs the injury done to the (lipoate) receptor in the pyruvate oxidase system by lewisite.

Organophosphates.—The action of organophosphates and carbamates causing the inhibition of acetylcholinesterase (AChE) in mammals, the kinetics of enzyme inhibition, and the role of antidotes in repairing the damage done to the enzymic receptor sites have been thoroughly discussed already (chapters 4,5). Accordingly, the arguments concerned will not be repeated here, and the present treatment is concerned solely with a pronounced difference in acute oral toxicity that is shown by dogs and rats towards chlorfenvinphos (9). This has very little to do with the biotransformations of (9) in the species concerned[95] (chapter 8), and raises some interesting points.

[90] R. A. Peters, *Current Sci.*, 1936, **5**, 207.
[91] R. A. Peters, H. M. Sinclair, and R. H. S. Thompson, *Biochem. J.*, 1946, **40**, 516.
[92] R. A. Peters, *Bull. Johns Hopkins Hospital*, 1955, **97**, 1.
[93] I. C. Gunsalus, L. Struglia, and D. J. O'Kane, *J. Biol. Chem.*, 1952, **194**, 859.
[94] L. J. Reed, *Physiol. Rev.*, 1953, **33**, 544.
[95] D. H. Hutson, D. A. A. Akintonwa, and D. E. Hathway, *Biochem. J.*, 1967, **102**, 133.

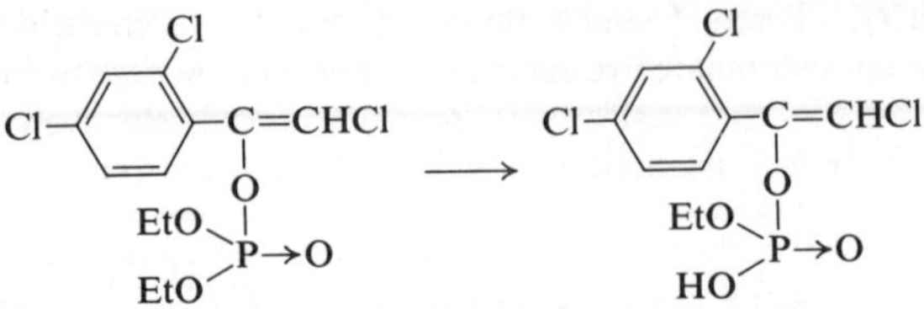

(9) (10)

It was considered that an interaction of several factors might account for the marked difference in acute oral toxicity between dogs and rats towards (9)[96] and, in this connection, the physiological and biochemical implications of relatively small differences in each of the parameters which may be involved would be relevant. In the peripheral blood of dogs the concentration of (9) was approximately one-fifth of that in rats, which had been given one-third of the dose level, and this indicates a fifteen-fold difference in the combined absorption–metabolism properties of the two species.[96] The very rapid detoxification and elimination of absorbed (9) as 2-chloro-1-(2′,4′-dichlorophenyl)vinyl ethyl hydrogenphosphate (10) in dogs, compared with the more complicated pattern of metabolism of (9) in rats[95], suggested that detoxification is more effective in dogs. A three-fold uptake of (9) by rat erythrocytes from rat plasma compared with that by dog erythrocytes from dog plasma is a valid measure of the different availabilities of the insecticide in the blood of the two species, as no difference in permeability is shown by the erythrocyte stroma of dogs and rats towards (9) dissolved in bovine albumin.[96]

Moreover, the brain is involved in chlorfenvinphos intoxication as EEG recordings during intoxication were consistent with (organophosphate) inhibition of neurohumoral transmission, and severe effects were associated with brain-uptake of (9). The toxic agent would appear to be (9) *per se*, and this is consistent with the non-toxicity of all of the (9) metabolites.[95] Thus, the mode of action of (9) would seem to be explicable in terms of its uptake by the brain and of its inhibitory action on the cerebral AChE. Whilst complicating symptoms in some animals may be due to peripheral effects, these were not investigated.[96]

A dose level of [^{14}C]-(9) that produced a lower concentration of unchanged (9) in the blood of rats than that of dogs yielded a two- to three-times higher brain-uptake of (9) in rats than in dogs, 1 h after dosing. [The workers[96] noted that this measure of difference may be too low since, whilst all of the radioactivity in the brain of rats may be attributed to unchanged (9), this could not be established in the dogs.]

There is a significant difference in the behaviour of the cerebral AChE of the dog and rat towards (9) *in vivo*, and work *in vitro* established that the rat-brain enzyme is ten times more sensitive than dog-brain enzyme. Incidentally, there would be a tendency *in vivo* for (9) to associate with those parts of the neurons which are rich in cerebral lipids, and only a small proportion of (9) in the brain would be available for reaction with neural AChE. This might account for the apparent insensitivity of dog cerebral AChE towards (9) *in vivo*, and for the fact

[96] D. H. Hutson and D. E. Hathway, *Biochem. Pharmacol.*, 1967, **16**, 949.

that, in rats, *in vivo* effects take several minutes to develop after an effective (9) concentration has accumulated in the brain. From another point of view, chlorfenvinphos would seem to fit the neural AChE receptor of rat brain better than that of the dog brain.

In rats and dogs, the concerted interaction of the proximate differences[96] in rates of absorption and metabolism, the availability in circulating blood, the rate of brain-uptake, and the sensitivity of brain AChE towards (9) *per se* would seem to account for a 900—1350 fold difference between the acute oral toxicities of the insecticide in the two species of animal.

There is a strong supposition[96] that the insensitivity of dog-brain AChE towards (9) is due to a recessive gene,[97] and that genetic considerations may apply also to the initial reactions of (9) which determine the course of its metabolism in dogs and rats.[95] Well-authenticated correlations between enzymic activity and genetic make-up in mammals might be important for the future, as they would help to predict the position of man from toxicological experiments made in animals.

Anti-coagulative Properties of Warfarin.—Present understanding of the anti-coagulative properties of 4-hydroxycoumarins, such as dicoumarol and the warfarin type of rodenticide, is incomplete, but action at a receptor is undoubtedly implied. The simple proposition[98] that warfarin (11) and vitamin K combine with a simple enzyme which is concerned with prothrombin synthesis now appears to be incorrect. Whilst vitamin K antagonizes the action of (11) both in a

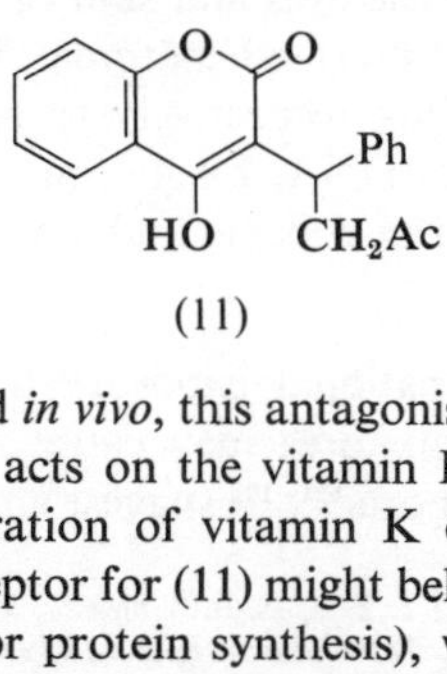

(11)

perfused liver preparation and *in vivo*, this antagonism is non-competitive. It has been suggested: (i) that (11) acts on the vitamin K-epoxide reductase system, thereby blocking the regeneration of vitamin K essential to the carboxylase system;[99] and (ii) that the receptor for (11) might behave as an allosteric modifier of the carboxylase system (for protein synthesis), which would accordingly be sensitive to changes in the concentration of (11) and of vitamin K.[100] In addition, the fact that warfarin-receptor protein reacts with (11) and with phylloquinone focuses attention on the influence of this receptor on vitamin K dependent carboxylation (*v. supra*):[101,102] the two systems might integrate in some way.

97 J. B. S. Haldane, in '*The Biochemistry of Genetics*,' George Allen and Unwin, London, 1965, pp. 63—85.
98 A. J. Quick and G. Collentine, *J. Lab. Clin. Med.*, 1950, **36**, 976.
99 R. G. Bell and J. T. Matschiner, *Nature*, 1972, **237**, 32.
100 S. R. Goodman, R. M. Houser, and R. E. Olson, *Biochem. Biophys. Res. Commun.*, 1974, **61**, 250.
101 J. A. Sadowski and J. W. Suttie, *Fed. Proc.*, 1976, **35**, 662.
102 R. M. Houser, J. P. Jones, A. Fausto, E. J. Gardner, F. C. Lee, and R. E. Olson, *Fed. Proc.*, 1976, **35**, 1353.

It ought to be said that haemorrhagic episodes affecting various organs constitute the toxic manifestations of (11) and the coumarin rat poisons. Vitamin K derivatives are specific antidotes to the poisoning, but a response is not immediate as sufficient time has to elapse for *de novo* synthesis of protein (chapter 5) to occur.

Diallate Toxicity.—In chapter 6, it was shown that 2-chloroacrolein (13) arose from diallate, *cis*- and *trans*-*S*-(2,3-dichloroallyl)di-isopropylthiocarbamate (12) (Scheme 6) through a [2,3] sigmatropic rearrangement followed by 1,2-elimination.[103,104] Since (13) is highly reactive and mutagenic, it is pretty clear that the

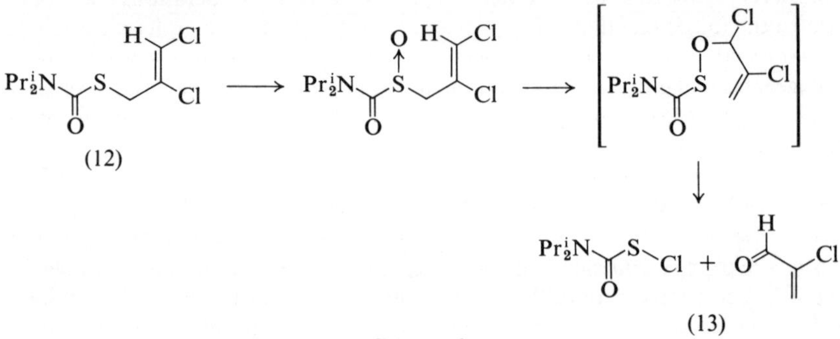

Scheme 6

irritational toxicity of (12) to the eyes and skin of guinea-pigs and rabbits[105,106] and the increased incidence of murine hepatomas[107–109] are due to formation of (13) and its subsequent binding respectively to skin plus eye cellular macromolecules and to parenchymal DNA. Excitation of the c.n.s. leading to clonic-tonic seizures, which is found in rodents and cats,[110] would seem to be caused by unchanged (12) *per se*.

Benzene Intoxication.—Occupational exposure to commercial benzene or to benzene-containing solvent mixtures may cause injury to the haematopoietic system. In fact, many case reports[111–122] suggest a relationship between exposure

[103] I. Schuphan, J. D. Rosen, and J. E. Casida, *Science*, 1979, **205**, 1013.
[104] I. Schuphan and J. E. Casida, *Tetrahedron Lett.*, 1979, 841.
[105] S. L. Doloshitsky, *Gig. Sanit.*, 1969, **34**, 21.
[106] M. I. Gzhegotsky and S. L. Doloshitsky, *Vrach. Delo*, 1971, **11**, 133.
[107] J. R. M. Innes, B. M. Ulland, M. G. Valerio, L. Petrucelli, L. Fishbein, E. R. Hart, A. J. Pallotta, R. R. Bates, H. L. Falk, J. J. Gart, M. Klein, I. Mitchell, and J. Peters, *J. Nat. Cancer Inst.*, 1969, **42**, 1101.
[108] NTIS 'Evaluation of Carcinogenic, Teratogenic and Mutagenic Activities of Selected Pesticides and Industrial Chemicals,' Carcinogenic Study, U. S. Department of Commerce, Washington D.C., 1968, vol. 1.
[109] 'Diallate,' IARC Monographs on the Evaluation of Carcinogenic Risks of Chemicals to Man, 'Some Carbamates, Thiocarbamates and Carbazides,' Lyon, France, 1976, vol. 12.
[110] A. G. Pestova, *Gig. Toksikol. Pestits. Klin. Oltravlenii*, 1966, **4**, 166.
[111] M. Aksoy, K. Dincol, T. Akgün, S. Erdem, and G. Dincol, *Br. J. Ind. Med.*, 1971, **28**, 296.
[112] M. Aksoy, K. Dincol, S. Erdem, and G. Dincol, *Am. J. Med.*, 1972, **52**, 160.
[113] M. Bowditch and H. B. Elkins, *J. Ind. Hyg. Toxicol.*, 1939, **21**, 321.
[114] R. L. DeGowin, *J. Am. Med. Assoc.*, 1963, **185**, 748.

to benzene and the induction of leukaemia, and a case-control study[123] supports this supposition.

It has been known for some time that benzene is metabolized in mammals into phenols (*ca.* 30% of the dose), including phenol itself (23.5%) as well as pyrocatechol, quinol, and hydroxyquinol plus the conjugate, L-phenylmercapturic acid (0.5%), and is degraded into the aliphatic compound, *trans,trans*-muconic acid[124–129] and CO_2, each of which account for a further 1.5% of the dose. Up to one-half of the dose is excreted unchanged in the exhaled air.[130,131] As long ago as 1949, Porteous and Williams[127] considered that the toxic effects of benzene were probably related to the formation of phenols.

It is very important that benzene should now have been found to react with DNA *in vivo*, although the reactive metabolite itself is unknown. Whilst one candidate compound would be benzene oxide, which rearranges slowly enough in an aqueous environment to give phenol for the reaction with DNA to be feasible, the metabolic formation of polyhydroxy aromatic compounds suggests the formation of phenol epoxide. In this case, the reactive intermediate would be a secondary metabolite, and this would concur with the example of benzo[*a*]pyrene, where a diol-epoxide has been found to be the ultimate carcinogen.[132] Experiment showed[133] the alkylating capacity of benzene towards liver DNA to be 3000 times lower than that of *N,N*-dimethylnitrosamine.

It follows that the causative mechanism for benzene induced leukaemia involves a reactive metabolite of benzene, probably phenol epoxide, and bone-marrow, lymphoid, or spleen[134] DNA. In this case, the damage done to the special receptors is incapable of antidotal repair, and therapy would have to do with the homeostasis of the blood-cell elements. In general, measurements in blood and bone marrow seem to support the foregoing suppositions. Thus: (i) whereas phenol was the main metabolite in bone marrow at the beginning of an exposure (500 p.p.m.) of rats to benzene vapour, pyrocatechol and quinol

[115] P. Delore and C. Borgomano, *J. Med. Lyon*, 1928, **9**, 227.
[116] R. Girard and L. Revol, *Nouv. Rev. Fr., Hematol.*, 1970, **10**, 477.
[117] A. Goguel, A. Cairgneaux, and J. Bernard, *Nouv. Rev. Fr. Hematol.*, 1967, **7**, 465.
[118] F. T. Hunter, *J. Ind. Hyg. Toxicol.*, 1939, **21**, 331.
[119] H. Ludwig and A. Werthemann, *Schweiz. Med. Wochenschr.*, 1962, **92**, 378.
[120] T. B. Mallory, E. A. Gall, and W. J. Brickley, *J. Ind. Hyg. Toxicol.*, 1939, **21**, 355.
[121] E. M. Tareeff, N. M. Kontchalovskaya, and L. A. Zorina, *Acta Unio. Int. Contra Cancrum*, 1963, **19**, 751.
[122] E. C. Vigliani and G. Saita, *N. Engl. J. Med.*, 1964, **271**, 872.
[123] T. Ishimaru, H. Okada, T. Tomiyasu, T. Tsuchimoto, T. Hoshino, and M. Ichimaru, *Am. J. Epidemiol.*, 1971, **93**, 157.
[124] J. C. Drummond and I. L. Finar, *Biochem. J.*, 1938, **32**, 79.
[125] M. Jaffe, *Z. physiol. Chem.*, 1909, **62**, 58.
[126] M. Nencki and P. Giacosa, *Z. physiol. Chem.*, 1880, **4**, 325.
[127] J. W. Porteous and R. T. Williams, *Biochem. J.*, 1949, **44**, 56.
[128] O. Schultzen and B. Naunyn, *Arch. Anat. Physiol., Leipzig*, 1867, 349.
[129] S. H. Zbarsky and L. Young, *J. Biol. Chem.*, 1943, **151**, 487.
[130] M. Nencki and P. Sieber, *Pfluegers. Arch. Gesamte Physiol. Menschen Tiere*, 1883, **31**, 319.
[131] D. V. Parke and R. T. Williams, *Biochem. J.*, 1953, **54**, 231.
[132] P. Sims, P. L. Grover, A. Swaisland, K. Pal, and A. Hewer, *Nature*, 1974, **252**, 326.
[133] W. K. Lutz and C. Schlatter, *Chem.-Biol. Interact.*, 1977, **18**, 241.
[134] R. G. Macfarlane and A. H. T. Robb-Smith, '*Functions of the Blood*,' Academic Press, London and New York, 1961, pp. 170—270 and 350—418.

dominated subsequently and remained both in the blood and bone marrow for at least 9 h after exposure had ended;[135] (ii) work with rat-liver microsomes in the presence of an NADPH-generating system showed that a further biotransformation product of phenol was responsible for binding to microsomal protein rather than a primary metabolite of benzene *per se*;[136] (iii) the binding of benzene metabolites to mouse-liver and rabbit-bone-marrow microsomes has been investigated;[137] and (iv) a study has been made of the biotransformations of benzene by rabbit-bone-marrow microsomes.[138] With reference to the industrial connotation, the metabolic interaction of benzene and toluene affects the rate of metabolism of the two components, which is slower in admixture than separately.

Thalidomide Teratogenicity.—Thalidomide (14) teratogenicity illustrates some important features: (i) daily administration p.o. of 25—200 mg kg^{-1} was

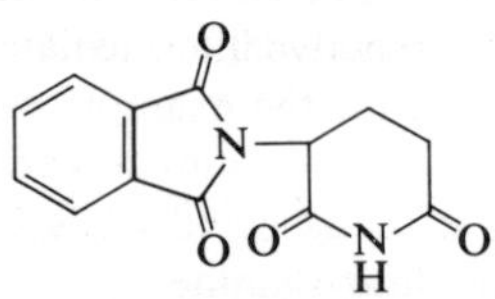

(14)

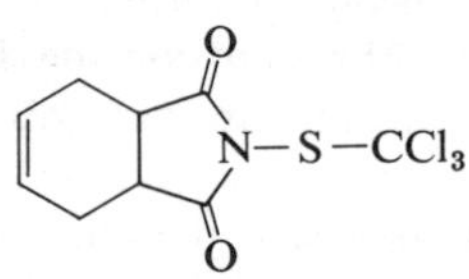

(15)

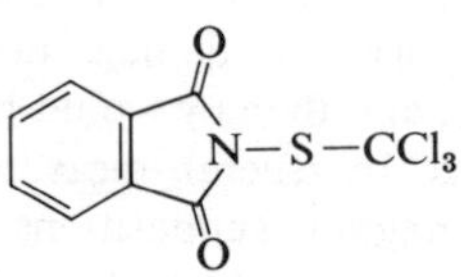

(16)

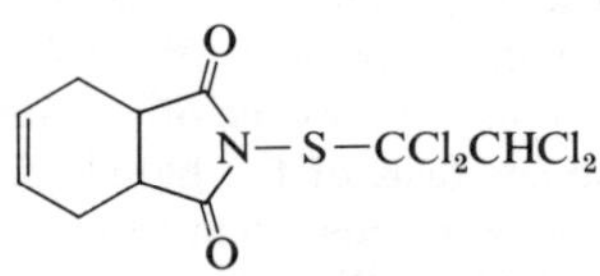

(17)

markedly teratogenic in rabbits, but only marginally in rats; (ii) after i.v. injection, (14) was four times more powerful as a teratogen in rabbits (2.5 mg kg^{-1}) than in rats (10 mg kg^{-1}), but these findings suggest that (14) administered i.v. might have a similar potency in the two species of animal if the dose were calculated in terms of surface area rather than of animal weight; (iii) in the case of human beings with a surface area to body-weight ratio of *ca.* one-seventh that of rats, (14) caused malformations at an oral dose of 100 mg, *i.e.* of *ca.* 2 mg kg^{-1};[143] (iv) the New Zealand white rabbit was first discovered as an

[135] D. E. Rickert, T. S. Baker, J. S. Bus, C. S. Barrow, and R. D. Irons, *Toxicol. Appl. Pharmacol.*, 1979, **49**, 417.
[136] A. Tunek, K. L. Platt, P. Bentley, and F. Oesch, *Mol. Pharmacol.*, 1978, **14**, 920.
[137] R. Snyder, E. W. Lee, and J. J. Kocsis, *Res. Commun. Chem. Pathol. Pharmacol.*, 1978, **20**, 191
[138] L. S. Andrews, H. A. Sasame, and J. R. Gillette, *Life Sci.*, 1979, **25**, 567.
[139] A. Sato and T. Nakajima, *Toxicol. Appl. Pharmacol.*, 1979, **48**, 249.
[140] P. Mikulski, R. Wiglusz, E. Galuszko, and G. Delag, *Bull. Inst. Marin. Trop. Med. Acad. Gdansk*, 1979, **30**, 89.
[141] P. Mikulski, R. Wiglusz, E. Galuszko, and G. Delag, *Bull. Inst. Marin. Trop. Med. Acad. Gdansk*, 1979, **30**, 77.
[142] T. Nakajuma and A. Sato, *Sangyo Igaku*, 1978, **20**, 34.
[143] W. Lenz, *Lancet*, 1962, **i**, 45.

experimental model for the teratogenic effects found in humans,[144] and was used fairly extensively[145–151] although it suffered from the disadvantage of becoming rapidly obese; (v) the Himalayan rabbit proved to be a better model than the New Zealand white because of its high fertility, its lower weight-gain and the fact that all doses of (14) produced malformations; (vi) in the case of Himalayan rabbits, both the abnormalities and the rate of resorption showed a dose-dependent increase;[152] (vii) malformations included fixation of the paw in an inwardly rotated position, abnormalities in the first digit, hypoplasia and aplasia of the radius and tibia, synosteosis of the sternebrae or additional sternal centres, disorientation of the distal tail vertebrae, and duplication of the gall-bladder;[152] and (viii) susceptibility to thalidomide teratogenic effects was confirmed in the rhesus monkey, *Macaca rhesus*, and in the stump-tailed macaque, *Macaca arctoides*.

Although (14) underwent spontaneous hydrolysis under physiological conditions, the rate of degradation was greater in rabbit liver, and high levels of thalidomide metabolites in the liver suggested that enzymic metabolism contributed to the (non-enzymic) chemical fate of the drug in these animals.[153a] However, arguments about metabolites may be irrelevant, as no teratogenic effects have ever been attributed to the administration of any of the polar (14) metabolites to a susceptible species of animal, and as species differences in the rate of formation and excretion of (14) metabolites are unrelated to species differences in teratogenic potency. Alternatively, the (14) acids would be likely to sequester Ca^{2+}, and the effect of their intracellular formation on limb-budding and growth would consequently differ profoundly from that of oral dosing where little (if any) of the (14)-acids would be absorbed.

Besides the thalidomide metabolites, other substances that are structurally related to thalidomide, such as captan (15), folpet (16), and difolatan (17), are also non-teratogens,[153b] and only (14) *per se* and its phthalidophthalimide analogue[153a] produce the teratogenic effects. Thus, this represents a unique case of structure–activity, which is highly suggestive of receptor involvement (chapter 2). Injection of (14) into rats was followed by irreversible binding to liver DNA, RNA, histones, and phospholipids.[153a] It was concluded [153a] (i) that, if teratogenesis is mediated through irreversible binding, species differences in teratogenicity may involve differences in the rate of acylation of an unidentified substance which is concerned with the regulation of organ development, and (ii) that an absence of binding to rat nucleic acids by (14) *per se* implies that the teratogenic effects in question are entirely unrelated to direct modification of the

144 G. F. Somers, *Lancet*, 1962, **i**, 912.
145 H. P. Drobeck, F. Coulson, and D. Cornelius, *Toxicol. Appl. Pharmacol.*, 1965, **7**, 165.
146 S. Fabro and R. L. Smith, *J. Pathol. Bacteriol.*, 1966, **91**, 511.
147 J. H. Pearn and T. H. Vickers, *Br. J. Exp. Pathol.*, 1966, **47**, 186.
148 P. B. Sawin, D. Crary, R. R. Fox, and H. M. Wuest, *Experientia*, 1965, **21**, 672.
149 M. J. Seller, *Lancet*, 1962, **ii**, 249.
150 G. F. Somers, *Proc. Eur. Soc. Study Drug Toxicity*, 1963, **1**, 49.
151 H. M. Wuest, J. Fratta, and E. B. Sigg, *Life Sci.*, 1966, **5**, 393.
152 H. Lehmann and A. Niggeschulze, *Toxicol. Appl. Pharmacol.*, 1971, **18**, 208.
153 (*a*) H. Schumacher, D. A. Blake, and J. R. Gillette, *J. Pharmacol.*, 1968, **160**, 201; (*b*) S. Fabro, R. L. Smith, and R. T. Williams, *Food Cosmet. Toxicol.*, 1966, **3**, 587.

genome. These data really confirm what is now largely predictable, although this may not have been the case 15 years ago when the experiments were carried out.

Other evidence[154,155] showed that (14) affected the incorporation of precursors into nucleic acids, suggesting increased nucleic acid biosynthesis, particularly of DNA. Actinomycin D inhibited thalidomide-stimulated thymidine incorporation, and those authors[154,155] concluded that the stimulation was concerned with the DNA-directed DNA synthesis. Thalidomide affects isotope incorporation into the brain, kidneys, liver, and spleen proteins of rats dosed with [^{14}C]formate and into the liver and plasma proteins of the foetus where the dams were given [^{14}C]glycine; but, on account of a low incorporation of [^{14}C]lysine, it was concluded[155] that the effect of (14) on protein biosynthesis was of a secondary nature. However, the present writer considers the disturbance in glycine incorporation into foetal protein at a critical stage in organogenesis to be very significant, as one of the characteristics of the almost unique mammalian structural protein, collagen, is its high glycine content.

Some consideration ought to be given as to how the biochemical effects of thalidomide may integrate with the development of congenital malformation. Since the processes of proliferation and differentiation to a strictly pre-determined time schedule make up the main biological function of foetal cells, it follows that any diversion or deviation from the work of these cells might upset the normal course of foetus development. Thus, the acceleration of DNA synthesis which has been found suggests a more rapid cell proliferation, which might project them into another level of differentiation without the provision of the requisite regulation. Under these circumstances, such cells may be incapable of fulfilling their strictly pre-determined role in (normal) differentiation. The sort of phenomenon which may arise in such a situation would be the elaboration of an enzyme complement, for example for nucleic acid synthesis to occur at a stage in cell differentiation when it may be usually absent.

The early investigations seem to show that the conditions for embryotoxic action in mammalian species are very complicated from the experimental biochemical point of view. The arguments (*v. supra*) themselves are tenuous. It is very difficult to learn very much about the complicated inter-relationships between developmental metabolic processes and the drug action unless extensive investigations are made of the biochemical reactions at the time when they occur, and when they are modified within the developing mammalian embryo. Some of the relevant biochemical parameters would seem to be covered by studies of (i) growth rate and cell division; (ii) nucleic acid metabolism; (iii) the energetics of cellular processes; (iv) the elaboration and laying down of the structural elements in the cells.

This approach constitutes an extension of the search for the primary 'biochemical lesion' in toxicology (chapter 9) and in pathology.[156] This approach is the most promising for elucidating the nature of the teratogenic lesion in

[154] B. Bakay and W. L. Nyhan, *J. Pharmacol.*, 1968, **161**, 348.
[155] B. Bakay and W. L. Nyhan, *J. Pharmacol.*, 1970, **171**, 109.
[156] Ref. 73, pp. 1—170.

molecular terms. It is relevant that investigations made by Neubert *et al.*[157,158] are in line with the foregoing propositions. Embryotoxic effects have been found with (i) a dose of 6-aminonicotinamide, equivalent to one-half of that necessary to cause adverse signs in the dams; (ii) a dose of cyclophosphamide, equivalent to one-tenth to one twentieth of the dose causing severe harm to the mother; and (iii) thalidomide in sensitive species of animal at doses which are two orders of magnitude lower than those which adversely affect the dams. This illustrates the importance of attempting to identify the biochemical factor, which is essential for the production of embryotoxic effects in the case of thalidomide.

Accordingly, the effect of thalidomide has been investigated *in vitro*[157,158] on guinea-pig embryo protocollagen prolinhydroxylase,[159] which is a complicated mixed-function oxidase, and which was the most strongly inhibited enzyme by thalidomide of any of the enzyme systems that have been studied hitherto. Thalidomide produces a dose-dependent inhibition over a range of acceptably low concentrations, but no inhibition and increased enzyme activity at higher concentrations of (14). Thus, optimal inhibition is limited to a narrow range of (14) concentrations. The scheme is complicated further by the fact that optimal inhibition varies very considerably, depending on the concentration of such other factors as ascorbic acid, α-oxoglutarate, and Fe^{2+}. A considerable degree of variance was found with the iso-enzyme of different mammalian species and even with ones belonging to different embryonic tissues of the same species, and this suggests an extremely variable degree of sensitivity. Thus, a definite degree of inhibition depends critically on the concentration of (14), ascorbic acid, α-oxoglutarate, and Fe^{2+} as well as on the special iso-enzyme peculiarities. Were inhibition of this enzyme system to be connected with the teratogenic action of thalidomide, and this hypothesis seems to be attractive in the light of other findings[155] (*v. supra*), then it might be assumed that there would be a large degree of variability depending on the ratio of the various factors which have been explored. Further work may be necessary, possibly *in vivo*, to establish the mode of action of thalidomide (and of other embryotoxic substances).

The Cleft-palate Lesion.—Three strands of inter-related evidence have to do with the induction of cleft-palate in the progeny of treated females.[160—163]

(i) Where cleft-palate was produced through the administration *in utero* to a 13-day-old rat embryo of benzhydrylpiperazine analogues, the polyelectrolyte-binding capacity of cartilage may have been implicated.[160]

157 D. Neubert and S. Teske, in 'Sonderforschungsbereich 29: Embryonale Entwicklung und Differenzierung (Embryonal-Pharmacologie),' Freie Universitat, Berlin, Jahresbericht 1969/1970, pp. 203—206a.

158 D. Neubert, H.-J. Merker, E. Köhler, R. Krowke, and H. J. Barrach, in 'Advances in the Biosciences 6,' Schering Symposium on Intrinsic and Extrinsic Factors in Early Mammalian Development, Venice 1970, ed. G. Raspé, Pergamon Press-Vieweg, Oxford, 1971, pp. 576—621.

159 J. J. Hutton, A. L. Tappel, and S. Udenfriend, *Anal. Biochem.*, 1966, **16**, 384.

160 A. L. Wilk, A. J. Steffek, and C. T. G. King, *J. Pharmacol.*, 1970, **171**, 118.

161 F. C. Fraser, *Science*, 1967, **158**, 1603.

162 B. E. Walker and F. C. Fraser, *Embryol. Exp. Morphol.*, 1956, **4**, 176.

163 K. S. Larson, *Exp. Cell. Res.*, 1960, **21**, 498.

(ii) Fine dissection of the palate from 15—20-day-old rat embryos and their immediate incubation with [^{14}C]glucose *in vitro* showed[164] that where the antimetabolite, 6-aminonicotinamide (8 mg kg^{-1}), had been administered to the dams on day 15 of pregnancy, the uptake of ^{14}C (at 10 h) was very markedly diminished in the foetal lipids, RNA, mucopolysaccharides, DNA, and the structural proteins, but although some of these disturbed distributions normalized later (at 24 h) in the incubation period, there remained a significant arrest of the intermediates which contributed to the lipid and RNA fractions.

(iii) Whilst experiments[165] showed that aspirin, salicylate,[166–170] and the metal-chelating agent EDTA[171,172] were teratogenic in rats and that, unlike EDTA, neither aspirin nor salicylate disturbed the mineral excretion or foetal uptake, the authors[165] argued nevertheless that salicylate might bind minerals within the foeto-placental environment.

In (i), the binding of the nitrogenous bases as well as of Na^+ and Ca^{2+} account collectively for the cation-binding capacity of the cartilage, as all three ion types bind to the same sites. However, whether the benzhydrylpiperazine-teratogen binding to and altering of embryonal polyelectrolyte relates to the induction of cleft-palate by these drugs is obscure, although it would certainly have a significant effect on rapidly differentiating cartilage and therefore may account for the accompanying limb malformation.[160] In the case of cleft-palate, a gross rotational movement of the palatal shelves from the vertical to a horizontal plane precedes fusion,[161] and different sets of ideas are thought to account for events leading up to that rotation. Thus, according to one set,[162,163] a network of elastin fibres and the presence of sulphated mucopolysaccharide initiate rotation, but another set[161] implicates mechanical force and the straightening of the flexure of the cranial base. This work seems to imply that mucopolysaccharide might play a critical role, and any change therefore to this connective tissue component might impede or prevent rotation, and so inhibit closure of the palate.

In (ii), DNA synthesis was normal at 24 h in the incubation period. These results[164] are most interesting, and it would seem to be relevant to investigate what may happen in such experiments after the implantation of cortisone, which also causes cleft-palate.

In (iii), despite the *prima facie* interpretation of the experimental evidence,[165] the authors[165] considered that salicylate might well bind (or solvate with) the minerals concerned within the foeto-placental environment, thus reducing their availability, which in turn might be insufficient for the usual biochemistry of foetal development. [Structure–activity considerations eliminate many analogues and metabolites, and this seems to be another case (*v. supra*), where salicylic

164 K. Pielsticker and D. Neubert, ref. 157, pp. 226—229.
165 R. P. Koshakji and A. R. Schubert, *Biochem. Pharmacol.*, 1973, **22**, 407.
166 J. Warkany and E. Takacs, *Am. J. Pathol.*, 1959, **35**, 315.
167 K. S. Larson, H. Boström, and B. Ericson, *Acta Paediat.* (*Uppsala*), 1963, **52**, 36.
168 K. S. Larson, B. Ericson, and H. Boström, *Acta Morphol. Neerl.-Scand.*, 1964, **6**, 35.
169 E. Takacs and J. Warkany, *Teratology*, 1968, **1**, 109.
170 D. G. Trasler, *Lancet*, 1965, **i**, 109.
171 H. Tuchmann-Duplessis and L. Mercier-Parot, *C.R. Acad. Sci.*, 1956, **243**, 1064.
172 H. Sweneston and L. S. Hurley, *Science*, 1971, **173**, 62.

acid (in this instance) is structure-specific with regard to the teratogenic effect.]

An outstanding limitation on the investigation of the mode of action of a teratogen is the confirmation of whether in fact the biochemical disturbance that has been studied belongs to the causative mechanism for the teratogenic effects. Clearly, complication arises in this biological situation (i) from the time-scale of pregnancy, (ii) from intra-uterine development, and (iii) from the fact that defects in organogenesis are completely irreversible once the relatively short critical periods of time concerned have elapsed.

3 Mechanisms Not Specifically Related to Enzyme Inhibition

There is no ready overall correlation in the case of the chloroalkanes between activity, for example, the anaesthetic properties, and structure.

In fact, not unexpectedly,[44,173,174] chemical reactivity conforms with a separate relationship for each of the structural classes, RCH_2Cl, RCH_2Cl_2, and $RCCl_3$ and Salmon *et al.*[175] have given attention to electron densities, calculated by the MINDO/3 method, in molecules for which dechlorination data were available (see also ref. 176). Predictably, the reactivities of the structural types were significantly different: $RCHCl_2 \gg RCH_2Cl > RCCl_3$, and within the structural classes dechlorination showed a specificity consistent with enzyme-catalysed reaction processes. In the case of the reductive dechlorination of CCl_4, the toxic effects of the compound are believed to result from the dechlorination reaction which generates reactive radicals (*v. supra*) (chapter 9). Where this reaction process occurs, for example, in the case of hexachloroethane, this may give similar toxicity,[175] whereas dechlorination reaction processes for the $RCHCl_2$ and RCH_2Cl classes, where an H atom and a Cl atom reside on the same C atom, are not necessarily deleterious in this way, and the rate of dechlorination is unrelated to toxicity. It will be clear that the degree of toxicity depends on the types of intermediate produced, for example, by cytochrome P-450 mediated metabolism *in vivo*.[175,177] Thus, 1,1,1-trichloroethane is metabolized slowly by cytochrome P-450 *in vitro*,[177] it does not give reactive metabolites, and it is not mutagenic/carcinogenic, whereas 1,1,2-trichloroethane and 1,1,2,2-tetrachloroethane are metabolized more rapidly by cytochrome P-450 *in vitro* into acyl chlorides,[177] which are mutagenic and carcinogenic.[178–181]

In connection with the foregoing considerations concerning the halogenoalkanes, the volatile anaesthetic, halothane ($CF_3{\cdot}CHBrCl$) (*v. infra*), belongs to the $RCHX_2$ broad category, ethyl chloride and bromide to the RCH_2X

[173] R. O. Recknagel and E. A. Glende, *CRC Crit. Rev. Toxicol.* 1973, **2**, 263.
[174] G. Paulet, *Eur. J. Toxicol., Supplement*, 1976, **9**, 385.
[175] A. G. Salmon, R. B. Jones, and W. C. Mackrodt, *Xenobiotica*, 1981, **11**, 723.
[176] R. A. Van Dyke and C. G. Wineman, *Biochem. Pharmacol.*, 1971, **20**, 463.
[177] K. M. Ivanetich and L. H. van den Houert, *Carcinogenesis*, 1981, **2**, 697.
[178] S. Rosenkranz, *Environ. Health Perspect.*, 1977, **21**, 79.
[179] U. Rannug, A. Sundvall, and C. Ramel, *Chem.-Biol. Interact.*, 1978, **20**, 1.
[180] N.C.I. Bioassay of 1,1,2-trichloroethane for possible carcinogenicity, CAS No. 79-00-5, *Gov. Rep. Announc. Index*, 1978, **78**, 112.
[181] N.C.I. Bioassay of 1,1,2,2-tetrachloroethane for possible carcinogenicity, CAS No. 79-34-5. *Gov. Rep. Announc. Index*, 1978, **78**, 106.

category, and chloroform to the $RCCl_3$ category. These and other volatile anaesthetics, such as diethyl ether and nitrous oxide which are not halogenoalkanes, express their (anaesthetic) activity through a physico-chemical mechanism. Ferguson[182] noticed that the conditions in Meyer and Hemmi's experiments[183] with gaseous and volatile substances approximated to equilibrium conditions, as the animals were maintained for some time in a steady state of depression. Although the concentration of the anaesthetic in the biophase was not measured, the chemical potential in all of the phases would be the same at equilibrium, and thus the chemical potential in the biophase would be the same as that in the inhaled mixture of gases.

Now, chemical potential is defined as

$$\mu = \left(\frac{\partial G}{\partial n}\right)_{T,p}$$

where G is the Gibbs Free Energy, and n the number of molecules, and T and p, the temperature and pressure, are constant.

If the chemical potential in a standard state is μ_0, the chemical potential, μ, of this substance, which is present in the inhaled mixture with a partial pressure of p_t, would be

$$\mu = \mu_0 + RT \ln (p_t)$$

The value $RT \ln (p_t/p_s)$, where p_t is the partial pressure in the anaesthetic mixture and p_s the saturation vapour pressure of the compound at the temperature of the experiments, would indicate the difference in Gibbs Free Energy between the molecule in the standard state and the molecule in the biophase.

Whence, Ferguson[182] used the fraction p_t/p_s as an indication of the 'thermodynamic activity' of a particular compound, and he found that this fraction was relatively constant. Hence, the biological activity of these substances depends primarily on their thermodynamic activity, and this means that ΔG, the difference in Gibbs Free Energy between the standard and biologically active states, is approximately the same for most compounds, irrespective of the absolute values of G.

In the development of a new general anaesthetic, halothane, Suckling[184] made use of the more or less constant value of the fraction p_t/p_s. Fluorinated hydrocarbons, the Arctons and Freons, were used in refrigerators, and it was feasible to use them as non-inflammable, volatile anaesthetics. From the value of p_s for these compounds or even from their boiling points, he[184] was able to predict the value of p_t and thus the concentration which would effect narcosis.

Up to this stage, the discussion has concerned the compounds in the gaseous state, and it is more difficult to be very specific about the action of drugs in solution, where the chemical potential, μ, at the concentration, C, which produces depression may be defined by:

$$\mu = \mu_0 + RT \ln (aC)$$

[182] J. Ferguson, *Proc. Roy. Soc.*, 1939, **127B**, 387.
[183] K. H. Meyer and H. Hemmi, *Biochem. Z.*, 1935, **277**, 39.
[184] C. W. Suckling, *Br. J. Anaesthesia*, 1957, **29**, 466.

where *a* is the activity coefficient. The value of *a* in the gaseous phase, *i.e.* the fugacity, may be omitted (*v. supra*), but for substances in solution in the body fluids, the values for the activities are preferred to those for the concentrations, and there is considerable uncertainty about these values. However, a great deal of evidence[185] suggests that, in certain tissues, the actions of various unspecific and 'inert' molecules in solution may depend, as in the gas phase, on their thermodynamic activity, and thus may be dependent on chemical structure, but it is uncertain how this action is brought about.

Trialkyltin and Lead Neurotoxicity.—In mammals, acetoxytrialkyltins[186] and acetoxytrialkyl-leads[187] cause neuropathological lesions and behavioural changes. This is reminiscent of the structure–activity considerations relating to mammalian and fungicidal toxicities of the trialkyltins which have been attributed to the inverse interaction of their ionisations and lipophilicities, where the ionisation is the dominating parameter[188] (chapter 2). Thus, this mechanism is clearly unrelated to enzyme inhibition, there being no suspicion of receptor involvement.

Calcium Oxalate Irritational Nephrotoxicity.—Several disparate types of industrial chemical appear to cause nephrotoxicity in mammals and, in this connection, there might be mentioned butadiene, cyclopentadiene, diethylene glycol, ethylene glycol and its commercially important esters, as well as propane-1,3-diol. The microsomal metabolism of butadiene (18) has been investigated,[189] and this is very interesting, because of the chemical capacity of (18) for 1,4-addition. However, neither butane-1,4-diol (19) nor but-2-ene-1,2-diol (20) was formed,

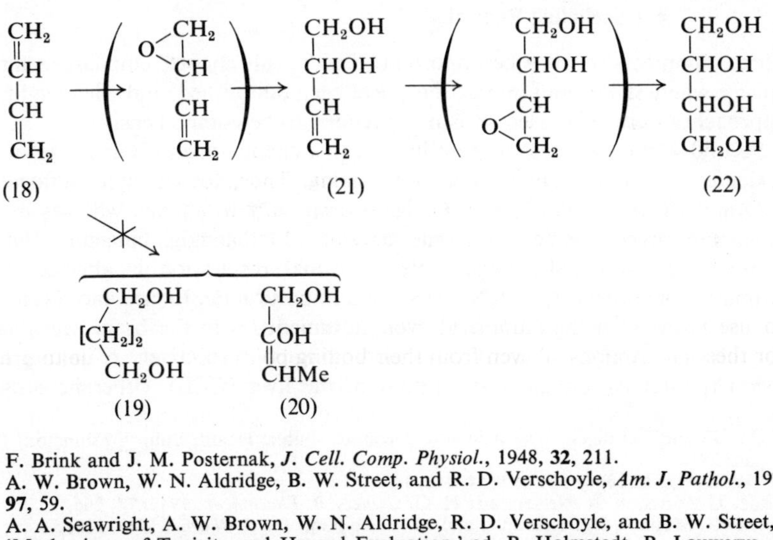

(18) (21) (22)

(19) (20)

[185] F. Brink and J. M. Posternak, *J. Cell. Comp. Physiol.*, 1948, **32**, 211.
[186] A. W. Brown, W. N. Aldridge, B. W. Street, and R. D. Verschoyle, *Am. J. Pathol.*, 1979, **97**, 59.
[187] A. A. Seawright, A. W. Brown, W. N. Aldridge, R. D. Verschoyle, and B. W. Street, in 'Mechanisms of Toxicity and Hazard Evaluation,' ed. B. Holmstedt, R. Lauwerys, M. Mercier, and M. Roberfroid, Elsevier North-Holland Biomedical Press, Amsterdam, 1980, pp. 71—74.
[188] D. E. Hathway, *Chem.-Biol. Interact.*, 1982, **42**, 1.
[189] W. P. Herschleb and K. C. Leibman, *Fed. Proc.*, 1972, **31**, 559.

but the products were but-3-ene-1,2-diol (21) and 1,2,3,4-tetrahydroxybutane (22), presumably a mixture of erythritol and threitol. Thus, in microsomal oxygenation, the two olefinic groups of (18) behave independently.[189] It is feasible that one of the products might be expected to undergo further degradation to yield a very small proportion of the well-known kidney irritant, oxalic acid.

In general, only those polyols which give rise to oxalic acid or malonic acid seem to be nephrotoxic. Thus, of a dose of ethylene glycol, perhaps only 2% is excreted as oxalic acid.[190] Bladder stones from rats, given 2% of ethylene glycol in their diet for 2 years, contain 80% of calcium oxalate,[191,192] and both ethylene glycol and its ester acetate afford calcium oxalate in the renal tubules and cause haematuria,[193] but oral administration of sodium oxalate is alleged[194] not to invoke nephrotoxicity. It is evident that where ethylene glycol is dosed chemically to animals, the consequent nephrotoxicity seems to be due, at least in part, to oxalic acid formation. Another possibility may be glyoxal.

Diethylene glycol, $HO_2CH_2CH_2OCH_2CH_2OH$, also affords oxalic acid, and is nephrotoxic,[195] whereas triethylene glycol, $HO_2CH_2CH_2OCH_2CH_2OCH_2CH_2OH$ is much less toxic, and carbitol, $EtOCH_2CH_2OCH_2CH_2OH$ is excreted principally as the glucuronide.[196] In the case of the triols, propane-1,2-diol participates in intermediary metabolism and produces no effects, but propane-1,3-diol gives malonic acid[197,198] which is nephrotoxic through the analogous formation of calcium malonate. Glycerol is a glycogen precursor *in vivo* and, amongst the tetraols, erythritol and threitol are excreted largely unchanged.

4 Concluding Remarks

Three comments seem to be important. Firstly, this chapter emphasizes mechanisms where the overall interactions have been established, and where valuable approaches have been used. It is not intended to be comprehensive.

Secondly, the mechanisms described in this chapter span a fair range of the toxicities encountered in toxicological testing. Thus, for example, suffocation (CO and CO_2) through lack of O_2 leads eventually to anoxia, whereas in O_2-poisoning, hyperoxemic symptoms develop. Methaemoglobinaemia (NO_2^-, aniline, *etc.*) is readily diagnosable. Terminal respiration is affected, with dramatic consequences, by CN^-, HS^-, and fluoroacetate. Interference (Telodrin and dieldrin) with the citric acid cycle intermediates in the brain precipitates convulsions. Actions akin to O_2-poisoning cause respectively a unique lung lesion (paraquat) and fatty infiltration of the liver (CCl_4). Other hepatogens

[190] W. F. von Oettingen, 'The Aliphatic Alcohols,' Public Health Bull., Washington, 1943, no. 281.
[191] W. Doerr, *Virchows Arch.*, 1944, **313**, 137.
[192] H. J. Morris, A. A. Nelson, and H. O. Calvery, *J. Pharmacol.*, 1942, **74**, 266.
[193] M. G. Mulinos, L. Pomerantz, and M. E. Loijkin, *Am. J. Pharm.*, 1943, **115**, 51.
[194] W. Doerr, *Sitzungsber. Akad. Wiss. Heidelberg, Math. Naturwiss. Kl.*, 1949, **7**, 112 pp.
[195] O. G. Fitzhugh and A. A. Nelson, *J. Ind. Hygiene.*, 1946, **28**, 40.
[196] J. K. Fellows, F. P. Luduena, and P. J. Hanzlik, *J. Pharmacol.*, 1947, **89**, 210.
[197] J. Scholz, *Klin. Wochenschr.*, 1950, **28**, 69.
[198] W. van Winkle, *J. Pharmacol.*, 1941, **72**, 227.

include CS_2 and the phosphorodithionates. Action on the c.n.s. affects neuro-humoral transmission (organophosphates and carbamates), and causes anaesthesia (the chloroalkanes including halothane) and neurotoxic effects (trialkyltins and trialkyl-leads). Disturbance of the haematopoietic system (benzene) leads eventually to the induction of leukaemia. Vesication and erythema of the skin are caused by the War gases. Anti-coagulatives (warfarin and 4-hydroxycoumarin rodenticides) produce haemorrhagic episodes. Uncoupling agents, such as DNOC, cause fever (chapter 5). Finally, teratogenicity is provoked by thalidomide (arrested limb-budding) and by salicylate, cortisone, *etc.* (cleft palate). Thirdly, in the second part of the chapter, receptors do not seem to be involved (i) in the neurotoxic effects of acetoxytrialkyltins (chapter 2) and acetoxytrialkyl-leads; (ii) in the nephrotoxicity of some simple aliphatic compounds; and (iii) in the anaesthesia caused by chloroalkanes, halothane, and some other compounds, which can be explained in terms of the 'thermodynamic activity' of the molecules themselves.

Part VI
Chemical Carcinogenesis

Chapter 10 Importance of Chemical Non-enzymic Reactions *in vivo*

1 Introduction

Evidence, derived from the fate of selected drugs and pesticides, attests that mechanistically and kinetically favoured (non-enzymic) chemical reaction processes compete and interact with biochemical reactions *in vivo*, and so contribute to the overall metabolism of these foreign compounds in mammals. The fact that chemical reactions play a very considerable role in chemical carcinogenesis is illustrated by: (i) the rearrangement of reactive halogenoalkene epoxide metabolites; (ii) the activation of some $HOH_2C{\cdot}NMe{\cdot}N{=}R$, $HOH_2C{\cdot}NH{\cdot}NMeR'$, and $R''N(OH){\cdot}C(O)Me$ systems; and (iii) the reaction of ultimate chemical carcinogens with nucleic acid through both mono- and bi-molecular mechanisms.

Whilst the tacit assumption is made that foreign compound metabolism in mammals is brought about through the operation of biochemical reactions, and the demonstration of enzyme-catalysed mechanisms both for foreign compound and intermediary metabolism strongly supports this supposition, consideration of the literature on drug and pesticide metabolism[1] showed that some metabolites of notable compounds were extremely unlikely to result from biotransformations alone.[2] Nevertheless, such products, which may be detected by their unusual structure and by the unlikelihood of their arising from

[1] 'Foreign Compound Metabolism in Mammals,' ed. D. E. Hathway, Specialist Periodical Reports, The Royal Society of Chemistry, London, 1970—1981, vols. 1—6.
[2] D. E. Hathway, *Chem. Soc. Rev.*, 1980, **9(1)**, 63.

enzyme-catalysed reactions, might be generated by mechanistically and kinetically favoured (non-enzymic) chemical reaction processes, consistent with the prevailing physiological conditions. It ought to be clearly stated at the beginning of this chapter that many of the reaction steps in the schemes that follow (*q.v.*) should be regarded as speculative or reasonable chemical possibilities, and that these steps, for which there is no direct supporting experimental evidence, are marked with an asterisk. Another caveat is that, despite the chapter heading, the substances mentioned in the first five paragraphs, *viz.*(1)—(19), are *not* carcinogens, and their inclusion is meant to exemplify (*v. supra*) the underlying concept concerned.

For example, in the mammalian metabolism of hydralazine, 1-hydrazinophthalazine (1) (Scheme 1), it is suggested[2] that the product of bioacetylation,

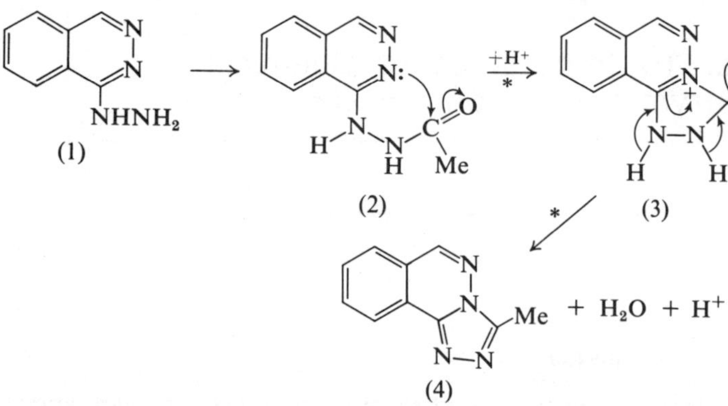

Scheme 1

1-(2-acetylhydrazino)phthalazine (2) undergoes simultaneously proton-induced enolization of the acetyl C═O and ring-closure followed by proton loss plus loss of the elements of water [(2)→(4)]. This reaction sequence accounts for methyl-*s*-triazolo[3,4-*a*]phthalazine (4); bioacetylation of (1) is rate-limiting *in vivo*.

Similarly, the human metabolism of proguanil (5) (Scheme 2) into the ten times more powerful dihydro-*s*-triazine anti-malarial (8) was considered[2] to proceed by elimination of the elements of water from the cytochrome P-450 mediated (ω-1) oxidation product (6) *via* the cyclic mechanism represented, followed by reverse cyclization of the bonds with ring-closure (7). Alternatively, although less likely in the author's opinion, attack by oxirene at the (ω-1) site of (5), followed by a rather similar elimination of the elements of water from (6′) to that postulated in the previous mechanism, would eventually lead to (8) through reverse cyclization of the bonds with ring-closure.

Again, in connection with trifluralin (9; R = Pr^n), profluralin (9; R = cyclopropylmethyl), and fluchloralin (9; R = CH_2CH_2Cl) (Scheme 3), which afford a common *N*-dealkylation product (10) and another metabolite (11) with a reduced nitro group, it is reasonable to suppose that (11) might be the starting material for benzimidazole (15) biosynthesis; whence, cytochrome P-450

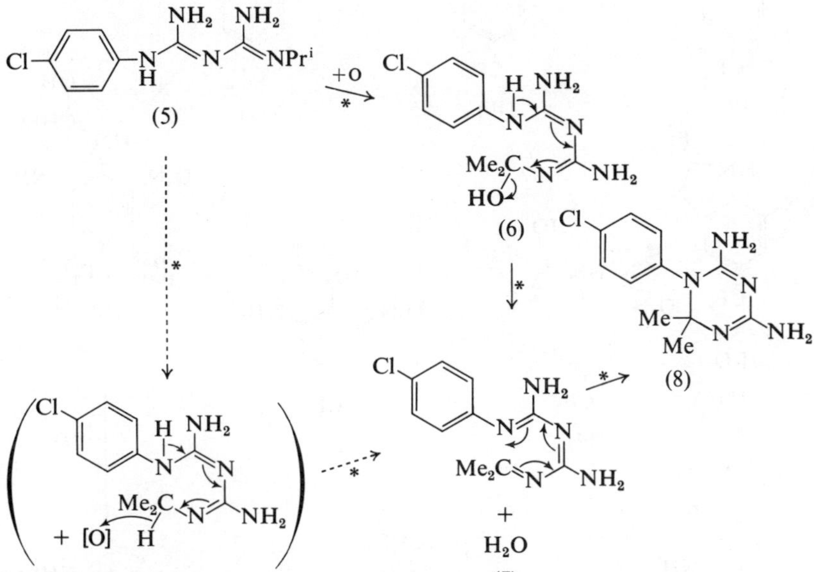

Scheme 2

oxidation of (11) would yield a reaction intermediate (12) and ring-closure of the corresponding amide (13) oxidation product, rather than of (12) *per se* which would have led [(12)→(a)→(b)] to the dihydrobenzimidazole derivative (15) itself *via* dehydration of the *gem*-hydroxy reaction intermediate (14). This appears to be the preferred mechanism, although enzymic dehydrogenation of (c) cannot be ruled out. Another unusual metabolite of (9; R = CH_2CH_2Cl), the quinoxaline (19), might be derived by nitro-reductase (17) from the known metabolite (16), followed by loss of the elements of HCl with ring-closure to give (18) and then by aromatization.

The chemical reactions that are represented in Schemes 1–3 account for the origin and orientation of the unusual metabolites, and predictions for the kinetics are matched by the corresponding product analyses. All of these simple chemical steps would be expected to occur under gentle reaction conditions which are consistent with the *in vivo* situation. Furthermore, in those examples where the purely chemical reactions yielding some of the metabolites of a particular drug are quite distinct from the biochemical ones leading to other metabolic products, only the corresponding proportions of the latter were found[2] to be altered through the induction and inhibition of the hepatic drug-metabolizing enzymes in the living animal.

The scientific basis of each suspected contribution of chemical reactions to foreign compound metabolism needs to be judged in its own right and, for example, the alleged tautomerism of 2-naphthylamine (20) in aqueous solution to afford a small proportion of the imino form (21),[3] which is supposed

[3] L. L. Poulsen, B. S. S. Masters, and D. M. Ziegler, *Xenobiotica*, 1976, **6**, 481.

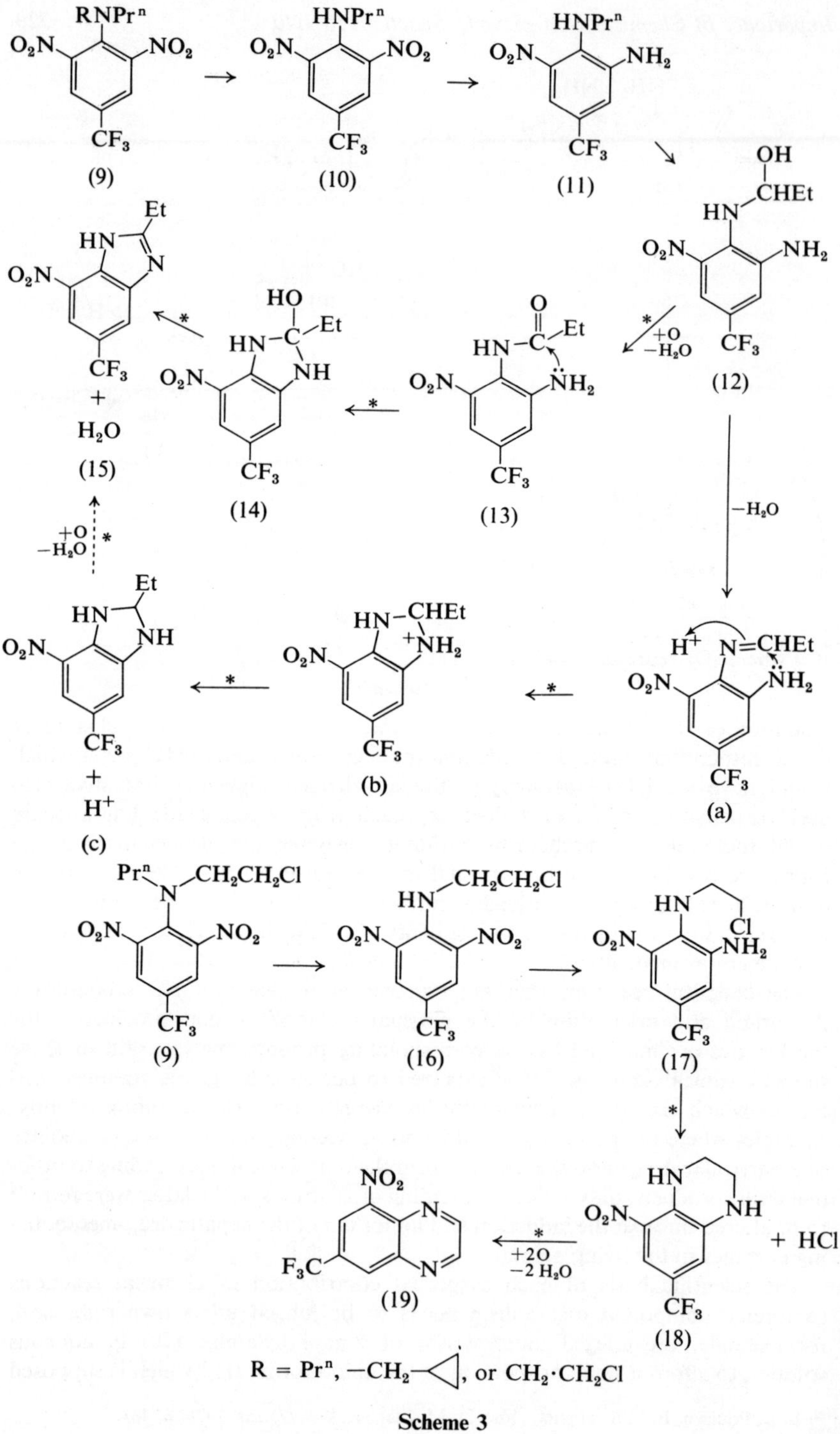

Scheme 3

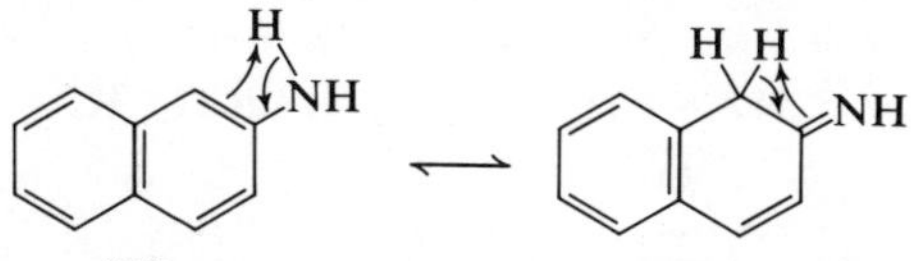

(20) (21)

to account[3] for the action of flavoprotein oxidase on (20), but not on the isomeric 1-naphthylamine, seems to be superfluous. A considerable difference in basicity between 1- and 2-naphthylamines (*inter al.* Guha and Zahradnik[4]) correlates with the conjugative effect of the unsubstituted nucleus (Robinson's[5] inductive effect) and facilitates delocalization of the lone pair of electrons on the N-atom of 1-naphthylamine. In the author's opinion, the oxidase preference for (20) is likely to correspond to an enzyme specificity for a substrate with the dissociation properties of that amine. In any case, the aromaticity of the unsubstituted aromatic nucleus would act against enamine–imino tautomerism[6] in the other nucleus of 2-naphthylamine.

Chemical reaction processes *in vivo* are nowhere more important than in the field of cancer mechanisms, and the possibility that they may contribute to this subject has been implied occasionally before. Such illustration arises out of the investigation (*inter al.* Ross[7]) of chemical reactivity in relation to the carcinogenic potential of direct alkylating agents such as mustard gas [bis(2-chloroethyl) sulphide], nitrogen mustard HN2 [bis(2-chloroethyl)methylamine], dimethyl sulphate, ethyl and methyl methanesulphonates, β-propiolactone, glycidol, and phosphates such as cyclophosphamide, which implies that these substances react *in vivo* in much the same way as they do *in vitro*. However, it now seems unlikely that the full implications of the occurrence *in vivo* of chemical reaction processes as distinct from biochemical ones were appreciated, even in those cases.[7] In fact (non-enzymic) chemical reaction processes are involved, for example, (i) with the rearrangement of the reactive halogenoepoxide metabolites of the halogenoalkenes; (ii) with the activation, for example, of the oxidation products of dimethylnitrosamine (DMN), 3,3-dimethyl-1-(2,4,6-trichlorophenyl)triazene, and 1,2-dimethylhydrazine, as well as of *N*-acetyl-2-fluorenylhydroxylamine; and (iii) with the reaction of ultimate carcinogens and nucleic acid. Thus it will be evident that they play a very considerable role in the mechanisms of chemical carcinogenesis.

2 Rearrangement of Reactive Halogenoalkene Epoxides

Vinyl chloride-derived chloroethylene oxide (22) or its rearrangement product, chloroacetaldehyde (23) (Scheme 4), reacts with calf-thymus DNA at pH 4.5 to give a modified DNA which afforded amongst the products of enzymic

[4] S. Guha and R. Zahradnik, *Coll. Czech. Chem. Commun.*, 1967, **32**, 2448.
[5] R. Robinson, 'Outline of an electrochemical (electronic) theory of the course of organic reactions,' The Institute of Chemistry of Great Britain and Ireland, London, 1932.
[6] J. W. Baker, 'Tautomerism,' George Routledge and Sons, London, 1934, pp. 121—125.
[7] W. C. J. Ross, 'Biological Alkylating Agents,' Butterworths, London, 1962.

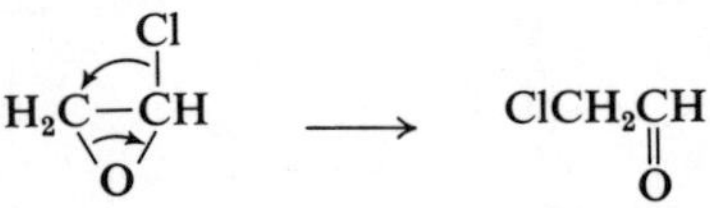

(22) (23)

hydrolysis 9-(β-D-2′-deoxyribofuranosyl)imidazo[2,1-*i*]purine ('etheno-deoxyadenosine') and 1-(β-D-2′-deoxyribofuranosyl)imidazo[1,2-*c*]pyrimidin-2(1*H*)-one ('etheno-deoxycytidine') (chapters 10 and 11); these were also identified in the enzymic hydrolysates of the modified DNA extracted from the liver of rats that had been exposed long-term to vinyl chloride in their drinking water.[8]

Irrespective of whether [1-^{14}C]dichloroethylene (vinylidene dichloride) or [1-^{14}C]chloroacetic acid (26) was administered to rats,[10] 1 mol equiv. of the resulting [1-^{14}C]thiodiglycolic acid (27) yielded by electrolysis *ca.* 1 mol equiv. of $^{14}CO_2$, which is interpreted in terms of the labelling of one of the carboxylic acid groups of (27).[9] This is consistent with the transformation of dichloroethylene oxide (24) into (26) by a mechanism which involved migration of one Cl atom and loss of the other, and this obtains only where the halogenoalkene is converted into the corresponding halogenoepoxide (24), which rearranges into chloroacetyl chloride (25).

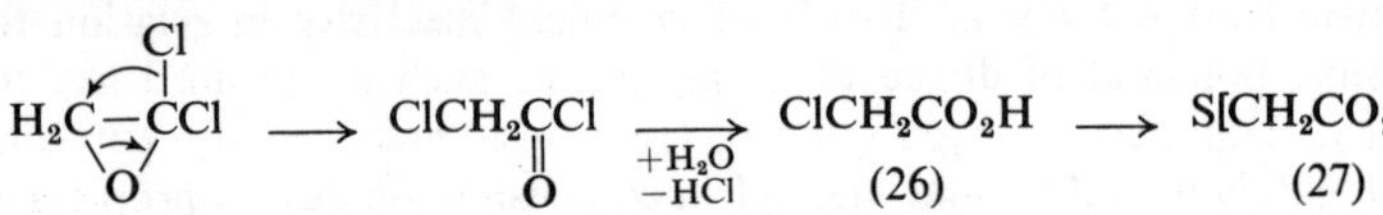

(24) (25) (26) (27)

Scheme 4

In both of these cases (Scheme 4), the rearrangement of the biochemically generated halogenoepoxide is a chemical reaction process, and the rearrangement products form sequences with those from complex series of subsequent biochemical reactions.[10–13]

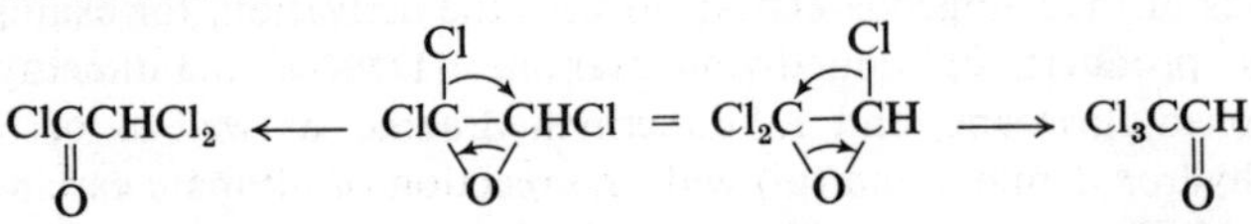

(29) (28) (30)

Scheme 5

The fact that chloral (30) (Scheme 5) is the authenticated rearrangement product of 1,1,2-trichloroethylene-derived 1,1,2-trichloroethylene oxide (28) *in vivo*, although in aqueous solution *in vitro* dichloroacetyl chloride (29)-derived dichloroacetic acid is formed exclusively, suggested to Hathway[14] that

[8] T. Green and D. E. Hathway, *Chem.-Biol. Interact.*, 1978, **22**, 211.
[9] G. H. Walker and D. E. Hathway, *Biochem. J.*, 1977, **167**, 505.
[10] B. K. Jones and D. E. Hathway, *Chem.-Biol. Interact.*, 1978, **20**, 27.
[11] T. Green and D. E. Hathway, *Chem.-Biol. Interact.*, 1975, **11**, 545.
[12] T. Green and D. E. Hathway, *Chem.-Biol. Interact.*, 1977, **17**, 137.
[13] B. K. Jones and D. E. Hathway, *Br. J. Cancer*, 1978, **37**, 411.
[14] D. E. Hathway, *Cancer Lett.*, 1979, **8(3)**, 263.

the usual rearrangement of (28) into (30) *in vivo* may occur in hepatocyte smooth endoplasmic reticulum (SER) in contact with a catalytic site simulating a Lewis acid (a haem prosthetic group). Fast cytosol biotransformation of (30) would facilitate its egress from the SER. In mice, on the other hand, rearrangement of (28) into (30) seems to be hindered, as in that species the greater cytochrome P-450 activity in the liver and kidneys would accelerate epoxidation and saturate sites for rearrangement, and there would also be a tendency towards the lower activity of the murine cytosol enzymes, responsible for (30) disposition, to become rate-limiting. Under these circumstances, (30) would accumulate, and with continuing formation of (28), some of it might be transformed at the cytosol surface into (29). Identification of some dichloroacetic acid in the presence of a large amont of trichloroacetic acid in the urine of 1,1,2-trichloroethylene-treated mice strongly supports the foregoing concept (*v. supra*) of a spill-over model for 1,1,2-trichloroethylene metabolism in mice.[14] Of the theoretically possible mechanisms of rearrangement for (28), that involving migration of hydrogen is unlikely,[15,16] and the one leading to (29) through rearrangement of Cl, which involves CO heterolysis and implicates a carbonium ion destabilized by a directly bound Cl-atom, is preferred, although a synchronous mechanism[17] cannot be entirely excluded. The less favoured rearrangement of (28) into (30) proceeds through a carbonium ion with two directly bound Cl atoms.

3 Chemical Activation of $HOH_2C.NMe.N{=}R$, $HOH_2C.NH.NMeR'$ and $R''N(OH).C(O)Me$ Systems

In the case of the indirectly acting dimethylnitrosamine (31) (Scheme 6), derivation of the reactive form (33) has been considered[18] to proceed by elimination

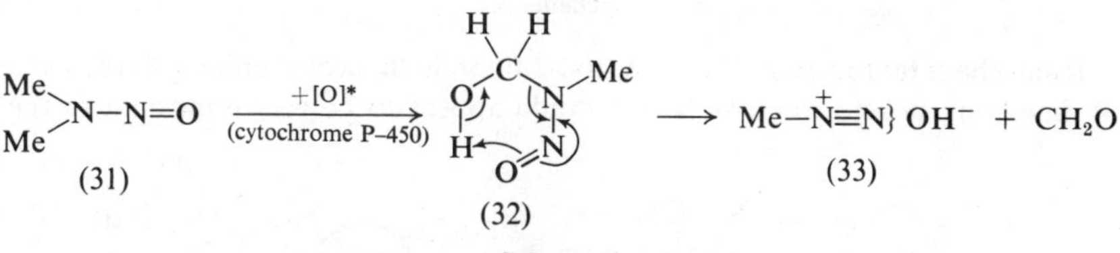

Scheme 6

of the elements of formaldehyde from the cytochrome P-450 mediated ω oxidation product (32) *via* the cyclic mechanism represented. The same reactive form (33) would appear to be generated by: (i) similar elimination of the elements of formaldehyde from the cytochrome P-450 mediated ω oxidation product (35) (Scheme 7) of 3,3-dimethyl-1-(2,4,6-trichlorophenyl)triazene (34) *via* the cyclic

15 R. N. McDonald and R. N. Steppel, *J. Am. Chem. Soc.*, 1969, **91**, 782.
16 K. Griesbaum, R. Kibar, and B. Pfeffer, *Annalen*, 1975, 214.
17 G. Köbich, J. Grosser, and W. Werner, *Chem. Ber.*, 1973, **106**, 2610.
18 H. Bartsch, G. P. Marginson, C. Malaveille, A. M. Camus, G. Brun, J. M. Margison, G. F. Kolar, and M. Wiessler, *Arch. Toxikol.*, 1977, **39**, 51.

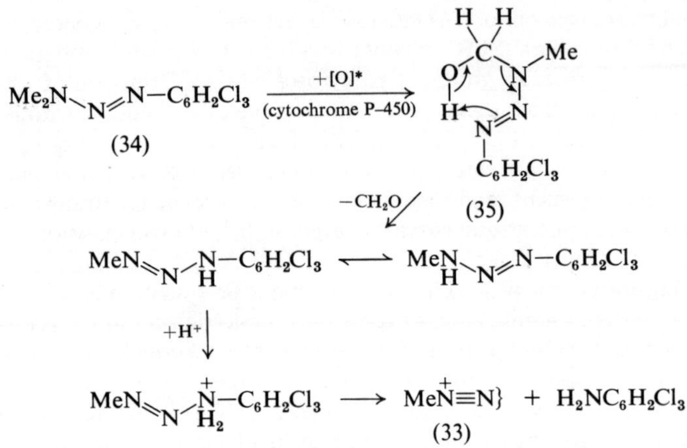

Scheme 7

mechanism represented, and (ii) proton loss plus loss of the elements of formaldehyde from the cytochrome P-450 mediated oxidation product (37) (Scheme 8) of 1,2-dimethylhydrazine (36), again through the cyclic mechanism that is shown.

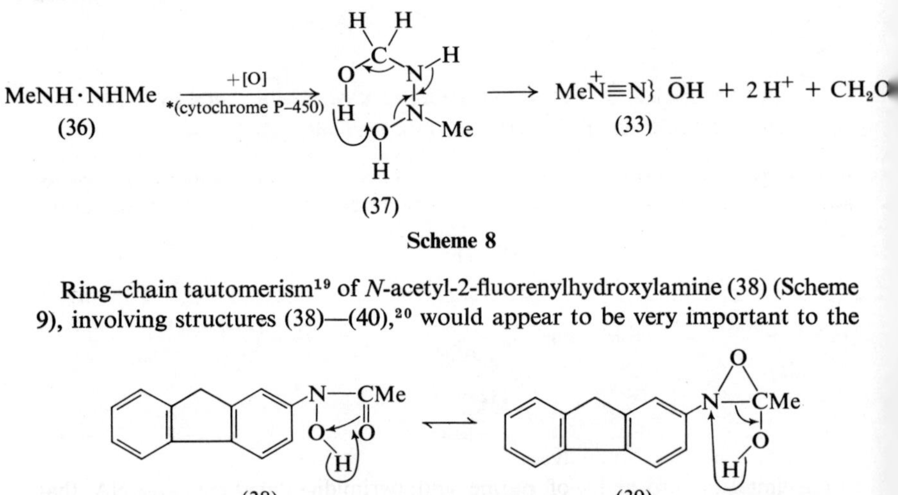

Scheme 8

Ring–chain tautomerism[19] of *N*-acetyl-2-fluorenylhydroxylamine (38) (Scheme 9), involving structures (38)—(40),[20] would appear to be very important to the

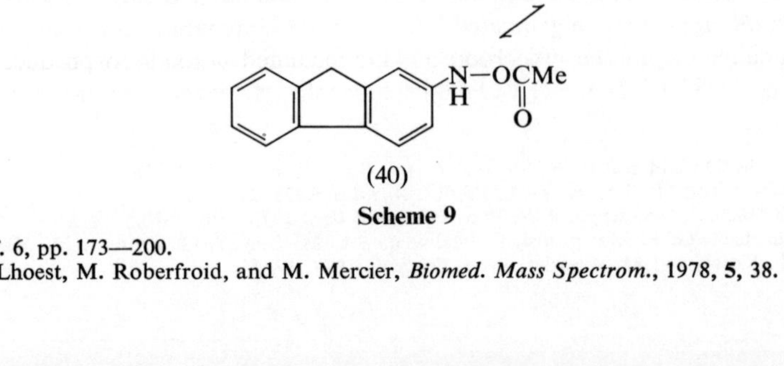

Scheme 9

[19] Ref. 6, pp. 173—200.

[20] G. Lhoest, M. Roberfroid, and M. Mercier, *Biomed. Mass Spectrom.*, 1978, **5**, 38.

further activation of the *N*-hydroxylation product[21] of the indirectly acting 2-fluorenylacetamide (2-AAF) bladder carcinogen.

4 Reaction of Ultimate Chemical Carcinogens and Nucleic Acid

Formation of the same product (*v. supra*), by reaction of vinyl chloride-derived chloroethylene oxide (22) or its rearrangement product, chloroacetaldehyde (23) (see Scheme 4), with DNA *in vitro*[8] and of vinyl chloride with rat-liver DNA *in vivo*,[8] implied a common reaction mechanism. In both of these cases, initial alkylation would occur at the most nucleophilic ring-nitrogen [N-1 of the deoxyadenosine residues (41) (Scheme 10) and N-3 of the deoxycytidine ones],

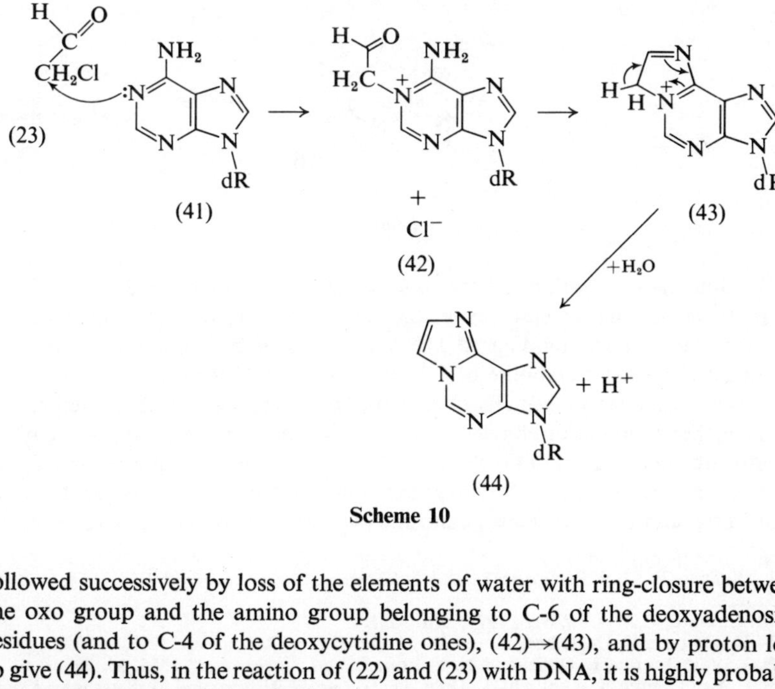

Scheme 10

followed successively by loss of the elements of water with ring-closure between the oxo group and the amino group belonging to C-6 of the deoxyadenosine residues (and to C-4 of the deoxycytidine ones), (42)→(43), and by proton loss to give (44). Thus, in the reaction of (22) and (23) with DNA, it is highly probable that an S_N2 reaction is involved.

The imidazo-cyclization of purine and pyrimidine residues in DNA that has been established for vinyl chloride *in vivo*[8] (Scheme 10) appears to be an important biochemical lesion. Thus, for example glycidaldehyde, which contains both an aldehyde and an alkylating function, reacts with deoxyguanosine at weakly alkaline pH to effect imidazo-cyclization between the N-1 position and the C-2 amino group.[22,23] Whilst Van Duuren *et al.*[23] did not identify their product and proposed the alternative formulae (A) and (B) (Scheme 11), irrespective of the

[21] J. A. Miller, J. W. Cramer, and E. C. Miller, *Cancer Res.*, 1960, **20**, 950.
[22] B. M. Goldschmidt, T. P. Balzej, and B. L. Van Duuren, *Tetrahedron Lett.*, 1968, 1583.
[23] B. L. Van Duuren, *Ann. N.Y. Acad. Sci.*, 1969, **163**, 633.

exact structure, bimolecular alkylation at the ring-nitrogen would appear to take place initially (Scheme 11). In this connection, imidazo-cyclization would seem to account for glycidaldehyde mutagenicity[24–26] and carcinogenicity[27–30] and possibly for the carcinogenicity in rodents of glycidyl esters.[31]

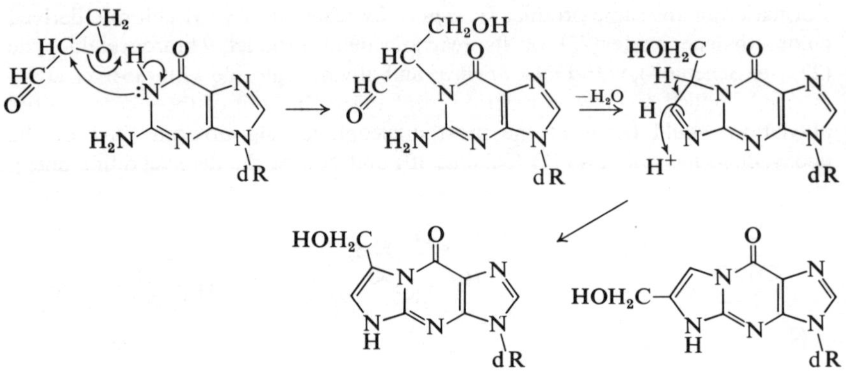

(A) (B)

Scheme 11

The imidazo-cyclization of the purine and pyrimidine residues of DNA attributable to chloroacetaldehyde and chloroethylene oxide[8] would account also for the covalent binding to DNA that has been found for the reactive bromoacetaldehyde metabolite of 1,2-dibromoethane[32] as well as for the mutagenicity[33–37] and carcinogenicity in rodents[38] observed for 1,2-dibromoethane.

In another connotation, however, the reactive form of the naturally occurring hepatocarcinogen safrole (45) (Scheme 12), *viz.* safrole 1′-sulphate (46), reacts both *in vitro* and *in vivo* with deoxyguanosine residues of target-organ DNA to afford O^6-(isosafrol-3′-yl)deoxyguanosine (47), which was characterized both by

24 J. McCann, E. Choi, E. Yamasaki, and B. N. Ames, *Proc. Natl. Acad. Sci., USA*, 1975, **72**, 5135.
25 M. C. Izard, *C.R. Acad. Sci.*, 1973, **276**, 3037.
26 T. H. Corbett, C. Heidelberger, and W. F. Dove, *Mol. Pharmacol.*, 1970, **6**, 667.
27 B. L. Van Duuren, L. Orris, and N. Nelson, *J. Natl. Cancer Inst.*, 1965, **35**, 707.
28 B. L. Van Duuren, L. Langseth, L. Orris, G. Teebor, N. Nelson, and M. Kuschner, *J. Natl. Cancer Inst.*, 1966, **37**, 825.
29 B. L. Van Duuren, L. Langseth, L. Orris, M. Baden, and M. Kuschner, *J. Natl. Cancer Inst.*, 1967, **39**, 1213.
30 B. L. Van Duuren, L. Langseth, B. M. Goldschmidt, and L. Orris, *J. Natl. Cancer Inst.*, 1967, **39**, 1217.
31 D. Swern, R. Wieder, M. McDonogh, D. R. Meranze, and M. B. Shimkin, *Cancer Res.*, 1970, **30**, 1037.
32 D. L. Hill, T.-W. Shih, T. P. Johnston, and R. F. Struck, *Cancer Res.*, 1978, **38**, 2438.
33 B. N. Ames, *Chem. Mutagens*, 1971, **1**, 267.
34 H. Brem, A. B. Stein, and H. S. Rosenkranz, *Cancer Res.*, 1974, **34**, 2576.
35 W. Buselmaier, G. Röhrborn, and P. Propping, *Mutat. Res.*, 1973, **21**, 25.
36 R. B. Cumming and M. F. Walton, *Food Cosmet. Toxicol.*, 1973, **11**, 547.
37 H. V. Malling and H. V. De Serres, *Genetics*, 1969, **61**, 39.
38 W. A. Olson, R. T. Habermann, E. K. Weisburger, J. M. Ward, and J. H. Weisburger, *J. Natl. Cancer Inst.*, 1973, **51**, 1973.

n.m.r. spectroscopy[39] and by mild acid degradation yielding 3′-hydroxyisosafrole (48).[40] The reaction between the reactive safrole (45) metabolite, (46), which is a benzylic ester, and the deoxyguanosine residues of DNA (*v. supra*) is most appropriately described by the S_N1 mechanism that is shown in Scheme 12.

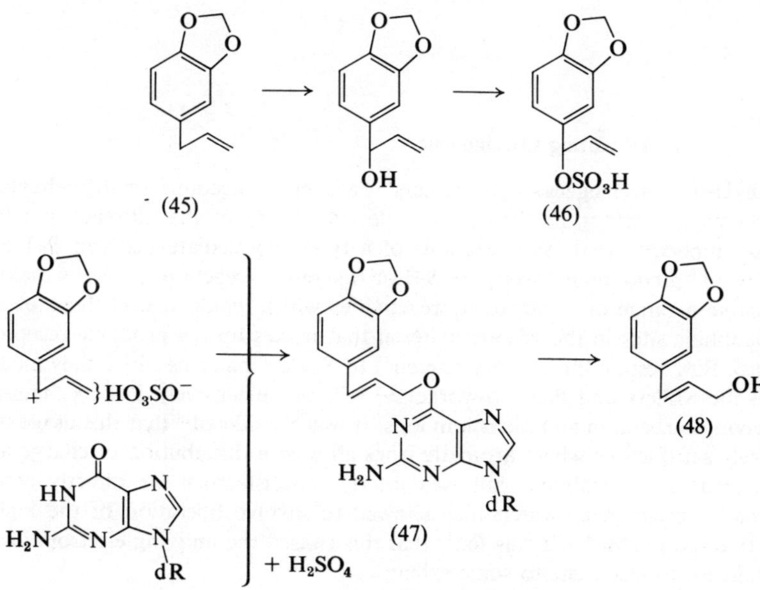

Scheme 12

[39] P. Borchert, P. G. Wislocki, J. A. Miller, and E. C. Miller, *Cancer Res.*, 1973, **33**, 575.
[40] P. G. Wislocki, P. Borchert, J. A. Miller, and E. C. Miller, *Cancer Res.*, 1976, **36**, 1686.

Chapter 11 Possible Mechanisms of Carcinogenesis and their Biological Significance

1 Alkylating Carcinogens

Methylating Carcinogens.—The Millers'[1,2] attempt to account for the behaviour of chemical carcinogens through the electrophilicity of the ultimate, reactive forms implied[2–4] that 'S_N2 reactions of a type intermediate between S_N1 and S_N2 would predominate over pure S_N1 or free radical reactions', thereby making available a range of electrophilic reactivities which would match those of the nucleophilic sites in the genetic material that makes up the probable receptors *in vivo*. But, despite this cursory reference to S_N2 mechanisms which they made,[2] both the Millers and their co-workers[1,2,5–14] used extensively S_N1 mechanisms involving carbenium and nitrenium ions. It was considered[15] that this usage was entirely satisfactory where aromatic rings allowed a distribution of charge and conferred cation stability, but was utterly unsatisfactory for directly acting aliphatic carcinogens, which they showed to involve liberation of the highly reactive species Me^+.[2] It was felt[15] that this caused the unifying electrophilicity principle[1,2] to lose caste to some extent.

There are two groups of direct-acting methylating carcinogens. On the one hand, there are the non-nitrogen containing dimethyl sulphate (DMS), methyl methanesulphonate (MMS), and the methyl halides, which show low electrophilic reactivity, and which are typical Ingold S_N2 reagents where the transferable alkyl group is bonded through oxygen, sulphur, *etc.*; the values of the Swain–Scott substrate constants (s) are relatively high (for MMS, $s = 0.83$).[16]

On the other hand, other direct-acting methylating carcinogens such as *N*-methyl-*N*-nitrosourea (MNU), *N*-methyl-*N*′-nitrosoguanidine (MNNG), and

1 J. A. Miller, *Cancer Res.*, 1970, **30**, 559.
2 J. A. Miller and E. C. Miller, *J. Nat. Cancer Inst.*, 1971, **47**, v.
3 C. C. Price, *Ann. N. Y. Acad. Sci.*, 1958, **68**, 663.
4 C. C. Price, G. M. Gaucher, P. Koneru, R. Shibakawa, J. R. Sowa, and M. Yomaguchi, *Ann. N. Y. Acad. Sci.*, 1969, **163**, 593.
5 J. G. Westra, E. Kriek, and H. Hittenhausen, *Chem.-Biol. Interact.*, 1976, **15**, 149.
6 E. Kriek, J. A. Miller, U. Juhl, and E. C. Miller, *Biochemistry*, 1967, **6**, 177.
7 E. Kriek, *Chem.-Biol. Interact.*, 1969, **1**, 1.
8 P. D. Lotikar, J. D. Scribner, J. A. Miller, and E. C. Miller, *Life Sci.*, 1966, **5**, 1263.
9 J.-K. Lin, J. A. Miller, and E. C. Miller, *Cancer Res.*, 1975, **35**, 844.
10 J. A. Miller and E. C. Miller, *Prog. Exp. Tumor Res.*, 1969, **11**, 273.
11 J. D. Scribner, J. A. Miller, and E. C. Miller, *Biochem. Biophys. Res. Commun.*, 1965, **20**, 560.
12 L. A. Poirier, J. A. Miller, E. C. Miller, and K. Sato, *Cancer Res.*, 1967, **27**, 1600.
13 J.-K. Lin, J. A. Miller, and E. C. Miller, *Biochemistry*, 1968, **7**, 1889.
14 J.-K. Lin, J. A. Miller, and E. C. Miller, *Biochemistry*, 1969, **8**, 1573.
15 D. E. Hathway and G. F. Kolar, *Chem. Soc. Rev.*, 1980, **9(2)**, 241.

3-methyl-1-phenyltriazene (MPT) contain the R—N—N—O or R—N—N—N systems, and they show a co-ordination between the intermediate produced and the nucleophile which lies between that of Ingold's S_N1 and S_N2 categories,[17] with a Swain–Scott *s* value of 0.42.[18,19] A clue to their reactivity is afforded by the fact that any one of these carcinogens reacts with alkali to give diazomethane, and *in vivo* the hydrolytic formation of methyl diazonium ($Me—N_2^+$) ions (1) (Scheme 1) takes place. From MNU (2), production is catalysed by OH^-, from

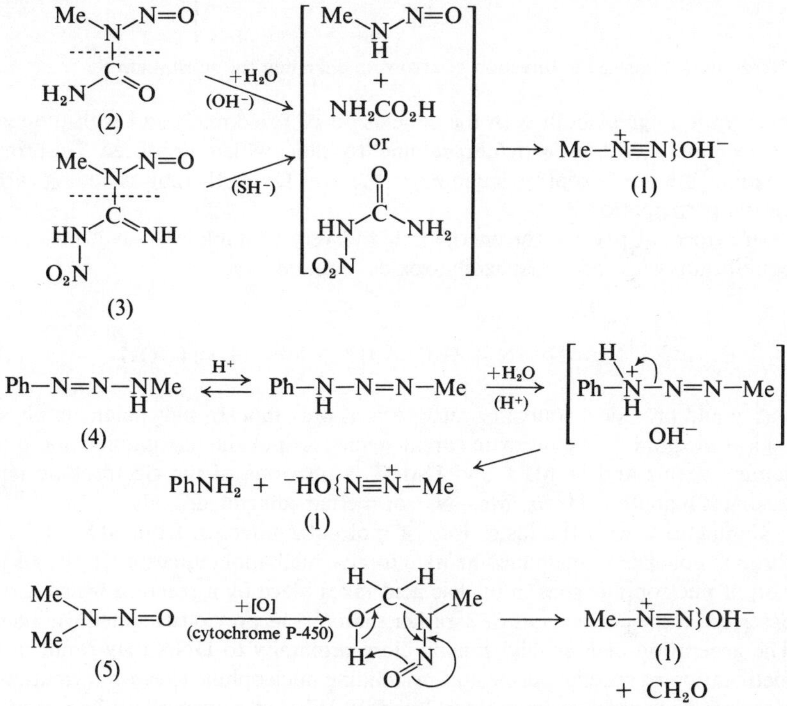

Scheme 1

MNNG (3) by cysteine or cysteinyl peptides,[20] and from MPT (4) by H^+ [21] and OH^-.[22] (Metabolic activation is not involved in any of these cases.) Theoretically, alkylation by agents which generate alkyldiazonium ions might be brought about through the alkyldiazonium cations *per se* or through the separate carbenium ions (Table), but methylation is most likely to occur by a mechanism involving $Me—N_2^+$ cations rather than the well-known highly reactive species Me^+. This

[16] S. Osterman-Golkar, L. Ehrenberg, and C. A. Wachtmeister, *Radiation Bot.*, 1970, **10**, 303.
[17] E. R. Garrett and S. Goto, *Chem. Pharm. Bull. Jpn.*, 1973, **21**, 1811.
[18] J. Veleminsky, S. Osterman-Golkar, and L. Ehrenberg, *Mutat. Res.*, 1970, **10**, 169.
[19] S. Osterman-Golkar, *Mutat. Res.*, 1974, **24**, 219.
[20] P. D. Lawley and C. J. Thatcher, *Biochem. J.*, 1970, **116**, 693.
[21] H. Bartsch, G. P. Marginson, C. Malaveille, A. M. Camus, G. Brun, J. M. Margison, G. F. Kolar, and M. Wiessler, *Arch. Toxikol.*, 1977, **39**, 51.
[22] R. J. Le Blanc and K. Vaughan, *Can. J. Chem.*, 1972, **50**, 2544.

Table *Reactivity of alkyldiazonium ions* $R-\overset{+}{N}\equiv N$

Reaction as R^{+}*		Reaction as $R-\overset{+}{N}\equiv N$
↓	Me	↑
	Et	
	Pr^{i}	
	Bu^{t}	

*Reactivity increased in direction of arrow on changing the substituent R.

observation agrees both with the conclusion of Friedman[23] and with the result of feeding *N*,*N*-di-n-propylnitrosamine to rats, which produced 7-n-propylguanine, but not 7-isopropylguanine, in the liver DNA, thereby excluding carbocation participation.[24]

In cytosol at pH 7.4, the energy-rich and very unstable $Me-N_2^{+}$ ions are in equilibrium with methanediazohydroxide (equation 1):

$$Me-\overset{+}{N}\equiv N + H_2O \rightleftharpoons H^{+} + Me-N=N-OH \qquad (1)$$

this would provide a source of carbocations only in a strongly acidic, unphysiological medium.[25] The ultimate carcinogenic form of the nitrosamide and nitrosamine agents and of MPT and DMPT is thus one of the electrophilic intermediates (equation 1), *viz.* $Me-N_2^{+}$ or methanediazohydroxide.

Competitive with the faster loss of molecular nitrogen from $Me-N_2^{+}$ ions through collapse of methanediazotate to give methanol (equation 1), the alkylation of nucleophilic sites in nucleic acid takes place by a reaction which is now described more correctly as S_N2, rather than S_N1 as previously stated[2] (*v. supra*). The generation of $Me-N_2^{+}$ ions in close proximity to DNA may result in the methylation of specific purine and pyrimidine nucleophilic sites *via* formation of transient intermediates (equations 2 and 3). Whence, concomitant loss of molecular nitrogen and collapse of the fugitive intermediates would transfer the methyl groups to the oxygen and nitrogen nucleophiles (equations 4 and 5).

$$Me-\overset{+}{N}\equiv N + ROH \rightarrow H^{+} + Me-N=N-OR \qquad (2)$$

$$Me-\overset{+}{N}\equiv N + NHRR' \rightarrow H^{+} + Me-N=N-NRR' \qquad (3)$$

$$Me-N=N-OR \rightarrow MeOR + N_2 \qquad (4)$$

$$Me-N=N-NRR' \rightarrow MeNRR' + N_2 \qquad (5)$$

[23] L. Friedman, 'Carbonium Ion Formation from Diazonium Ions,' in 'Carbonium Ions', ed. G. A. Olah and P. von R. Schleyer, John Wiley and Sons, New York, 1970, Vol. 2, pp. 655—711.
[24] K. K. Park, M. C. Archer, and J. S. Wishnok, *Chem.-Biol. Interact.*, 1980, **29**, 139.
[25] R. A. Moss, *Acc. Chem. Res.*, 1974, **7**, 421.

There is plenty of analogy for the various chemical reaction processes represented, for diazoethers have been isolated from other coupling reactions,[26–28] the coupling to nitrogen is well-known, and MPT decomposes to give *N*-methylaniline,[29] but crucial experimental evidence is missing and the underlying concept in this paragraph must be regarded as a speculative or reasonable chemical possibility. In its favour, order would be restored (*v. supra*) to Millers' great unifying principle.[1,2]

Product analysis sheds light on reactivity considerations, and it is interesting to follow the course of the reactions which have been suggested from this point of view. Thus, whilst the reaction of DMS or MMS with DNA yields a relatively small proportion of *O*-alkylation products, the ratio of O^6-methylguanine to 7-methylguanine being *ca.* 0.004[30] (and the proportion of phosphotriesters in the methylation product being *ca.* 0.01[31]), MNU and MNNG give relatively high yields of *O*-alkylation products, the ratio of O^6-methylguanine to 7-methylguanine being *ca.* 0.11 (and the proportion of phosphotriesters being about 0.2[32,33]). In the case of MPT, the ratio of O^6-methylguanine to 7-methylguanine ranges from 0.08 for liver DNA, through 0.12 for DNA from the kidney and lungs to 0.15 for that from the brain which is one of the chief target organs for tumour induction.[21] Thus, the (S_N2) DMS and MMS reagents react more exclusively at *N*-7 of guanine than the Me—N_2^+ generating MNU, MNNG, and MPT ones. Reaction of DMS or MMS with DNA seems to give relatively more of the minor products, 1- and 3-methyladenine (so that the ratio of 3-methyladenine to 7-methylguanine is *ca.* 0.2) and 3-methylpyrimidines, and a relatively smaller proportion of 7-methyladenine and 3-methylguanine than MNU and MNNG (which give a ratio of 3-methyladenine to 7-methylguanine of *ca.* 0.13).[34–36] Reaction of MPT with DNA *in vivo* also yields 3-methyladenine and 3-methylpyrimidines.[37]

In the case of the indirectly acting *N,N*-dimethylnitrosamine (DMN) (5) (Scheme 1), generation of the reactive form (1) involves an oxidative *N*-demethylation step[21] (chapter 10). The pattern of DNA methylation products derived from DMN *in vivo*[38–40] parallels that given by chemically activated MNU (*v. supra*), and thus reflects the common methylation mechanisms *via* Me—N_2^+ ions (1). Moreover, the relative amounts of methylated bases formed by MPT[37]

[26] A. Ginsberg and J. Goerdeler, *Chem. Ber.*, 1961, **94**, 2043.
[27] H. T. Bucherer, *Ber.*, 1909, **42**, 47.
[28] E. Müller and H. Haiss, *Chem. Ber.*, 1962, **95**, 1255.
[29] G. F. Kolar, unpublished work, cited in ref. 15.
[30] P. D. Lawley and S. A. Shah, *Chem.-Biol. Interact.*, 1972, **5**, 286.
[31] P. Bannon and W. G. Verly, *Eur. J. Biochem.*, 1972, **31**, 103.
[32] J. V. Frei and P. D. Lawley, *Chem.-Biol. Interact.*, 1976, **13**, 215.
[33] D. H. Swenson, P. B. Farmer, and P. D. Lawley, *Chem.-Biol. Interact.*, 1976, **15**, 91.
[34] P. D. Lawley, *Mutat. Res.*, 1974, **23**, 283.
[35] P. D. Lawley, in 'Screening Tests in Chemical Carcinogenesis,' I.A.R.C. Scientific Publications no. 12, ed. R. Montesano, H. Bartsch, and L. Tomatis, Lyon, France, 1976, pp. 181—208.
[36] A. E. Pegg, *Adv. Cancer Res.*, 1977, **25**, 195.
[37] G. P. Marginson, A. J. Likhachev, and G. F. Kolar, *Chem.-Biol. Interact.*, 1979, **25**, 345.
[38] P. J. O'Connor, M. J. Capps, and A. W. Craig, *Br. J. Cancer*, 1973, **27**, 153.
[39] V. M. Craddock, *Biochim. Biophys. Acta*, 1973, **312**, 202.
[40] J. M. Nicholl, P. F. Swann, and A. E. Pegg, *Chem.-Biol. Interact.*, 1977, **16**, 301.

were essentially similar to those given by the indirectly acting 3,3-dimethyl-1-phenyltriazene (DMPT).[41] This observation implies that both DMPT and MPT react with DNA through the Me—N_2^+ species (chapter 10), and that oxidative *N*-demethylation of DMPT *in vivo* affords MPT (chapter 10) as a relatively stable transport form.

As there is no relationship between the capacity to form 7-methylguanine in DNA and carcinogenicity,[42] *prima facie* the feasible correlation of carcinogenic potency with chemical reactivity is very confusing. Nevertheless, in general, nitroso compounds and alkylaryltriazenes are powerful carcinogens, whereas the (S_N2) non-nitrogen containing alkylating agents are poor ones. The direct-acting nitrosamides, which are transformed into reactive forms without metabolic activation (*v. supra*), induce tumours in numerous organs as well as at the site of administration, and at any rate the action of the *N,N*-dialkylnitrosamines is modulated by those organs which metabolize them into reactive forms.[43–46] *sym-N,N*-Dialkylnitrosamines afford hepatomas at the main site of metabolism, but *asym-N,N*-dialkylnitrosamines (such as *N*-methyl-*N*-pentylnitrosamine and *N*-methyl-*N*-phenylnitrosamine), which are metabolized through relatively stable intermediates that can be transported from the site of metabolism to another organ where they are metabolized further into R—N_2^+ cations, are oesophageal carcinogens.[44] DMPT and its MPT transport form are non-hepatic carcinogens.

On the other hand, i.v. injection of MNU, which causes a high incidence of brain tumours in animals, also methylates rat-brain DNA to afford a relatively large yield of *O*-alkylation products,[47] the ratio of O^6-methylguanine to 7-methylguanine being *ca.* 0.12; however, when MMS, which these workers[47] claimed did not induce brain tumours (*v. infra*), was used instead of MNU, no O^6-methylguanine resulted.[47] Separate investigation[39] of the liver DNA of rats that were given either the DMN hepatocarcinogen or MMS, which does not induce liver cancer, afforded a ratio of O^6-methylguanine to 7-methylguanine of *ca.* 0.12 in the case of DMN. In the two sets of experiments,[39,47] the two types of alkylating agent gave the same minor products of DNA alkylation, *viz.* 1- and 3-methyladenine and 3-methylcytosine. Thus, there is a strong supposition that formation of the miscoding O^6-methylguanine base[48,49] in DNA provides a possible relationship between the carcinogenic potency and the reactivity of these methylating agents. Other experiments[38,47,50–59] with nitrosamides and nitrosamines in hamsters, mice, and rats endorse this correlation. However, reinvestigation (*v. supra*) showed that in fact MMS caused some tumours in the c.n.s,[45,46] but this result can be reconciled with the very small amounts of O^6-methylguanine formed in the brain by MMS,[53] which may be sufficient as the nervous system of the developing rat is particularly sensitive to carcinogenesis by alkylating agents.[43–46]

41 P. Kleihues, G. F. Kolar, and G. P. Marginson, *Cancer Res.*, 1976, **36**, 2189.
42 P. F. Swann and P. N. Magee, *Biochem. J.*, 1968, **110**, 39.
43 P. N. Magee and J. M. Barnes, *Adv. Cancer Res.*, 1967, **10**, 163.
44 H. Druckrey, R. Preussmann, S. Ivankovic, and D. Schmähl, *Z. Krebsforsch.*, 1967, **69**, 103.

The fact that O^6-methylguanine, of all of the possible methyl purine or pyrimidine analogues, is the only one which persists for a very much longer time in the DNA of tissues that are especially susceptible to tumours than in other tissues which are resistant to tumour induction, infers that its formation in DNA belongs to the causative cancer mechanism. It is relevant that such persistence studies have been used to investigate the biological significance of nucleoside analogues resulting from the alkylation of DNA *in vivo*, and this theme will be taken up later in this section of the chapter (*v. infra*).

Ethylating Carcinogens.—Nucleic acid is alkylated in smaller proportions by ethylating- than by methylating-agents, and phosphotriesters may comprise up to 70% of the ethylation products.[50,51,60] The difference in reactivity between the two types of alkylating carcinogen, which was discussed in the case of the methylating agents (section 1), applies also to ethylating agents. Thus, typical Ingold S_N2 ethylating carcinogens have relatively high *s* values: $s = 0.64$ for diethyl sulphate (DES) and $s = 0.67$ for ethyl methanesulphonate (EMS).[16] On the other hand, *N*-ethyl-*N*-nitrosourea (ENU), *N*-ethyl-*N′*-nitro-*N*-nitrosoguanidine (ENNG), and *N,N*-diethylnitrosamine (DEN), which have low *s* values of *ca.* 0.26,[18,19,61] afford alkyl—N_2^+ ions (section 1), and would be expected to react through a mechanism involving Et—N_2^+ ions *per se.*[23] Whilst EMS produced a significant amount of O^6-ethylguanine in DNA, the ratio of O^6-ethylguanine to 7-ethylguanine being 0.03,[60] ENU and DEN have ethylated DNA in which the ratio of O^6-ethylguanine to 7-ethylguanine ranges from 0.48 to at least 0.70.[60] After 7-ethylguanine and O^6-ethylguanine, 3-ethyladenine is the third most abundant product of DNA ethylation.[50,51,60]

The capacity of alkylating agents to form the miscoding O^6-alkylguanine bases in the DNA of target tissues correlates with their carcinogenic potency (section 1), and the formation of O^6-ethylguanine agrees with this concept.

45 P. N. Magee, R. Montesano, and R. Preussmann, in 'Chemical Carcinogens,' A.C.S. Monograph no. 173, ed. C. E. Searle, American Chemical Society, Washington, D.C., 1976, pp. 491—625.
46 R. Montesano and H. Bartsch, *Mutat. Res.*, 1976, **32**, 179.
47 P. Kleihues and P. N. Magee, *J. Neurochem.*, 1973, **20**, 595.
48 A. Loveless, *Nature*, 1969, **223**, 206.
49 P. J. Abbott and R. Saffhill, *Br. J. Cancer*, 1977, **36**, 404.
50 R. Goth and M. F. Rajewsky, *Proc. Nat. Acad. Sci., USA*, 1974, **71**, 639.
51 R. Goth and M. F. Rajewsky, *Z. Krebsforsch.*, 1974, **82**, 37.
52 P. Kleihues and G. P. Marginson, *J. Nat. Cancer Inst.*, 1974, **53**, 1839.
53 P. Kleihues, K. Patzschke, G. P. Marginson, L. A. Wegner, and C. Mende, *Z. Krebsforsch.*, 1974, **81**, 273.
54 L. Den Engelse, *Chem.-Biol. Interact.*, 1974, **8**, 329.
55 J. V. Frei and P. D. Lawley, *Chem.-Biol. Interact.*, 1975, **10**, 413.
56 V. M. Craddock, *Chem.-Biol. Interact.*, 1975, **10**, 323.
57 G. P. Marginson, J. M. Margison, and R. Montesano, *Biochem. J.*, 1976, **157**, 627.
58 J. W. Nicholl, P. F. Swann, and A. E. Pegg, *Nature*, 1975, **254**, 261.
59 A. E. Pegg, J. W. Nicholl, P. N. Magee, and P. F. Swann, *Excerpta Med. Int. Congress Series*, 1976, **376**, 39.
60 L. Sun and B. Singer, *Biochemistry*, 1975, **14**, 1795.
61 A. E. Pegg and J. W. Nicholl, in 'Screening Tests in Chemical Carcinogenesis,' I.A.R.C. Scientific Publications no. 12, ed. R. Montesano, H. Bartsch, and L. Tomatis, Lyon, France, 1976, pp. 571—590.

Thus, doses of ENU and DEN, which gave the same incidence of kidney tumours as that given by MNU or DMN, afforded a smaller amount of 7-alkylguanine in kidney nucleic acids than the analogous methyl reagents,[62] but the relative proportion of O^6-alkylguanine to 7-alkylguanine formed by ENU and DEN exceeds that given by MNU and DMN, which in turn exceeds by far that produced by DES and DMS. The apparent anomaly, that rats produce kidney tumours after three closely spaced i.p. injections of EMS[62] is explicable in terms of the small amounts of O^6-ethylguanine that are formed through reaction of EMS with kidney DNA in these animals. In fact, the *s* value for EMS (0.67) lies between that (0.42) for MNU and for MMS (0.83).

Metal Carcinogens.—Although chromium, nickel, and cadmium are suspected of being associated with industrial cancer, the reactive forms are largely unknown. However, in the case of chromium, the fact that Cr^{VI} is a mutagen in standard test systems,[63–66] whereas Cr^{3+} is non-mutagenic,[63,64] provides strong evidence for the reaction of Cr^{VI} with DNA, but the significance of the recent finding[67] that Cr^{VI} reacts with ribonucleotides to give Cr^{V}[68] is unknown. The basis for nickel carcinogenicity has not been investigated.

cis-Diamminodichloroplatinum(II) is a mutagen in standard test systems,[69–71] and platinum S_N2 electrophiles show approximately the same specificity[72,73] towards DNA nucleophilic sites, *i.e.* guanine> adenine> cytosine, as the DES, DMS, and MMS alkylating agents considered in section 1.[74] Under neutral conditions, they alkylate preferentially *N*-7 of guanine, *N*-1 of adenine, and *N*-3 of cytosine. There is no crystallographic evidence for bidentate binding of these Pt electrophiles to guanine residues of DNA[73] (*cf.* ref. 75).

Pearson's Soft and Hard Acids and Bases.—Some of the conclusions (*q.v.*) about the reactivities of alkylating carcinogens for the various nucleophilic sites in DNA might have been made had consideration been given alternatively to Pearson's principle of soft and hard acids and bases.[76–78] By means of[79]

[62] P. F. Swann and P. N. Magee, *Biochem. J.*, 1971, **125**, 841.
[63] S. Venitt, *Nature*, 1974, **250**, 493.
[64] F. L. Petrilli and S. de Flora, *Appl. Environ. Microbiol.*, 1977, **33**, 805.
[65] H. Nishioka, *Mutat. Res.*, 1975, **31**, 185.
[66] H. Nishioka, *Jpn J. Genetics*, 1975, **50**, 485.
[67] D. M. L. Goodgame, P. B. Hayman, and D. E. Hathway, *Polyhedron*, 1982, **1**, 497.
[68] K. W. Jenette, *J. Am. Chem. Soc.*, 1982, **104**, 874.
[69] D. J. Beck and R. R. Brubaker, *Mutat. Res.*, 1975, **27**, 181.
[70] C. Monti-Bragadini, M. Tarano, and E. Banfi, *Chem.-Biol. Interact.*, 1975, **11**, 469.
[71] P. Lecointe, J.-P. Macquet, J.-L. Butour, and C. Paoletti, *Mutat. Res.*, 1977, **48**, 139.
[72] S. Mansy, G. Y. H. Chu, R. E. Duncan, and R. S. Tobias, *J. Am. Chem. Soc.*, 1978, **100**, 607.
[73] D. M. L. Goodgame, I. Jeeves, F. L. Phillips, and A. C. Skapski, *Biochim. Biophys. Acta*, 1975, **378**, 153.
[74] B. Singer, *Prog. Nucleic Acid Res. Mol. Biol.*, 1975, **15**, 219.
[75] J. J. Roberts and A. J. Thomson, *Prog. Nucleic Acid Res. Mol. Biol.*, 1979, **22**, 71.
[76] R. G. Pearson, *J. Am. Chem. Soc.*, 1963, **85**, 3533.
[77] R. G. Pearson, *Science*, 1966, **151**, 172.
[78] R. G. Pearson and J. Sonstad, *J. Am. Chem. Soc.*, 1967, **89**, 1827.
[79] R. F. Hudson, paper presented at a symposium on S.H.A.B., Cyanamid European Research Institute, Geneva, May 1965: *Chem. Eng. News*, 1965, **43** [no. 22], pp. 102, 103.

the hardness–softness principle,[76–78] the site of reaction in an ambident nucleophile with alternative hard and soft sites may be deduced and, for example, considerable attention has been given[80–84] to the problem of *C versus O* alkylation; in the case, for example, of deoxyguanosine, the donor *N*-7 atom is a softer base than the donor *O*-8 atom. Hence, the harder alkyldiazonium (alkyl—N_2^+) cations would be expected to react with deoxyguanosine to afford a larger proportion of O^6-alkylation products relative to that of the *N*-7 ones) than the softer alkyl groups belonging to the DES, DMS, and MMS agents. This prediction agrees with the foregoing experimental evidence (section 1). In contrast to the harder (acid) alkyl—N_2^+ cations, the softer $(N_3N)_2Pt^{2+}$ cations, for which the simple Me—Hg^+ is an archetype,[85] would be expected to react with deoxyguanosine residues of DNA to bring about almost exclusive platination at *N*-7 and again this supposition agrees with the previously presented experimental evidence.

DNA Repair.—In general, the tissue with the greatest susceptibility to the induction of tumours by alkylating carcinogens is the one in which the repair system for the O^6-alkylguanine lesion in DNA is least effective (see chapter 13). At any rate, the persistence of this promutagenic lesion in DNA would tend to increase the opportunity for miscoding events to occur during DNA synthesis and, thus, would predispose the tissue in question to malignancy. Thus, after the administration of such a (single) dose of ENU as would cause an high incidence of c.n.s tumours in new-born rats,[50] the extent of O^6-alkylation of the guanosine residues was very similar in all of the tissues investigated, but loss of O^6-ethylguanine from brain DNA was much slower than from non-target organ DNA.[50] Similarly, in other sensitive species of animal, O^6-alkylguanine was detectable for a very much longer period in the DNA of tissues that are particularly susceptible to tumour induction than in the DNA of non-target tissues, but in some cases there were complicating factors. Thus, for example, in two strains of mouse with different susceptibilities to the induction of liver tumours by DMN, the liver DNA was methylated to a similar extent,[54] but the proliferative response, measured in terms of DNA synthesis, was much more extensive in susceptible strain hepatocytes than in the resistant ones.[86] In the event, a high incidence of brain tumours, a low incidence of kidney tumours, and the lack of hepatic response, which was produced in rats dosed chronically with MNU correlated with the retention of O^6-methylguanine by the DNA of the various tissues.[87] Similarly, chronic administrations of DMPT[88] and of DMN[89] to

[80] A. L. Kurts, N. K. Genkina, A. Macias, I. P. Beletskaya, and O. A. Reutov, *Tetrahedron*, 1971, **27**, 4777.
[81] W. J. Le Noble and H. F. Morris, *J. Org. Chem.*, 1969, **34**, 1969.
[82] W. S. Murphy and D. J. Buckley, *Tetrahedron Lett.*, 1969, 2975.
[83] J. A. Campbell and J. F. Wolfe, *Org. Prep. Proc. Int.*, 1971, **3**, 303.
[84] J. P. Boisset, J. Boyer, and J. Rouzand, *C. R. Acad. Sci. Ser. C*, 1966, **263**, 1253.
[85] G. Schwarzenbach, paper presented at a symposium on S.H.A.B., Cyanamid European Research Institute, Geneva, May 1965: *Chem. Eng. News*, 1965, **43** [no. 22], p. 92.
[86] H. K. De Munther, L. Den Engelse, and P. Emmelot, *Chem.-Biol. Interact.*, 1979, **24**, 299.
[87] G. P. Marginson and P. Kleihues, *Biochem. J.*, 1975, **148**, 521.
[88] H. K. Cooper, E. Hauenstein, G. F. Kolar, and P. Kleihues, *Acta Neuropathol.* (*Berlin*), 1978, **43**, 105.
[89] J. W. Nicholl, P. F. Swann, and A. E. Pegg, *Chem.-Biol. Interact.*, 1977, **16**, 301.

rats led to the greatest accumulation of O^6-methylguanine in brain DNA[88] and in kidney DNA[89] respectively, the target organs for the alkylating carcinogens concerned. On the other hand, chronic DMN treatment, which was intended to induce liver tumours, led to the retention of O^6-methylguanine in kidney and lung DNA,[90] and to the augmentation of the already high capacity of the liver[89–91] to remove O^6-methylguanine from (liver) DNA. It is noteworthy in this context that the induction and inhibition of DNA repair suggests that this system, which effects O^6-methylguanine repair, may act as well on higher alkyl derivatives[92,93] and other types of DNA injury.[92]

The mechanism by which O^6-alkylguanine is removed from tissue is not clear, as its removal and that of other methylpurines from MNU-methylated DNA by *E. coli* endonuclease 11 *in vitro*[94] was not adopted *in vivo* where the liberation of methanol inferred the participation of an *O*-demethylating enzyme.[95] Two systems may operate in the removal of O^6-methylguanine from DNA in rats, as more of that produced in liver DNA by low doses of DMN was removed than of that by higher doses; this suggests that one system may be saturated by small amounts of this base whereas a less efficient system may have a much greater capacity for effecting its removal.[96,97] Much the same applies in the case of Syrian hamsters, and the greater sensitivity of the hamster to tumour induction by DMN[57,98] may be due to the much smaller capacity of this animal than of the rat to remove O^6-methylguanine after high doses of DMN.[57,98]

In addition, enzymes remove 3-methyladenine from tissue DNA,[99,100] but unlike the excision of O^6-methylguanine, such eliminative mechanisms are not modified *in vivo*.[99] On the other hand, phosphotriesters are not removed enzymically from tissue DNA and thus may afford 'markers' in the assessment of potential injury after low-level exposure to alkylating carcinogens.[101–104]

RNA repair has received comparatively little attention.

Miscoding Incurred in Nucleic Acid Synthesis by Alkylation.—Various attempts to explain the mutagenicty of *N*-nitroso compounds depend on the possibility that particular alkylated bases may interfere with the H-bonding of the (dA–dT)

90 G. P. Marginson, J. M. Margison, and R. Montesano, *Biochem. J.*, 1977, **165**, 463.
91 E. Scherer, A. P. Steward, and P. Emmelot, *Chem.-Biol. Interact.*, 1978, **19**, 1.
92 P. Kleihues and G. P. Marginson, *Nature*, 1976, **259**, 153.
93 A. E. Pegg, *Chem.-Biol. Interact.*, 1978, **22**, 109.
94 D. M. Kirtikar and D. A. Goldthwait, *Proc. Nat. Acad. Sci., USA*, 1974, **71**, 2022.
95 A. E. Pegg, *Biochem. Biophys. Res. Commun.*, 1978, **84**, 166.
96 A. E. Pegg, *J. Nat. Cancer Inst.*, 1977, **58**, 681.
97 A. E. Pegg and G. Hui, *Biochem. J.*, 1978, **173**, 739.
98 R. Stumpf, G. P. Marginson, R. Montesano, and A. E. Pegg, *Cancer Res.*, 1979, **39**, 50.
99 G. P. Marginson and P. J. O'Connor, 'Nucleic acid Modification by *N*-Nitroso Compounds,' in 'Chemical Carcinogens and DNA,' ed. P. L. Grover, C. R. C. Press, West Palm Beach, Florida, 1979, vol. **1**, pp. 111—159.
100 G. P. Marginson and P. J. O'Connor, *Biochim. Biophys. Acta*, 1973, **331**, 349.
101 K. V. Shooter and T. A. Slade, *Chem.-Biol. Interact.*, 1977, **19**, 353.
102 K. V. Shooter, T. A. Slade, and P. J. O'Connor, *Chem.-Biol. Interact.*, 1977, **19**, 363.
103 B. G. J. Floot, E. J. Philippus, A. A. M. Hart, and L. Den Engelse, *Chem.-Biol. Interact.*, 1979, **25**, 229.
104 K. V. Shooter, *Nature*, 1978, **274**, 612.

and (dC–dG) base pairs in the Watson–Crick double helix for DNA,[48,105–111] and a great deal of the work on miscoding (abnormal base pairing) properties has involved DNA and RNA synthesizing systems that employ bacterial DNA or RNA polymerases acting on DNA- or RNA-like polymer templates which contain varying proportions of the modified bases. Whilst templates containing a single modified base, prepared by the reaction of polynucleotide phosphorylase and the relevant mixture of ribonucleoside diphosphates, are used with RNA polymerase, those prepared by direct alkylation,[112,113] which will obviously contain more than one modified base, are employed with DNA polymerase; with its high degree of accuracy, involving only about one error compared with 100 000 for RNA polymerase,[114] and with its realistic double-stranded template, this latter incurs outstanding advantage. This facilitates the detection of very low levels of misincorporation consequent upon the presence of small amounts of miscoding base.

With regard to the DNA and RNA synthesizing systems, O^6-ethyl- and O^6-methyl-guanine lead to misincorporation,[113,115] which agrees with the miscoding properties that have been proposed for these bases.[48] O^4-Methylthymine also causes error with DNA polymerase,[112] whereas 3-methylguanine, 1-, 3-, and 7-methyladenines, 3-methylthymine, and the phosphotriesters do not afford any significant misincorporation of wrong nucleotides.[112,113] Hence, miscoding with DNA polymerase takes place only where it is possible to construct a stable H-bonded base pair, *viz.* (6)—(8) (Scheme 2), involving the modified base and that of the nucleotide which is in process of being incorporated.[116] Despite the feasibility of an H-bonded base pair involving O^2-methylthymine and guanine, because of the steric interaction between the O^2-methyl group and the deoxyribose residue of the nucleotide[117] the O^2-methyl group cannot take up the requisite planar configuration with the bases within the limitations imposed by the Watson–Crick double helix for DNA.

[105] B. Singer, *Nature*, 1976, **264**, 333.
[106] P. D. Lawley and P. Brookes, *Nature*, 1961, **192**, 1081.
[107] D. R. Krieg, *Genetics*, 1963, **48**, 561.
[108] D. B. Ludlum and R. C. Wilhelm, *J. Biol. Chem.*, 1968, **243**, 2750.
[109] B. Singer and H. Fraenkel-Conrat. *Biochemistry*, 1970, **9**, 3694.
[110] P. D. Lawley, D. J. Orr and S. A. Shah, *Chem.-Biol. Interact.*, 1971/1972, **4**, 431.
[111] P. D. Lawley, D. J. Orr, S. A. Shah, P. B. Farmer, and M. Jarman, *Biochem. J.*, 1973, **135**, 193.
[112] P. J. Abbott and R. Saffhill, *Nucleic Acids Res.*, 1977, **4**, 761.
[113] P. J. Abbott and R. Saffhill, *Biochim. Biophys. Acta*, 1977, **562**, 51.
[114] L. A. Loeb, L. A. Weymouth, T. A. Kunkel, K. P. Gopinathan, R. A. Beckman, and D. K. Duke, in 'Cold Spring Harbor Symposia on Quantitative Biology,' 1979, Volume XLIII.
[115] L. L. Gerchman and D. B. Ludlam, *Biochim. Biophys. Acta*, 1973, **308**, 310.
[116] P. J. O'Connor, R. Saffhill, and G. P. Marginson, '*N*-Nitroso Compounds: Biochemical Mechanisms of Action,' in 'Environmental Carcinogens,' ed. P. Emmelot and E. Kriek, Elsevier/North Holland Biomedical Press, Amsterdam, 1979, pp. 73—96.
[117] R. Saffhill and P. J. Abbott, *Nucleic Acids Res.*, 1978, **5**, 1971.

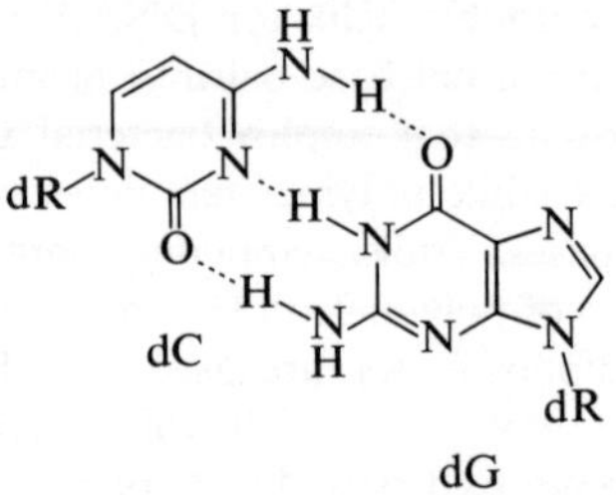

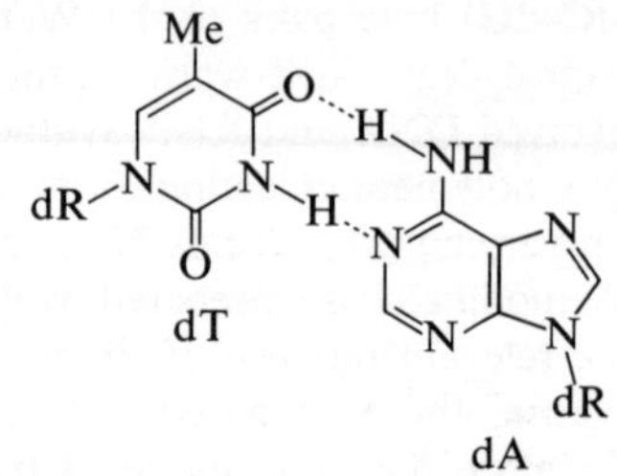

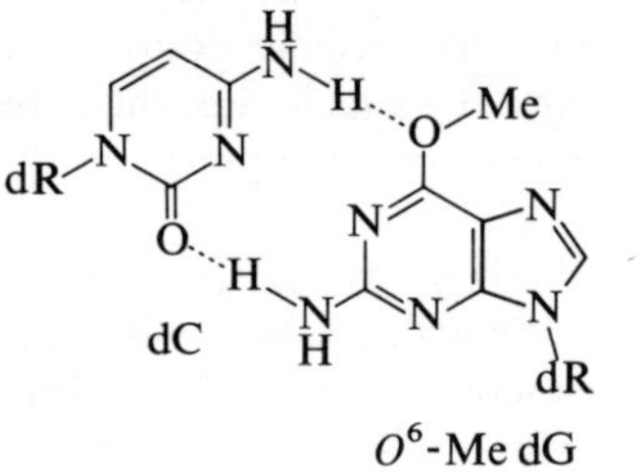

(6)

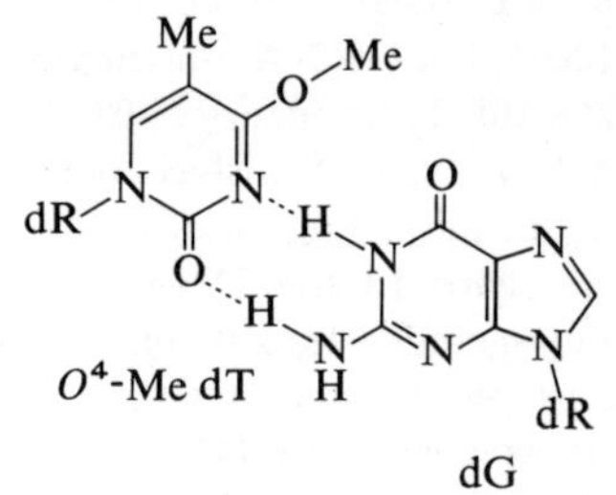

(8)

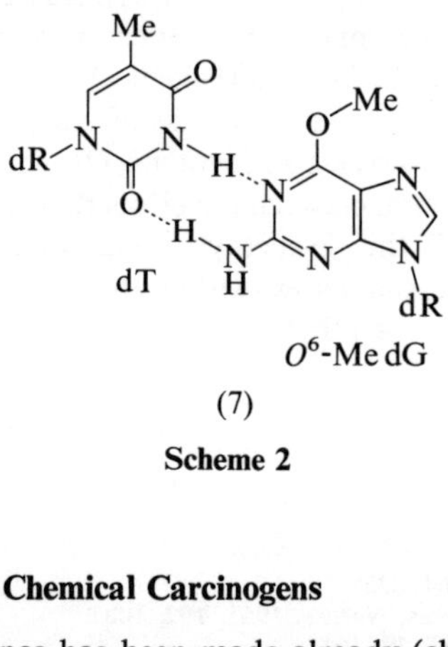

(7)

Scheme 2

2 Industrial Chemical Carcinogens

Vinyl Chloride.—Reference has been made already (chapter 10) to the reaction mechanism between vinyl chloride-derived chloroethylene oxide or its rearrangement product, chloroacetaldehyde, and DNA *in vitro* and to the fact that the same nucleoside analogues, *viz.* 9-(β-D-2′-deoxyribofuranosyl)imidazo[2,1-*i*]-purine (etheno-dA) and 1-(β-D-2′-deoxyribofuranosyl)imidazo[1,2-*c*]pyrimidin-2(1*H*)-one (etheno-dC), are formed both *in vitro* and in the liver DNA of rats exposed chronically to vinyl chloride in their drinking water. These results implied a common reaction mechanism, involving in both cases initial (S_N2) alkylation at the most nucleophilic ring-nitrogen (*N*-1 of the dA residues and *N*-3 of the dC ones) (chapter 10), and the authors[118] implicitly inferred that these

[118] T. Green and D. E. Hathway, *Chem.-Biol. Interact.*, 1978, **22**, 211.

results indicated a causal) relationship, *i.e.* that formation of etheno-dA and -dC may represent pro-mutagenic lesions in the extra-hepatocellular liver-tissue DNA of animals exposed to vinyl chloride. At the same time, Laib and Bolt[119,120] produced evidence for the presence of correspondingly modified ribonucleosides in fractions of the enzymic hydrolysates of the liver RNA of rats which had been exposed to a massive acute dose of [^{14}C]vinyl chloride, and they confirmed their results in incubations of rat-liver microsomes, [^{14}C]vinyl chloride, and the appropriate polynucleotide, fortified with NADPH.

Molecular models showed that: (i) the imidazole ring in vinyl chloride nucleoside analogues is co-planar or almost co-planar with the rest of the molecule;[121,122] (ii) the imidazole ring in these nucleoside analogues shields two normal H-bonding sites;[15] (iii) in the case of etheno-dC (or etheno-C), the second ring confers on the cytosine residue the dimensions of adenine, with the result that etheno-dC would be expected to simulate dA nucleosides/nucleotides in replication[123,124] and etheno-C the A ones in transcription;[125] (iv) the misincorporation envisaged in these biological processes would be facilitated by complex-formation involving base pairing (Scheme 3) of protonated molecular species which have been invoked[126] to extend the Watson–Crick concept for complementary base pairing; and (v) that the relatively bulky imidazole ring resembles an alkyl substituent and effectively blocks one of the available base-pairing sites.

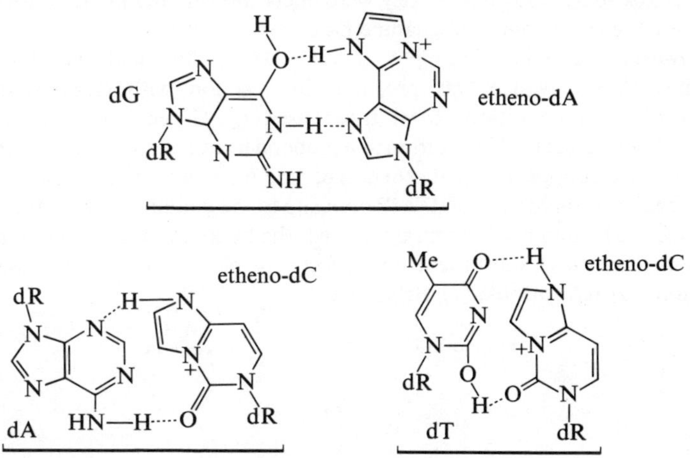

Scheme 3

119 R. J. Laib and H. M. Bolt, *Toxicology*, 1977, **8**, 185.
120 R. J. Laib and H. M. Bolt, *Arch. Toxikol.*, 1978, **39**, 235.
121 A. H. J. Wang, L. G. Dammann, J. R. Barrio, and I. C. Paul, *J. Am. Chem. Soc.*, 1974, **96**, 1205.
122 A. H. J. Wang, J. R. Barrio, and I. C. Paul, *J. Am. Chem. Soc.*, 1976, **98**, 7401.
123 J. A. Hall, R. Saffhill, T. Green, and D. E. Hathway, *Carcinogenesis*, 1981, **2**, 141.
124 A. Barbin, H. Bartsch, P. Leconte, and M. Radman, *Nucleic Acids Res.*, 1981, **9**, 375.
125 S. Spengler and B. Singer, *Nucleic Acids Res.*, 1981, **9**, 365.
126 M. D. Topal and J. R. Fresco, *Nature*, 1976, **263**, 285.

When DNA-like polymers poly(dA-dT) and poly(dC-dG), pre-treated with chloroacetaldehyde, were used as templates for *E. coli* DNA polymerase 1 in an *in vitro* assay,[123] replication was decelerated and increased levels of non-complementary nucleosides were incorporated. (Although DNA repair has never been studied *per se*, it is not entirely ignored in this work, as DNA polymerase 1 belongs to the repair system.) With the modified (dA-dT) templates, one dGMP was incorporated for every *ca.* 60 etheno-dA residues present, but no misincorporation of dCMP occurred, and with the poly(dC-dG) templates, one misincorporation of dAMP or dTMP occurred respectively in the presence of *ca.* 30 or 80 etheno-dC residues. The principal miscodings of dA may represent a potential pro-mutagenic lesion, which would be expected to lead to (dA-dT) → (dC-dG) transversions, and similarly those of etheno-dC would possibly induce (dC-dG) → (dA-dT) transversions. Nearest-neighbour analysis with modified poly(dC-dG) templates showed that 90% of the misincorporations of dAMP occurred opposite cytosine (or etheno-cytosine), and a small number of errors (*ca.* 10%) occurred opposite guanine bases, whereas dTMP seemed to be incorporated opposite both cytosine and guanine bases or their modifications. The authors[123] noted that, whilst a reaction product of chloroacetaldehyde and guanine, *viz.* N^2,3-ethenoguanine, had been described,[127] as it had been made under rather different conditions from the ones which they used to prepare the poly(dC-dG) templates,[123] they were uncertain whether in fact it was responsible for the errors opposite guanine bases.

However, the recent finding[128] (*cf.* ref 129) that the acid hydrolysates of a modified DNA, which was prepared by reaction with chloroacetaldehyde under different conditions from those used by Green and Hathway,[118] do contain some etheno-G in addition to a preponderance of etheno-A and etheno-C, supports the supposition that etheno-guanine may cause the misincorporations described[123] (*v. supra*), *i.e.* of dTMP opposite to the guanine bases in the modified poly(dC-dG) template. In this case as well, the bulky imidazo ring of etheno-dG resembles an alkyl substituent and effectively blocks one of the base-pairing positions (9) [*cf.* formula (7), Scheme 2].

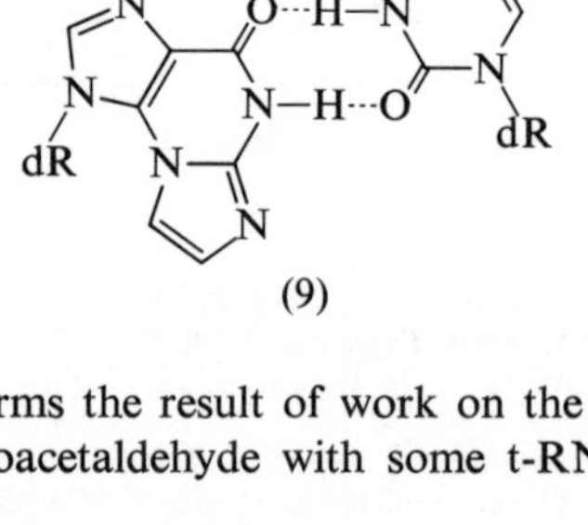

(9)

All this evidence confirms the result of work on the kinetics and selectivity of the reaction of chloroacetaldehyde with some t-RNA constituents, which

[127] P. D. Sattsangi, N. J. Leonard, and C. R. Frihart, *J. Org. Chem.*, 1977, **42**, 3296.
[128] F. Oesch and G. Doerjer, *Carcinogenesis*, 1982, **3**, 663.
[129] N. K. Kochetov, V. N. Shibaev and A. A. Kost, *Dokl. Acad. Nauk. SSSR*, 1973, **213**, 1327.

showed that no nucleoside analogues apart from imidazo-cyclization ones are formed.[130]

Induction of (dA-dT) → (dC-dG) and (dC-dG) → (dA-dT) transversions by etheno-dA, -dC, and -dG is consistent with the fact that chloroethylene oxide, chloroacetaldehyde, and metabolically activated vinyl chloride* induce base-pair substitution mutations in *Salmonella typhimurium* strains;[131–134] vinyl chloride is not a frame-shift mutagen. The fact that vinyl chloride and vinyl bromide[135] alkylate nucleic acid similarly means that the mechanism (*q.v.*) established (chapters 10 and 11) for vinyl chloride carcinogenicity applies also to its bromide analogue.

In this connection, the mechanism for vinyl chloride carcinogenicity is capable of further extension. Thus, the same imidazo-cyclization of the purine and pyrimidine residues of DNA as was attributable to chloroethylene oxide and chloroacetaldehyde in the case of vinyl chloride[118] would account for the covalent binding to tissue DNA of the 1,2-dibromoethane metabolite, bromoacetaldehyde,[136] and for the associated 1,2-dibromoethane mutagenicity[137–141] and carcinogenicity in rodents.[142,143]

$$\mathrm{BrCH_2CH_2Br} \xrightarrow[+\mathrm{O}]{} \mathrm{BrCH_2C(OH)HBr} \xrightarrow[-\mathrm{HBr}]{} \mathrm{BrCH_2CHO}$$

1,2-Dichloroethane has been found also to be carcinogenic to rodents[144–146] and metabolic study, involving ingenious mutagenicity testing,[147] showed that the bile of treated animals contained mutagen(s) 15—30 min after dosing,

* For ease of cross-reference, the metabolic fate of vinyl chloride was described in chapter 6, its mechanism of reaction with DNA was illustrated in chapter 10, and the tissue specificity of vinyl chloride cancer will be taken up in chapter 13.

130 J. Biennat, J. Ciesiolka, P. Górnicki, R. W. Adamiak, W. J. Krzyzosiak, and M. Wiewiorowski, *Nucleic Acids Res.*, 1978, **5**, 789.
131 U. Rannug, A. Johansson, C. Ramel, and C. A. Wachtmeister, *Ambio*, 1974, **3**, 194.
132 C. Malaveille, H. Bartsch, A. Barbin, A. M. Camus, and R. Montesano, *Biochem. Biophys. Res. Commun.*, 1975, **63**, 363.
133 J. McCann, V. Simmon, D. Streitwieser, and B. N. Ames, *Proc. Nat. Acad. Sci., USA.*, 1975, **73**, 3190.
134 R. A. Phillips, S. A. Zahler, and A. J. Garro, *Mutat. Res.*, 1980, **74**, 267.
135 H. Ottenwaelder, R. J. Laib, and H. M. Bolt, *Arch. Toxicol.*, 1979, **41**, 290.
136 D. L. Hill, T.-W. Shih, T. P. Johnston, and R. F. Struck, *Cancer Res.*, 1978, **38**, 2438.
137 B. N. Ames, *Chem. Mutagens*, 1971, **1**, 267.
138 H. Brem, A. B. Stein, and H. S. Rosenkranz, *Cancer Res.*, 1974, **34**, 2576.
139 W. Buselmaier, G. Röhrborn, and P. Propping, *Mutat. Res.*, 1973, **21**, 25.
140 R. B. Cumming and M. F. Walton, *Food Cosmet. Toxicol.*, 1973, **11**, 547.
141 H. V. Malling and H. V. de Serres, *Genetics*, 1969, **61**, 39.
142 W. A. Olson, R. T. Habermann, E. K. Weisburger, J. M. Ward, and J. H. Weisburger, *J. Nat. Cancer Inst.*, 1973, **51**, 1973.
143 Bioassay of 1,2-dibromoethane for possible carcinogenicity, *Gov. Rep. Announc. Index*, 1979, **79**(6), 81.
144 Bioassay of 1,2-dichloroethane for possible carcinogenicity CAS No. 107-06-2, *Gov. Rep. Announc. Index*. 1978, **78**(26), 84.
145 Current Intelligence Bulletin: 1,2-dichloroethane, DHEW (NIOSH) Publ., 1978, 78—149.
146 L. J. Bahlman, N. A. Leidel, J. C. Parker, H. P. Stein, A. W. Thomas, B. S. Woolf, and J. D. Miller, *Am. Ind. Hyg. Assoc. J.*, 1978, **39**, A35, A37, A39, A41, A43.
147 U. Rannug and B. Beije, *Chem.-Biol. Interact.*, 1979, **24**, 265.

but 2-chloroethanol was established as a non-mutagen. These results agree with the previously established metabolic activation of 1,2-dihalogenoethanes through their conjugation with glutathione and, in fact, *N*-acetyl-*S*-(2-chloroethyl)-L-cysteine and *S*-(2-chloroethyl)-L-cysteine are mutagenic in *S. typhimurium* TA1535 strain. Accordingly, there is considerable similarity between the metabolic fates of vinyl chloride (chapter 6) and 1,2-dihalogenoethanes (*q.v.*).

The important biochemical lesion described for vinyl chloride (*q.v.*) seems to apply to glycidaldehyde, which has been used commercially for tanning doe-skin gloving leather and which has been found to be mutagenic[148–150] and carcinogenic.[151–154] A mechanism (S_N2) involving imidazo-cyclization[155,156] with the *N*-1 position and the *C*-2 amino group has been described in chapter 10.

It will become increasingly apparent that, whilst the significance of the mechanisms of reaction between the ultimate, reactive carcinogens and DNA has been explored both with regard to the simple alkylating carcinogens and to vinyl chloride (*v. supra*), molecular biological investigation of the interactions between DNA and the aromatic amines, amino-azo dyes (section 2), and naturally occurring carcinogens (section 3) is strictly limited or non-existent.

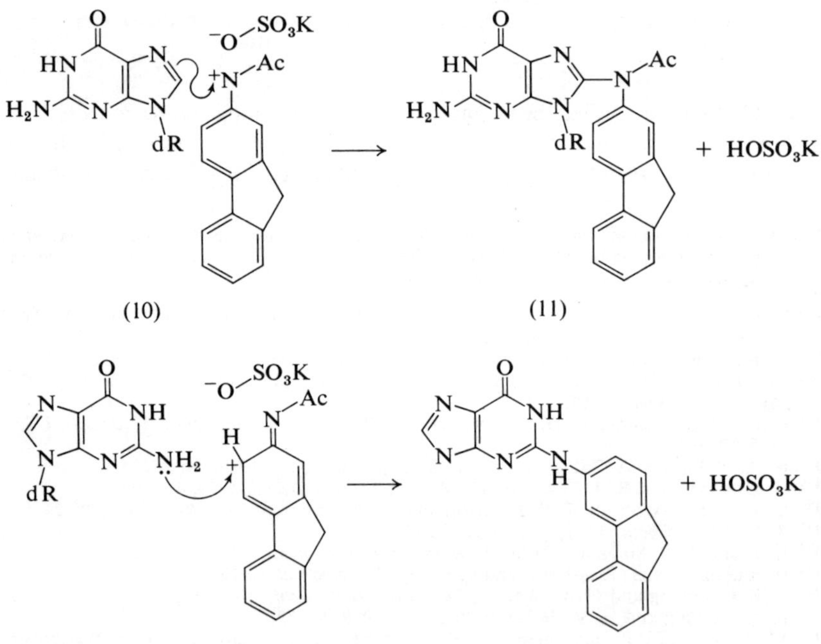

(10) (11) (12)

Scheme 4

Aromatic Amines.—In line with the ideas of the Millers,[1,2] deoxyguanosine reacted both *in vitro* and *in vivo* with the sites of the *N*-fluoren-2-ylacetamide derivative, *viz*. at the amido nitrogen and at C3, which were activated through esterification of the *N*-hydroxylation product.[5] Thus, gentle chemical reaction

(S_N1) between deoxyguanosine and the ultimate carcinogen of *N*-fluoren-2-yl-acetamide, *viz.* the *N* sulphate salt of *N*-fluoren-2-ylacetamide (10) (Scheme 4), gave *N*-deoxyguanosin-8-yl-*N*-fluoren-2-ylacetamide (11),[5] which had been identified previously as a reaction product,[6,157] and *N*-[3-(deoxyguanosin-N^2-yl) fluoren-2-yl]acetamide (12), identical with the product obtained from hydrolysates of the modified DNA, extracted from the liver of rats injected with *N*-hydroxy-*N*-fluoren-2-ylacetamide.[2,25,157]

A voluminous literature describes the biochemical data about the metabolism and activation of *N*-fluoren-2-ylacetamide, much of which is more or less relevant to the mode of its chemical carcinogenesis, and in this connection monumental papers by Dybing *et al.* might be instanced.[158–161] The importance of ring-chain tautomerism in chemical carcinogenesis has been discussed[162] and exemplified by *N*-fluoren-2-ylacetamide, *viz.* (13)—(15) (Scheme 5).

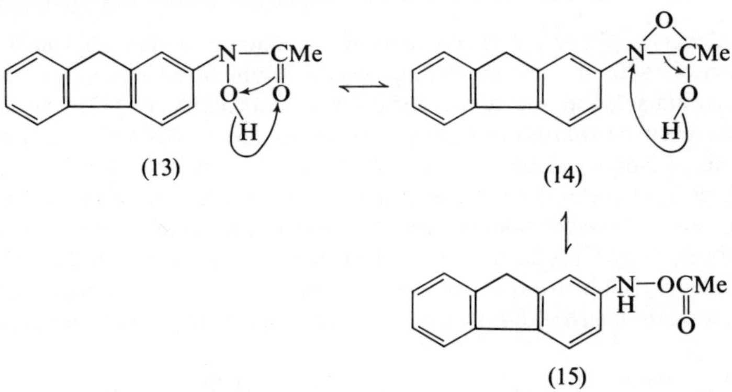

Scheme 5

Modified DNA, obtained by reaction of either 4-acetylamino-4′-fluorobiphenyl or 4-amino-4′-fluorobiphenyl with rat-liver and -kidney DNA, gave on hydrolysis either *N*-deoxyguanosin-8-yl-4-acetylamino-4′-fluorobiphenyl

148 J. McCann, E. Choi, E. Yamasaki, and B. N. Ames, *Proc. Nat. Acad. Sci., USA*, 1975, **72**, 5135.
149 M. C. Izard, *C. R. Acad. Sci.*, 1973, **276**, 3037.
150 T. H. Corbett, C. Heidelberger, and W. F. Dove, *Mol. Pharmacol.*, 1970, **6**, 667.
151 B. L. Van Duuren, L. Orris, and N. Nelson, *J. Nat. Cancer Inst.*, 1965, **35**, 707.
152 B. L. Van Duuren, L. Langseth, L. Orris, G. Teebor, N. Nelson, and M. Kuschner, *J. Nat. Cancer Inst.*, 1966, **37**, 825.
153 B. L. Van Duuren, L. Langseth, L. Orris, M. Baden, and M. Kuschner, *J. Nat. Cancer Inst.*, 1967, **39**, 1213.
154 B. L. Van Duuren, L. Langseth, B. M. Goldschmidt, and L. Orris, *J. Nat. Cancer Inst.*, 1967, **39**, 1217.
155 B. M. Goldschmidt, T. P. Balzeu, and B. L. Van Duuren, *Tetrahedron Lett.*, 1968, 1583.
156 B. L. Van Duuren, *Ann. N. Y. Acad. Sci.*, 1969, **163**, 633.
157 E. Kriek, *Chem.-Biol. Interact.*, 1969, **1**, 1.
158 E. Dybing, E. J. Soederlund, and L. T. Haug, *Cancer Res.*, 1979, **39**, 3268.
159 E. Dybing and E. J. Soederlund, in 'Proc. Symp. Conjugation Reactions in Drug Biotransformations,' ed. A. Aitio, Elsevier, Amsterdam, 1978, pp. 283—292.
160 D. L. Stout and F. F. Becker, *Cancer Res.*, 1979, **39**, 1168.
161 E. Dybing, C. von Bahr, T. Aune, H. Glaumann, D. S. Levitt, and S. S. Thorgeirsson, *Cancer Res.*, 1979, **39**, 4206.
162 G. Lhoest, M. Roberfroid, and M. Mercier, *Biomed. Mass Spectrom*, 1978, **5**, 38.

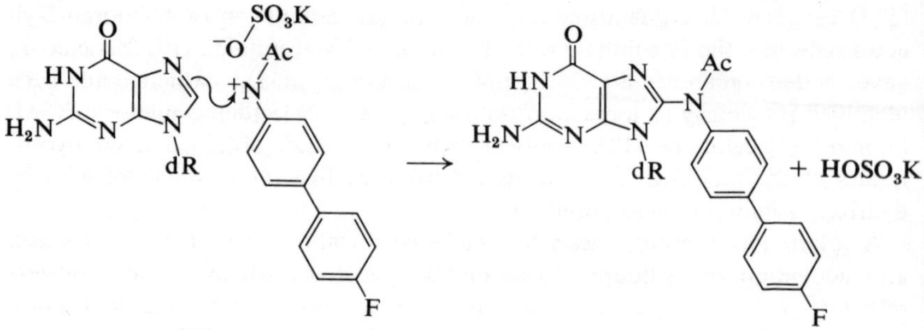

(17) (16)

Scheme 6

(16) (Scheme 6) or *N*-deoxyguanosin-8-yl-4-amino-4′-fluorobiphenyl.[163] In comparison with the corresponding acetylaminobiphenyl derivative synthetic *N*-potassium sulphate salt of 4-acetylamino-4′-fluorobiphenyl (17) proved to be twice as reactive towards the deoxyguanosine residues of DNA.[163] The attempted synthesis of 3-deoxyguanosin-N^3-ylarylamides was unsuccessful[163].

N-Acetoxy-4-acetamidostilbene reacted with cytidine to give the deamination product, 1-(4-acetamidophenyl)-1-(3-uridyl)-2-hydroxy-2-phenylethane (18) plus three minor products, with adenosine to give 1-(4-acetamidophenyl)-1-(N^6-adenosyl)-2-hydroxy-2-phenylethane (19) and 3-(β-D-ribosyl)-7-phenyl-8-(4-acetamidophenyl)-7,8-dihydroimidazo[2,1-*i*]purine (20), and with guanosine

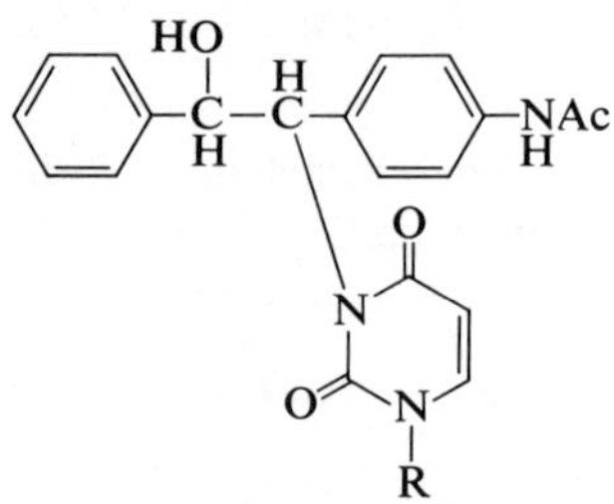

(18)

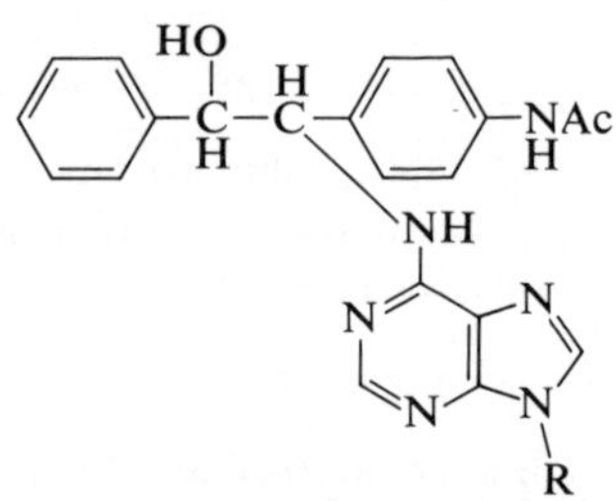

(19)

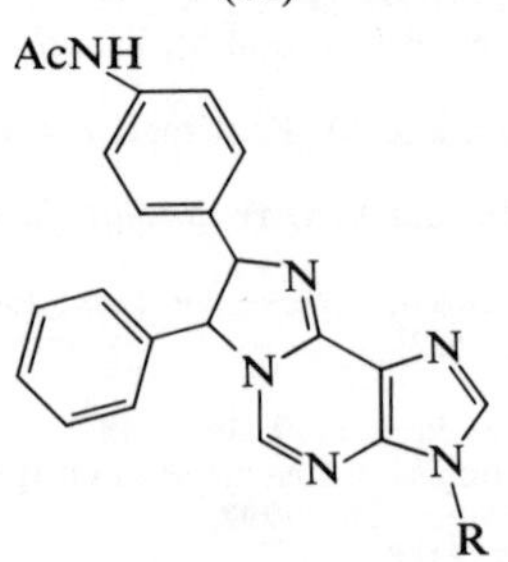

(20)

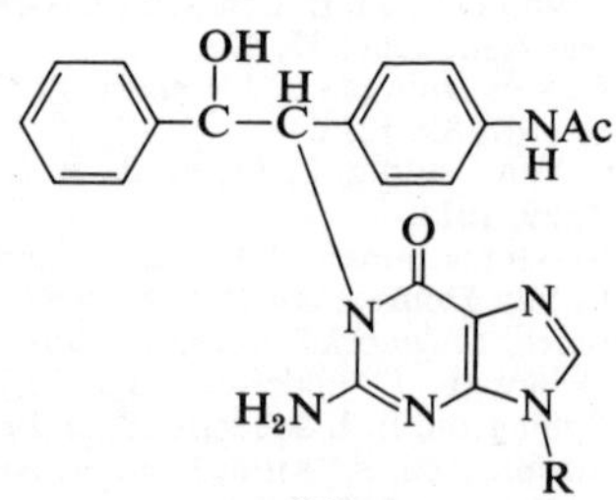

(21)

[163] E. Kriek and G. M. Hengeveld, *Chem.-Biol. Interact.*, 1978, **21**, 179.

to give 1-(4-acetamidophenyl)-1-(1-guanosyl)-2-hydroxy-2-phenylethane (21), a minor product which appeared to be also a guanosine *N*-1 derivative and two other minor products which on hydrolysis afforded 1-(4-acetamidophenyl)-2-phenylethane-1,2-diol, and thus appeared to be O^6-derivatives.[164] None of the guanine products which was isolated, had the properties of *N*-7, *C*-8, or N^2 adducts, and in this respect *N*-acetoxy-4-acetamidostilbene behaved more like a classical alkylating agent than like other previously studied *N*-acetoxy-*N*-arylacetamides.[164] In this connection, many of the adducts which had been formed through reaction of *N*-acetoxy-4-acetamidostilbene with nucleosides *in vitro* (*v. supra*), were obtained also through treatment of nucleic acids with the carcinogen.[165]

Although the foregoing illustrations cannot be said to have ever been bulk chemicals, they have a bearing on the interaction with genetic material of the industrial aromatic amines, *viz.* 4-aminobiphenyl, benzidine, and 1- and 2-naphthylamines, and their important derivatives.

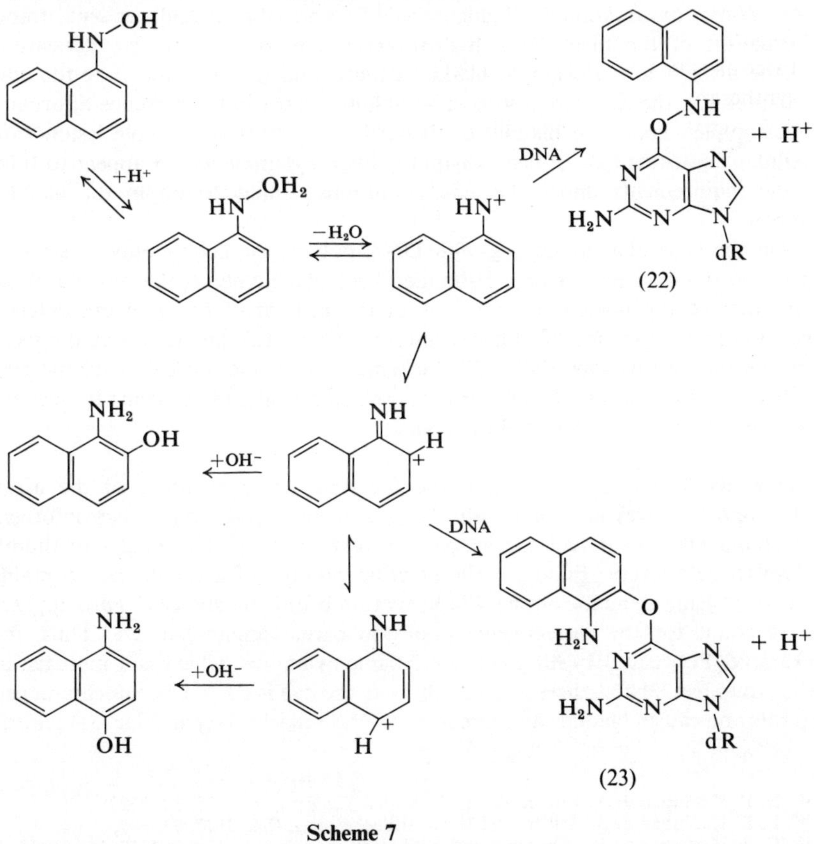

Scheme 7

[164] N. K. Scribner, J. D. Scribner, D. L. Smith, K. H. Schram, and J. A. McCloskey, *Chem.-Biol. Interact.*, 1979, **26**, 27.

[165] N. K. Scribner and J. D. Scribner, *Chem.-Biol. Interact.*, 1979, **26**, 47.

1-Naphthylhydroxylamine, the ultimate carcinogenic form of 1-naphthylamine, reacts (S_N1) with nucleic acids under slightly acidic conditions (pH 5) to form covalently bonded nucleoside analogues with 3—20 naphthyl residues/1000 monomer units, and the rates of reaction were first order both with respect to DNA and to 1-naphthylhydroxylamine.[166] These authors[166] identified the major adduct as *N*-deoxyguanosin-O^6-yl-1-naphthylamine (22) (Scheme 7), and two other adducts as 2-deoxyguanosin-O^6-yl-1-naphthylamine (23) and its decomposition product. Direct evidence for acid-dependent arylnitrenium ion formation was obtained by isotope exchange upon solvolysis of 1-naphthylhydroxylamine in acidic $H_2{}^{18}O$, and carbocation formation was indicated by the simultaneous formation of the solvolysis products, 1-amino-2-naphthol and 4-amino-1-naphthol. These experiments established formation of arylnitrenium ion and carbocation species from arylhydroxylamine[166] (Scheme 7).

The reaction mechanism (Scheme 7) has important biological implications for arylamine-induced urinary bladder carcinogenesis. If the hydrolysis of the *N*-hydroxyarylamine *N*-glucuronide[167] and the acid-dependent transformation of the liberated *N*-hydroxyarylamine to give reactive derivatives in the urine[166] are relevant to bladder cancer, and this appears to be the case (chapter 13), the electrophiles must be able to persist in the presence of urinary nucleophiles, enter the bladder epithelium, and induce a heritable lesion in a cellular constituent(s). In fact, 1-naphthylhydroxylamine would appear to fulfil these requirements under the acid conditions usually found in the bladder lumen.

On the basis that miscoding with DNA polymerase occurs only where it is possible to construct a stable H-bonded base pair involving the modified base and that of the nucleotide, which is in the process of being incorporated[116] (section 1), then the modified bases described,[166] *viz.* (22) and (23), would appear to interfere in this way, (24)—(29) (Scheme 8), with the normal Watson–Crick (dC-dG) base-pairing (*cf.* ref. 166). The resulting miscoding seems to account for the mutagenicity of 1-naphthylamine.

Amino-azo Dyes.—At first sight, the fact that some members of the array of amino-azo dyes are comparatively safe or even innocuous, whereas others are mutagens and potent carcinogens, is very puzzling. Three rules of thumb seem to be relevant. Firstly, if the reaction product of azo-reductase contains a carcinogenic aromatic amine, the formation of this substance *de novo* appears to account for the carcinogenicity of the parent amino-azo dye. Thus, for example, Ponceau 3R (30) yields 2,4,5-trimethylaniline, which is a mutagen in the Ames test,[168] and there is no doubt that the dye itself is a hepatocarcinogen in rats and causes bladder tumours in mice.[169] Similarly, Trypan Blue (31) affords

[166] F. F. Kadlubar, J. A. Miller, and E. C. Miller, *Cancer Res.*, 1978, **38**, 3628.
[167] F. F. Kadlubar, J. A. Miller, and E. C. Miller, *Cancer Res.*, 1977, **37**, 605.
[168] C. P. Hartman, A. W. Andrews, and K.-T. Chung, *Infect. Immunol.*, 1979, **23**, 686.
[169] IARC Monographs on the Evaluation of Carcinogenic Risk of Chemicals to Man, International Agency for Research on Cancer, Lyon, France, 1975, vol. 8, Ponceau 3R, pp. 199—204.

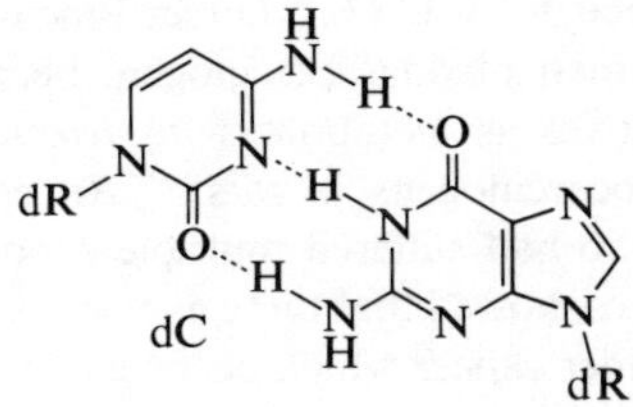

dC dG

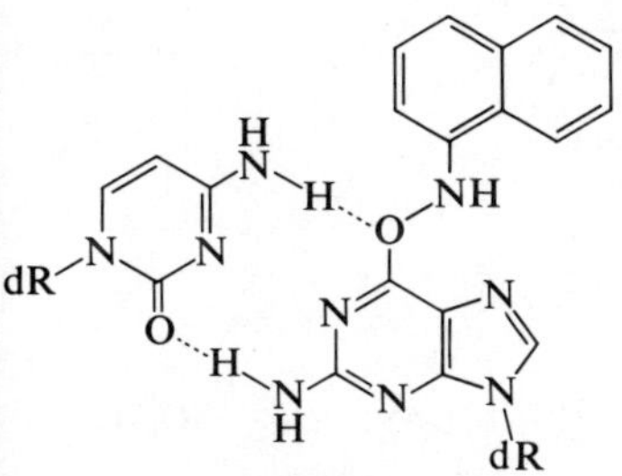

(24)

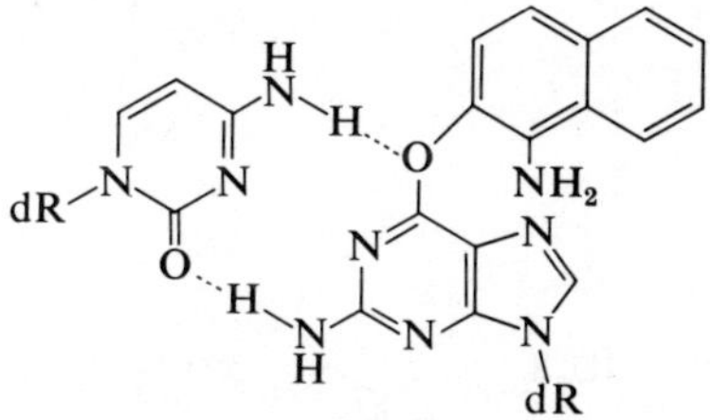

(25)

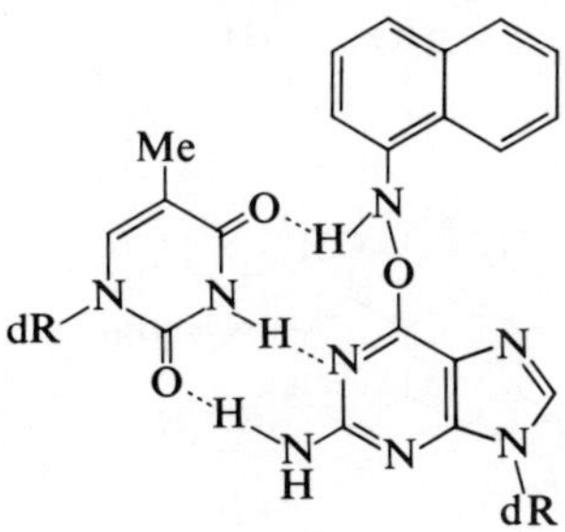

(26)

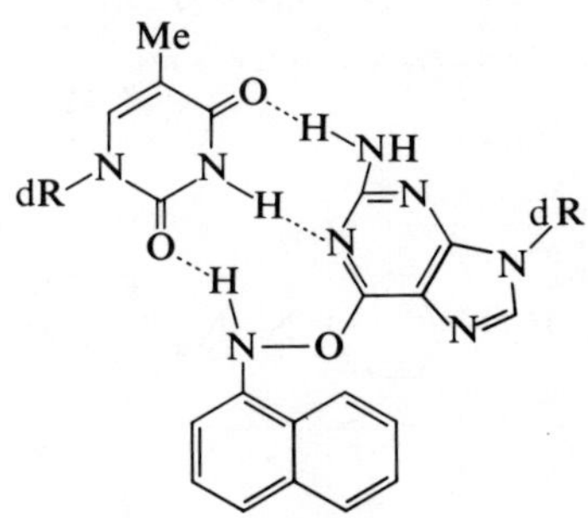

(27)

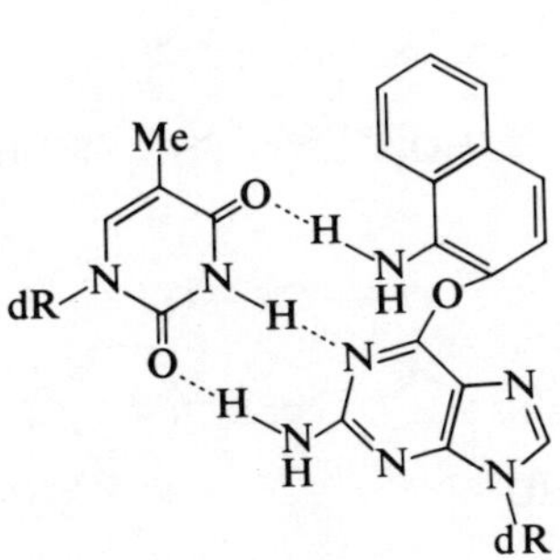

(28)

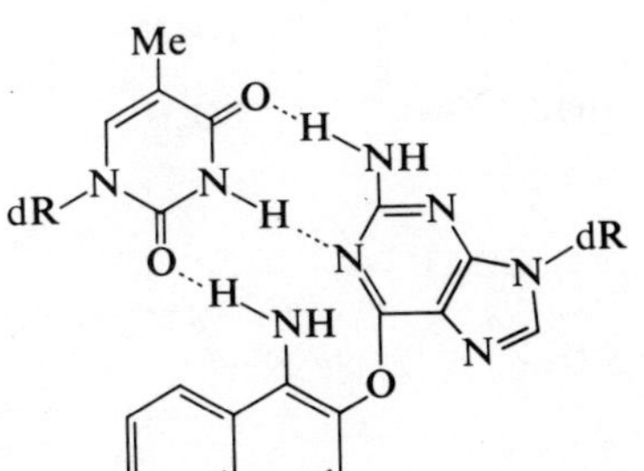

(29)

Scheme 8

o-tolidine, which is mutagenic in the Ames test,[170] and is itself a potent hepatocarcinogen in rats.[171] Direct Black 38 (32), Direct Blue 6 (33), and Direct Brown 95 (34) all afford the human bladder carcinogen, benzidine, and its *N*-acetyl and *N,N'*-diacetyl derivatives as metabolites *in vivo*, and all three amino-azo dyes are powerful hepatocarcinogens in rats.[172] An epidemiological study of silk dyers and painters who had suffered multiple exposure both to benzidine-based dyes and to other dyes showed that these exposures were strongly associated with the incidence of bladder cancer which occurred.[172] Secondly, in other cases

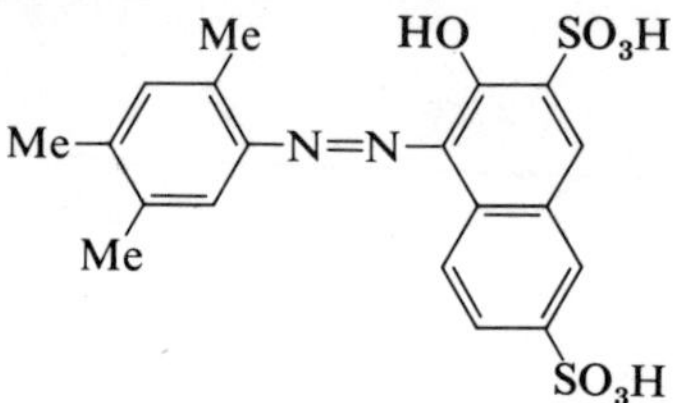

(30)

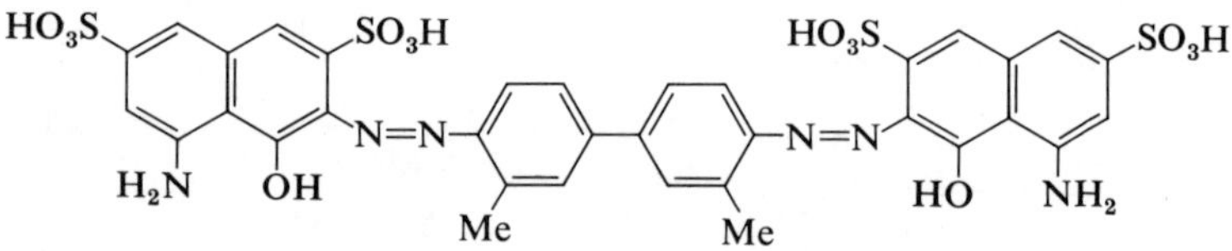

(31)

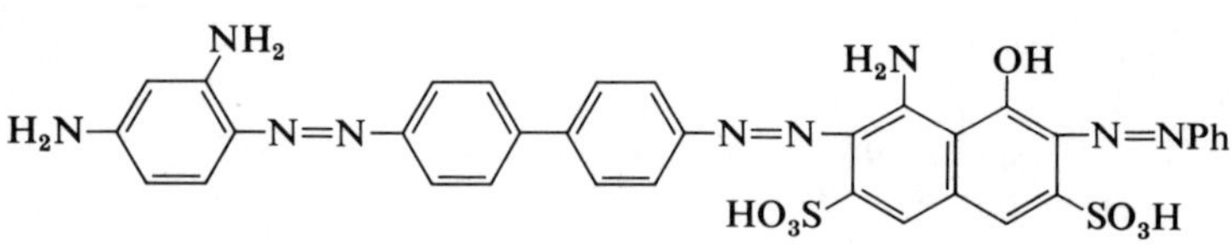

(32)

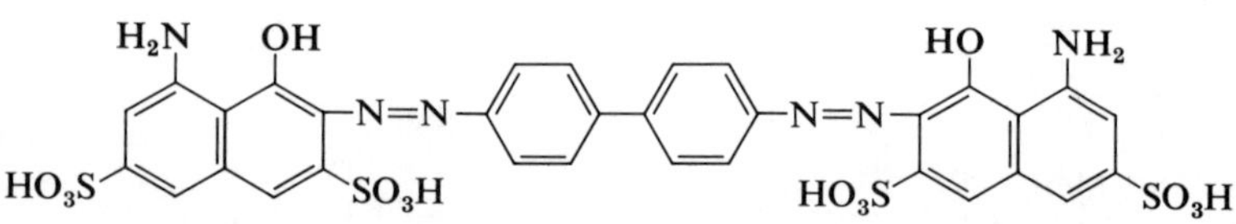

(33)

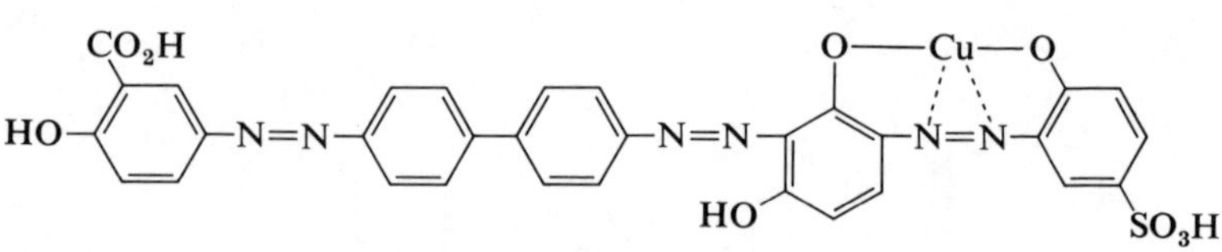

(34)

[170] C. P. Hartman, G. E. Fulk, and A. W. Andrews, *Mutat. Res.*, 1978, **58**, 125.
[171] Ref. 169; pp. 267—278.
[172] IARC Monographs on the Evaluation of Carcinogenic Risk of Chemicals to Man, International Agency for Research on Cancer, 'Direct Black 38, Direct Blue 6 and Direct Brown 95' Lyon, France, 1982, vol. 29, pp. 295—330.

where azoreductase does not yield carcinogenic aromatic amines, the carcinogenicity of the parent dyes may be attributable to direct *N*-hydroxylation of the dyes *per se*. In such cases, the lipophilicity of the compounds concerned

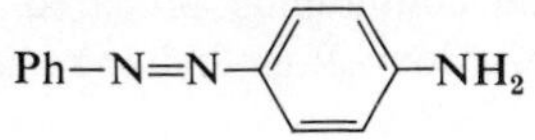

(35)

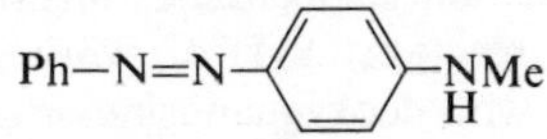

(36)

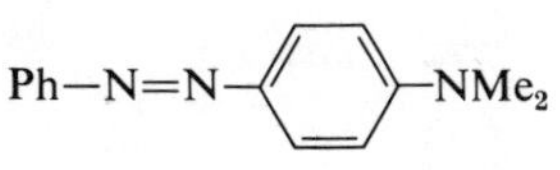

(37)

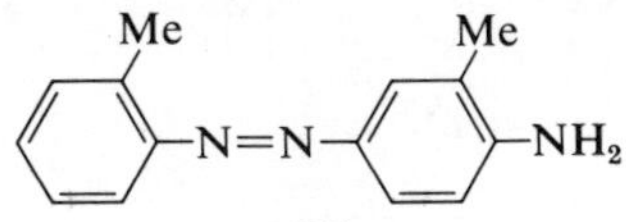

(38)

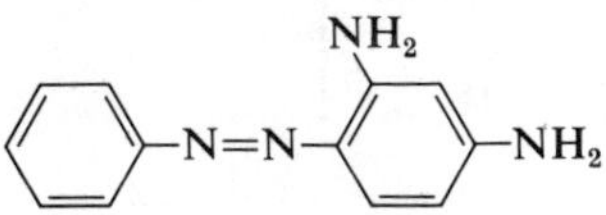

(39)

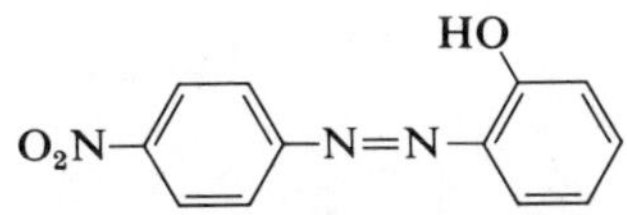

(40)

and their consequent tissue retention undoubtedly play a role. Exemplification is provided by the hepatocarcinogens,[173] *p*-aminoazobenzene (35), *p*-methylaminoazobenzene (36), *p*-dimethylaminoazobenzene (37), *o*-aminoazotoluene (38), chrysoidine (39), and para-Red (40). Thirdly, in other cases where there is a relatively high degree of sulphonation in comparison with molecular size, as in the case, for example, of Amaranth (41), of Sunset Yellow FCF (42), of Orange G(43), and of Ponceau SX (44),[174] detergent action mitigates against absorption and facilitates the elimination of unchanged dye from the body. Little, if any, risk attaches to the use of such substances.[174]

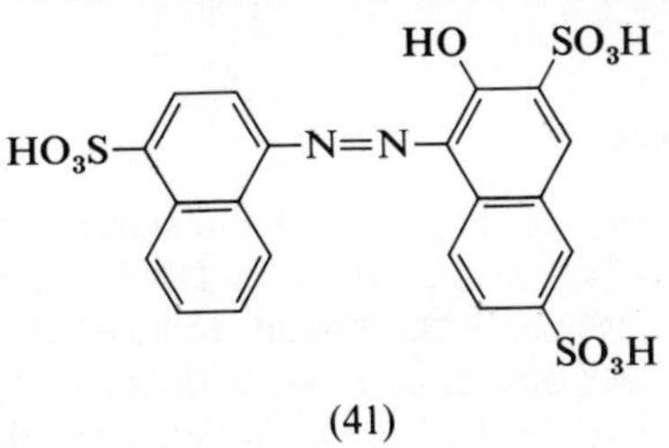

(41)

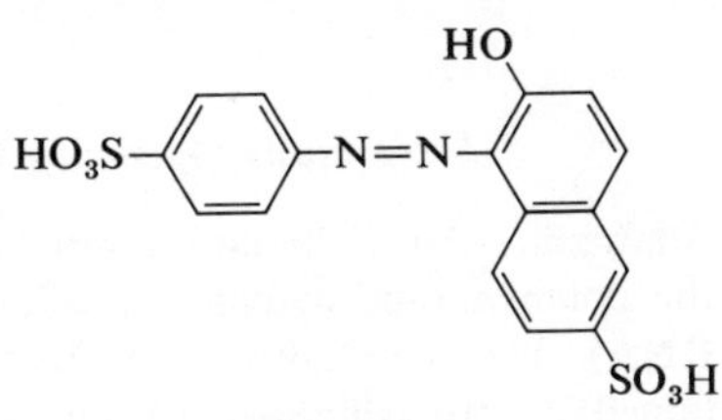

(42)

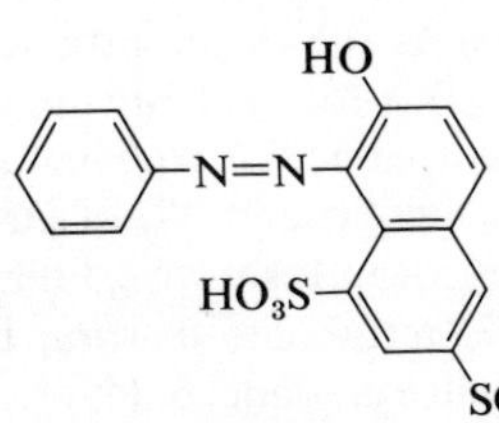

(43)

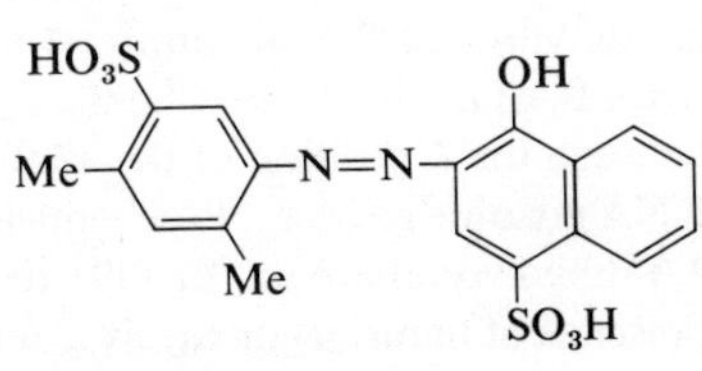

(44)

[173] Ref. 169; pp. 53—58, 61—69, 91—96, 125—146.
[174] Ref. 169; pp. 41—51, 181—187, 207—215, 257—266.

Degradation of the liver DNA and RNA from rats which had been injected with 4-(*N*-methylamino)azobenzene (36) (Scheme 9) gave respectively 4-[*N*-(deoxyguanosin-8-yl)-*N*-methylamino]azobenzene (45) and 4-[*N*-(guanosin-8-yl)-*N*-methylamino]azobenzene, identical with the compounds prepared by the chemical reaction (S_N1) of synthetic 4-(*N*-benzoyloxy-*N*-methylamino)azobenzene (46) with deoxyguanosine or guanosine.[9]

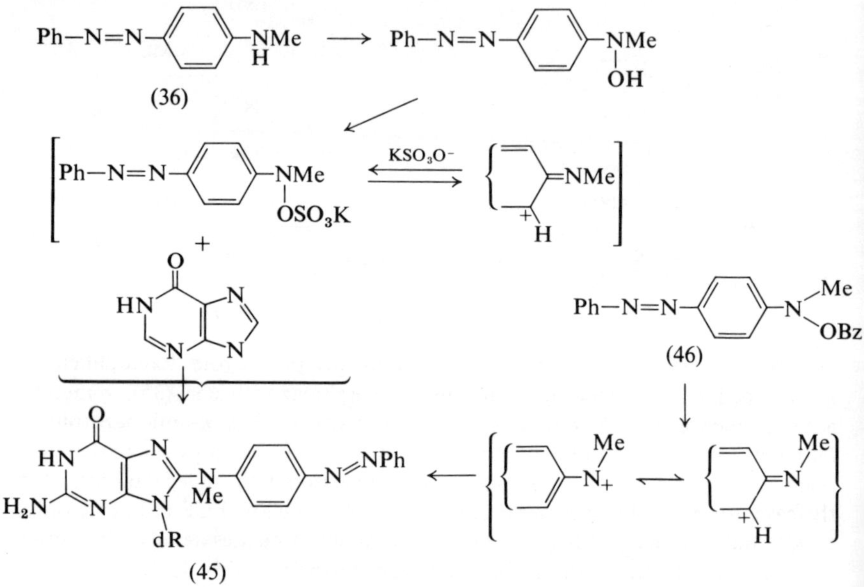

Scheme 9

3 Naturally Occurring Carcinogens

Aflatoxin.—An S_N2 mechanism would appear to apply to the reaction of the potent mould carcinogen, aflatoxin B_1 (47) (Scheme 10), with DNA (and RNA). The structure of the DNA- and ribosomal RNA-bound adducts obtained[175] from salmon-sperm DNA and rat-liver ribosomal RNA with fortified rat- and hamster-liver microsomes was inferred by hydrolysis, which yielded 2,3-dihydro-2-(7-guanyl)-3-hydroxyaflatoxin B_1 (48) as the major product and 2,3-dihydro-2-[(2,5,6-triamino-4-oxopyrimidin-N^5-yl)-*N*-formyl]-3-hydroxyaflatoxin B_1 as a minor one. Chemical reaction thus occurred both *in vitro* and *in vivo* between the 2-position of the aflatoxin B_1-epoxy metabolite and *N*-7 of DNA or RNA guanine residues. Biochemical study[176] has subsequently shown 2,3-dihydro-2,3-dihydroxyaflatoxin B_1 (49) to be a major (47) metabolite *in vitro*, in the presence of hamster- or rat-liver microsomes; negligible amounts of (49) resulted from (47) and rat-liver microsomes in the presence of DNA. This result[176]

[175] J.-K. Lin, J. A. Miller, and E. C. Miller, *Cancer Res.*, 1977, **37**, 4430.
[176] J.-K. Lin, K. A. Jennan, E. C. Miller, and J. A. Miller, *Cancer Res.*, 1978, **38**, 2424.

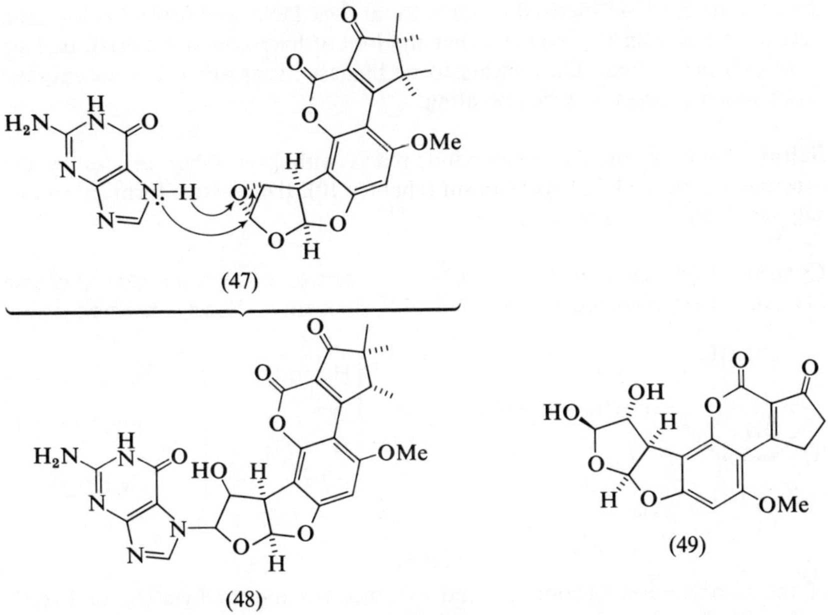

Scheme 10

substantiates the biotransformation in hamster and rat liver of (47) into aflatoxin B_1 2,3-epoxide, which would be expected to hydrolyse to yield (49).

Garner *et al.*[177] have identified the major aflatoxin G_1-DNA adduct, which is formed both *in vitro* and *in vivo* and after peracid oxidation, and have shown it to be the *trans*-9,10-dihydro-9-(7-guanyl)-10-hydroxyaflatoxin G_1 (50). Thus, (50) is similar to that, (48), obtained in exactly the same way from (47). Garner *et al.*[177] found: (i) that both aflatoxin B_1 (47) and G_1 bound more to rat-kidney and -liver DNA than to protein *in vivo*; (ii) that aflatoxin G_1 has a greater binding capacity than (47) for rat-kidney and -liver cellular macromolecules; (iii) that

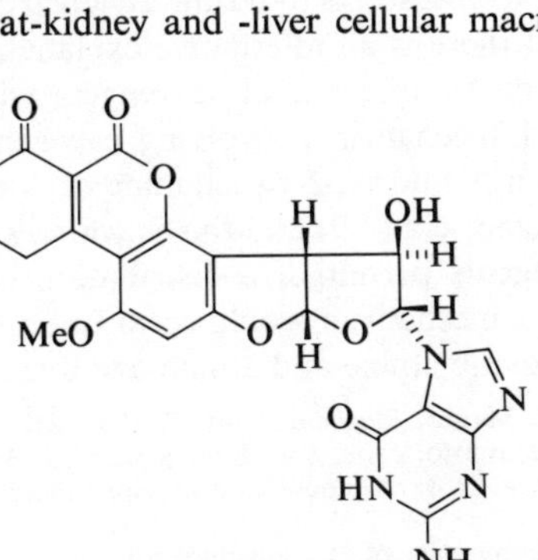

(50)

177 R. C. Garner, C. N. Martin, J. R. L. Smith, B. F. Coles, and M. R. Tolson, *Chem.-Biol. Interact.*, 1979, **26**, 57.

the persistence of (47)-derived material in rat-liver DNA and protein is less than that from aflatoxin G_1; and (iv) that the loss of liver-bound material, derived from (47) or aflatoxin G_1, appears to be biphasic, suggesting that an enzymic DNA-repair process may be operating.

Safrole.—Safrole, on the other hand, reacts with liver DNA *in vivo* by the previously described S_N1 mechanism (chapter 10), the reactive form safrole 1′-sulphate being a benzylic ester.

Cycasin.—Mutagenic and carcinogenic properties of cycasin (51) (Scheme 11) and other methylazoxymethanol (52) derivatives closely resemble those

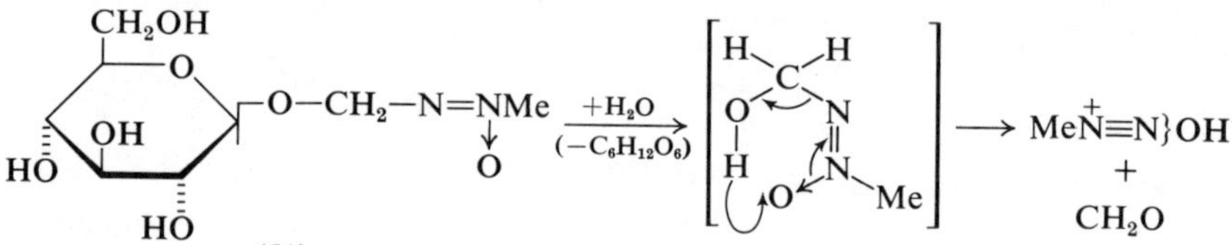

(51) (52)

Scheme 11

of the nitrosamines (section 1), and evidence for the methylation of liver[178] and brain[179] nucleic acids *in vivo* was obtained 10—15 years ago. Some work also with DNA chromatin preparations from carcinogen-treated animals and with *E. coli* RNA polymerase (miscoding sub-section, section 1) has been implemented.[180]

4 Concluding Remarks

(1) It will be seen that the Millers' concept (1970, 1971),[1,2] that reaction of chemical carcinogens with genetic material may be due to the electrophilicity of the ultimate reactive forms, seems to be universally true. Nucleophiles are non-carcinogenic,[181,182] and there is an alternative explanation[183,184] to the obvious one for the intervention of free-radical scavengers with carcinogenicity. The Millers[2] attributed S_N1 mechanisms involving carbenium and nitrenium ions to the reactions between *N*-fluoren-2-ylacetamide or *N*-methylaminoazabenzene and DNA *in vivo* (Schemes 6 and 9) and this is entirely satisfactory, as the aromatic rings of the reagents permit of a distribution of charge which confers cation stability. An S_N1 mechanism would seem to apply to the corresponding interactions of the aromatic amine and amino-azo dye carcinogens.

178 R. C. Shank and P. N. Magee, *Biochem. J.*, 1967, **105**, 521.
179 Y. Nagata and H. Matsumoto, *Proc. Soc. Exp. Biol. Med.*, 1969, **132**, 383.
180 D. J. Grab, M. S. Zedeck, N. I. Surslocki, and M. Sonenberg, *Chem.-Biol. Interact.*, 1973, **6**, 259.
181 L. A. Poirier, Thesis, University of Wisconsin-Madison.
182 Z. Hadidian, T. N. Fredrickson, E. K. Weisburger, J. H. Weisburger, R. M. Glass, and N. Mantel, *J. Nat. Cancer Inst.*, 1968, **41**, 985.
183 P. A. Craven and F. R. De Rubertis, *Cancer Res.*, 1977, **37**, 4088.
184 D. E. Hathway, in 'Foreign Compound Metabolism in Mammals,' ed. D. E. Hathway, The Chemical Society, London, 1979, vol. 5, pp. 190—243.

(2) In general, there is no clear relationship between the reactivity of the ultimate carcinogens and carcinogenic potency. Thus, it is considered that the mechanism of the initial reaction between metabolically activated vinyl chloride, chloroethylene oxide, or chloroacetaldehyde and the deoxyadenosine, deoxycytidine, or deoxyguanosine residues of DNA is S_N2, and that glycidaldehyde as well as the epoxy-metabolites of aflatoxin B_1 and G_1 react similarly with the deoxyguanosine residues. On the other hand, aromatic amines, reactive amino-azo dyes, and safrole have an S_N1 reaction mechanism with DNA deoxyguanosine residues.

(3) Amongst directly acting methylating carcinogens, DMS and MMS show low electrophilic reactivity and are typical S_N2 alkylating agents, whereas MNU, MNNG, and MPT show co-ordination between the intermediate produced and the nucleophile, and a reactivity somewhat between that of an S_N1 and an S_N2 mechanism. Methylation by the latter agents involves $Me—N_2^+$ ions or methanediazohydroxide rather than the highly reactive Me^+ species, and is bimolecular. A mechanism is discussed. Whilst DMS and MMS yield a relatively low proportion of *O*-alkylation products, the ratio of O^6-methylguanine to N^7-methylguanine being 0.004, MNU, MNNG, and MPT give relatively high yields of *O*-alkylation products, the ratio of O^6-methylguanine to N^7-methylguanine being *ca.* 0.12. Oxidative *N*-demethylation of DMN and DMPT occurs and alkylation involves $Me—N_2^+$ ions. Relatively stable transport forms of some *asym-N,N*-dialkylnitrosamines determine the site of tumour induction, where further metabolism into the powerful alkylating $R—N_2^+$ species takes place. The capacity of the agents to form O^6-methylguanine in target-tissue DNA correlates with their carcinogenic potency, and DES, DMS, and MMS fail to induce tumours in tissues where MNU, DMN, MPT, and DMPT are active carcinogens.

Nucleic acid is alkylated to a lesser extent by ethylating than by methylating agents. The typical S_N2 agent EMS affords an O^6-ethylguanine to N^7-ethylguanine ratio of 0.03, whereas ENU and DEN, which react through $Et—N_2^+$, give a ratio of from 0.48 to at least 0.70. DEN and ENU are much more powerful carcinogens than EMS.

(4) Evidence is cited for the chemical reaction of Cr^{VI} or Cr^{V} with DNA *in vivo*. *cis*-$[PtCl_2(NH_3)_2]$ reacts with DNA by an S_N2 mechanism.

(5) In summary, points (1)—(4) show that not many reactions between ultimate chemical carcinogens and nucleic acid can be described as S_N1, and the suggestion[2–4] that S_N2 reactions predominate over pure S_N1 reactions (*v. supra*) applies to the subject-matter of this chapter.

(6) The persistence in DNA of nucleoside analogues, formed by the reactive forms of carcinogens, enables DNA-repair to be investigated. This approach and work on the miscoding incurred by alkylation during nucleic acid synthesis facilitate appraisal of the biological significance of the presence of various nucleoside analogues in DNA with reference to tumour induction in the target tissues. Thus, the importance of O^6-alkylation of the deoxyguanosine residue of DNA becomes apparent. The same arguments as were used in the case of the simple alkylating carcinogens apply also to the miscoding adducts, for example

of vinyl chloride (Scheme 3) and of those afforded by 1-naphthylhydroxylamine (Scheme 8).

(7) Introduction of bulky substituents at sites on the back-side of the purine residues of DNA would tend to interfere with the stacking of the bases inside the double helix, and so lead to 'unstacking'[15] and formation of *N*-deoxyguanosin-8-yl-*N*-fluoren-2-ylacetamide and 4-[*N*-(deoxyguanosin-8-yl)-*N*-methylamino]azobenzene, and N^7-platination might exemplify such distortion; but the miscoding properties of these and of many other nucleoside analogues (or adducts) have yet to be investigated.

(8) Particularly in the past, progress in elucidating meaningful mechanisms of chemical carcinogenesis has been hampered severely by the methodology available. In much of the work even today methods are stretched to breaking-point, and in this context, for example, liquid scintillation counting, mass fragmentometry involving multiple-ion detection, the most sensitive n.m.r. spectroscopy, and spectrophotofluorimetry are used at the very limits of their sensitivity. Great advances in chemical/biochemical instrumentation have been made over the last three decades, and it would not have been possible to muster the present techniques at the time when the double helix structure for DNA was elucidated, in the early 1950s. Notable advances are being made currently in contiguous areas of molecular biology, and it is likely that the application of this new knowledge will give more meaning to the molecular studies which have been described in this chapter.

Chapter 12 Host Factors and Cellular Aspects

By R. Süss
Deutsches Krebsforschungszentrum, Heidelberg

1 Introduction

Chemical carcinogens have been best sellers in cancer research ever since the days of Yamagiwa[1] and Yoshida,[2] for good reasons. They are abundant in our environment, and although Ames' expression of 'a sea of carcinogens' may be a slight exaggeration, they can be very effective. Distillation workers handling β-naphthylamine in the old dye factories eventually succumbed to bladder cancer;[3] however, this high incidence seems to be rather the exception than the rule. Only one out of eight heavy smokers ends up with lung cancer, and although women whose mothers were treated with high doses of oestrogen during pregnancy may develop vaginal cancer, only four out of 100 000 do.[4]

In the last few years the emphasis has shifted in cancer research. The main question is no longer why people do get cancer but, why so many people do not. In other words, what keeps them surviving even in a 'sea of carcinogens'?

There is a trivial answer as well as a rather complex answer to this question. The trivial answer is that most carcinogens present in our environment occur in rather low concentrations, while the complex answer is that the host, that is the organism attacked by chemical carcinogens, can react to these agents. 'Host factors' thus increase or decrease the action of a carcinogen, and host defence is more than wishful thinking.

In this chapter, some of these host factors will be presented, more in an anecdotal than in a systematic way, as follows: (i) the host as modifier of chemical carcinogenesis. (ii) The targets with which the chemical carcinogens react; basic strategies of chemical carcinogens. (iii) Chemical carcinogenesis as a multi-step process. (iv) The winning cell; a few remarks on some sociocellular parameters.

2 Chemical Carcinogens and Their Host

If a chemical carcinogen and a host coincide, cancer is not the inevitable consequence. The carcinogen needs the co-operation of the host. Most convincing evidence for the host's involvement in chemical carcinogenesis comes from genetic experiments and observations.

[1] K. Yamagiwa and K. Ichikawa, *Mitt. Med. Fakulat Kaiserl.*, (*Tokyo*) 1915, **15**, 295.
[2] T. Sasaki and T. Yoshida, *Virchows Arch. Pathol. Anat.*, 1935, **295**, 175.
[3] E. Boyland, 'The Causes of Cancer,' in 'Aktuelle Probleme aus dem Gebiet der Cancerologie II,' (ed. H. Lettre and G. Wagner, Berlin, 1968, p. 3 (Figure 2).
[4] F. P. Li, 'Host factors in cancer in man,' in 'Abstracts of the 9th annual medical symposium on successes in cancer management today,' Boston, Mass., 1977 (quoted after cancerlit).

Genetic Evidence.—As an example, Boutwell's experiments may be referred to.[5] Boutwell induced skin cancer in mice using the so-called two-step procedure (see below). In breeding studies, he selected susceptible and resistant mice and finally obtained a wide spectrum of mouse strains with different susceptibilities. The most sensitive strain had 12 times more papilloma per mouse after 12 weeks than the original strain, while levels in the most resistant strain reached not more than 30% of this.

A second example stems from human epidemiology. Tokuhata observed that the risk for smokers from non-cancer families of developing lung cancer was 2.6 times smaller than for smokers from lung-cancer families.[6]

Boutwell's mice and Tokuhata's smokers were born with different sensitivities. Such differences, however, may be as much a consequence of environmental as of genetic influences.

Diet Factors.—Variations in diet appear to be an important environmental factor.[7] Liver cancer can be induced by azo dyes only when the rats are living on a low-protein diet.[2] Experiments with animals on low caloric diets[8] point in a rather different direction. In these animals, the induction of sarcomas by chemical carcinogens, for instance, is delayed. Fats have been accused of favouring the induction of colon and breast cancer.

Mammary gland tumours were induced by DMBA[9] and colon cancers by direct instillation of different carcinogens such as *N*-methyl-*N*-nitro-*N*-nitrosoguanidine, methylnitrosourea, or methylazoxymethanol.[10] The observations made in animals' systems with cancer, produced by chemical carcinogens, are supported by epidemiological evidence.

Vitamin A and its derivatives protect against epithelial tumours (bladder, lung, skin, and breast). This has prompted the daring adventure of a cancer-prevention programme with vitamin A pills.[11]

Selenium at trace element concentrations reduces the incidence of colon, liver, skin, and mammary-gland cancers induced by chemical carcinogens.[12]

The way in which dietary constituents modify chemical carcinogenesis may vary. The changing of the metabolism of chemical carcinogens may be the main mechanism by which diet factors act, and shifting metabolic consequences from activation to detoxification could be the strategic manoeuvre. To quote a

[5] R. K. Boutwell, 'Some biological aspects of skin carcinogenesis,' in Progress Exp. Tumor Res. IV,' (ed. F. Homburger) Basel, 1964, p. 207.

[6] G. K. Tokuhata, 'Cancer of the lung: Host and environmental interactions,' ed. H. T. Lynch, Cancer Genetics, Springfield, 1976, p. 213 (Table 4).

[7] 'Nutrition and Cancer,' ed. M. Winick, New York, 1977; A. Tannenbaum, 'Nutrition and Cancer,' in 'Physiopathology of Cancer,' ed. F. Hornberger, New York, 1959.

[8] F. Homburger, A. Treger, and J. R. Baker, *Cancer Res.* 1963, **23**, 1539.

[9] K. K. Caroll, and H. T. Khor, *Lipids* 1971, **6**, 415; P. C. Chan, and L. A. Cohen, *J. Natl. Cancer Inst.*, 1974, **52**, 25.

[10] M. S. Martin, *Bull. Cancer* (*Paris*), 1978, **65**, 49.

[11] M. B. Sporn, Prevention of Epithelial Cancer by Vitamin A and its synthetic analogues,' ed. H. H. Hiatt, *et al.* in 'Origins of Human Cancer, Book A,' Cold Spring Harbour 1977, p. 801.

[12] C. W. Welsch, *et al. Carcinogenesis*, 1981, **2**, 519.

rather recent observation, 'vitamin A and vitamin C reduce the binding of dimethylbenzanthracene to the DNA of mouse epithelial cells.'[13]

Formation of oestrogen hormones from the steroids of diets rich in fats by the intestinal flora has been suggested as a mechanism by which breast cancer may be promoted.[14]

In addition, even immunological defence mechanisms may be disturbed by nutritional imbalance.[15]

Hormonal Status.—The mammary gland is well known to be hormone sensitive and many tumours of this organ are hormone dependent as well. Chemical carcinogenesis of the mammary gland does not occur in castrated animals nor in hypophysectomized animals.[16]

More surprising is the dependency of liver tumours on some hormones. The induction of hepatomas by acetamidofluorene is only possible in the presence of thyroxine and testosterone. Removal of the gland by castration and thyroidectomy abolishes liver carcinogenesis by acetamidofluorene.[17]

Manipulating the immune system may have paradoxical results.[18–20] Procedures intended to enhance the immune defence may actually increase tumour growth (this phenomenon has been known for a long time as enhancement), but the reverse can be true as well. Splenectomy abolishes liver carcinogenesis by *p*-dimethylaminoazobenzene (see ref. 45). The removal of an important part of the immune system does not lead to the faster growth of tumours that may be expected, but it prevents chemical carcinogenesis.

Viral Status.—There are reports that chemical carcinogens can induce tumours only when a 'virus is present'. Discussion of the interactions of chemical carcinogens with tumour viruses is postponed until the next section.

Age of the Host.—Young animals are more susceptible to chemical carcinogens than older ones. The most dramatic case is pre-natal carcinogenesis. In studies by Ivancovic,[21] the dose which will produce tumours in the offspring is only 1/50 of that necessary to induce tumours in the adult animal.

Another matter is the increasing susceptibility towards cancer with age. It is sometimes believed that old age as such could be 'carcinogenic' and, in a sense, that surveillance mechanisms dwindle with old age, thereby allowing cancer cells to multiply freely. Indeed, age is a major factor in risk from cancer, as the risk increases dramatically with age. However, it is hard to decide whether

13 M. Shoyab, *Oncology*, 1981, **38**, 187.
14 B. Reddy and J. H. Wiesburger, *J. Natl. Cancer Inst.*, 1974, **52**, 507.
15 R. R. Chandra, *Fed. Proc. Fed. Am. Soc. Exp. Biol.*, 1980, **39**, 3088.
16 K. H. Clifton, and B. N. Sridaran, 'Endocrine Factors and Tumor Growth,' in 'Cancer.' ed. F. F. Becker, New York, 1975, vol. 3, p. 249.
17 M. D. Reuber, *J. Natl. Cancer Inst.*, 1969, **43**, 445.
18 T. H. Weisburger and G. M. Williams, 'Metabolisms of Chemical Carcinogens,' in 'Cancer,' ed. F. F. Becker, New York, 1975, vol. 1, p. 185.
19 R. W. Baldwin, *Adv. Cancer Res.*, 1973, **18**, 1.
20 R. Kroes, J. W. Weiss, and J. H. Weisburger, *Recent Results Cancer Res.*, 1975, **52**, 65.
21 S. Ivancovic, *Recent Results Cancer Res.*, 1974, **44**, 16.

this increased risk is the trivial consequence of accumulating doses of carcinogens, or whether it is the effect of age alone.

In an experiment carried out by Peto, no influence of age on chemical carcinogenesis was detected. The induction of skin cancer had always the same latency irrespective of whether it was induced in young or old adult animals.[22]

3 Basic Strategies for Chemical Carcinogens

What are the targets attacked by chemical carcinogens? Are cells directly transformed by chemical carcinogens, or are there more indirect ways? There would seem to be room for both of them.

Cells as Targets.—Since the pioneering work of Sachs,[23] there is no denying the fact that chemical carcinogens can transform normal cells into tumour cells in a test tube. Cells transformed *in vitro* may grow as other tumour cells do; criss-cross and piling up in tissue-culture plates, forming cell colonies in soft agar, or growing as tumours when transplanted into a suitable host. What is surprising is that what takes weeks or months in an animal is brought about in tissue culture in hours or days.[24] Transformation *in vitro* clearly demonstrates that chemical carcinogens can bring about transformation more or less directly, but this does not mean that such a direct way is followed *in vivo* as well.

Cancer as a Systemic Disease.—It is sometimes believed that cancer is in principle a systemic disease with local manifestations, but there are some puzzling observations:

(i) Todaro observed that fibroblasts isolated from patients pre-disposed to leukaemia are transformed more easily by a tumour virus than those from normal patients.[25] Fibroblasts (which have nothing to do with the later leukaemia) obviously suggest that a general alert has been given to the whole organism.

(ii) Azzarone made a similar observation,[26] *viz.* that the fibroblasts from lung cancer patients were more easily transformed *in vitro* than those from healthy patients. This suggests that the whole organism has a tendency for cancer, long before tumours arise at a specific site, as the fibroblasts were taken from the skin, far away from lung tumour sites.

(iii) Kopelovich discovered another parameter which would indicate the organism's susceptibility to cancer.[27] The cytoskeleton of tumour cells is of a different type from that of normal cells. Such tumour type cytoskeletons were found in fibroblasts from patients with adenomatosis of the colon and rectum. However, even symptomless children of these patients had these 'pre-cancer' fibroblast types.

[22] R. Peto, *et al., Br. J. Cancer*, 1975, **32**, 411.
[23] Y. Berward and L. Sachs, *J. Natl. Cancer Inst.*, 1965, **35**, 641.
[24] C. Heidelberger, *Ann. Rev. Biochem.*, 1975 **44**, 79.
[25] R. W. Miller and G. J. Todaro, *Lancet*, 1969, **1**, 81.
[26] Azzarone quoted after G. Mathe, 'Dossier Cancer,' Masson et Cie, Paris, 1977, p. 106.
[27] L. Kopelovich *et al., Proc. Natl. Acad. Sci. USA*, 1977, **74**, 3019.

Thus, a chemical carcinogen does not necessarily have to transform cells into neoplastic cells. In the instances quoted, the cells have already gone quite a long way in the direction of cancer. Chemical carcinogens just complete this process, and this seems to be true for another case. O-28 Mice have a genetically fixed lung-cancer incidence (about 30% after 12 months). If they are treated with diethylnitrosamine, predominantly a liver carcinogen, they go down with bronchus carcinomas to an extent of 90%.[28] Obviously the chemical carcinogen did not have to create tumour cells; it is more likely to release defensive mechanisms, which normally deplete the tumour yield.

At least one such defence system is known, *viz.* the immune system.

Carcinogens acting on the Immune System.—Chemical carcinogens suppress antibody production, and they do so even at the low concentrations necessary for cancer induction. But not only the humoral response is hampered; cellular immune reactions are also suppressed by chemical carcinogens. Graft rejection was inhibited, and sometimes graft survival was significantly retarded, after chemical carcinogen had been administered.[29]

There was a good correlation between this immunosuppressive action and the carcinogenicity of the chemical carcinogens tested. This might imply that the immunosuppressive action is an important parameter in the overall carcinogenic action.

Another set of experiments points in the same direction. Methylcholanthrene was found to be immunosuppressive only in those mouse strains which were sensitive to its carcinogenic action. Again, immunosuppression and carcinogenicity are closely related. However, it is difficult to believe that the immunosuppressive action of a chemical carcinogen alone would lead to cancer. According to the classical immune surveillance theory, tumour cells are formed continuously within the organism, but they are taken care of by the immune system. Shutting down this system would automatically allow these vagabonding tumour cells to multiply. If this were actually the main path by which chemical carcinogens produce tumours, it would be difficult to understand why so many different tumours are produced by so many different chemical carcinogens. Shutting down the immune system would allow tumour cells to grow independently of the type of carcinogen used.

Thus, the immunosuppressive 'side action' of chemical carcinogens appears rather as a supplementary feature within the carcinogenic process.

Activating Tumour Viruses.—Oncogenetic viruses can transform normal cells into tumour cells, and they do so by inserting their genome or at least part of it into the host's genetic material. As long as the strategic part of the tumour virus genome is integrated (commonly named sarc-gene in the case of RNA tumour viruses) the transformation works. The principle of viral transformation appears to be the transfer of a complete set of information from virus to cell (transfer of a 'cancer gene').

[28] J. Hilfrich, J. Althoff, and U. Mohr *Z. Krebsforsch.*, 1970, **75**, 240.
[29] See ref. 19.

This appears to be a completely different route to neoplasia than that taken by chemical carcinogens which interact with strategic targets in the cell until this target is suitably changed. The difference is similar to that between a prefabricated house and a house built from numerous bricks. However, there are strong indications that chemical carcinogens and tumour viruses may have something in common.

Lymphomas, originally induced by chemicals, can be propagated by cell-free extracts, that is by viruses.[30] This has been shown by Irino, experimenting with mice and methylcholanthrene. The chemical carcinogen seems to have activated a virus.

Using a special strain of a leukaemia virus (RadLV), Price was able to show that immunisation against this virus prevented the induction of sarcomas by methylcholanthrene.[31] Obviously the antibodies killed the virus, which was activated by the chemical carcinogen.

Fey, to quote a rather recent observation, also demonstrated the potentiating effect of tumour viruses and chemical carcinogens in producing tumours.[32] A cell-free extract (containing mouse leukaemia virus) produced neoplasms in 13% and nitrosomethylurea at suboptimal doses produced tumours in 9.7% of the mice. Cell-free extract followed by nitrosomethylurea however led to tumours in 48.6% of the animals treated.

There are signs that a chemical carcinogen can potentiate the effects of a tumour virus, if it is given before the virus is applied. In this case, the chemical carcinogen does not activate a virus, but it possibly facilitates the integration of the virus genome into the host's genome. However, in both cases, whether the chemical carcinogen prepares the way for reception of the tumour virus, or whether it activates a latent tumour virus, the virus appears to be the prime mover in carcinogenesis, with the chemical carcinogens relegated to an auxiliary role only. [There is a good explanation for all of the cases in which a chemical carcinogen alone brings about cancer, as the tumour virus genes, responsible for carcinogenesis (the oncogenes) are thought to be always present in more or less all of the cells of an organism.] However, the dominant role of tumour viruses has been challenged recently.

The Cancer Gene.—It is true that RNA tumour viruses carry a *sarc*-gene (a cancer gene), which is transferred to cells to make them neoplastic. However, very similar genes have been detected in normal cells as well. This leads to the idea that it is not the virus which brings the 'cancer gene' to a cell, but that this gene is present in the cell from the beginning. The virus, according to this view, is an innocent carrier.[33] A slight irritation remains. What is special about tumour viruses bringing cancer genes to cells which already have them? Why should the viral cancer gene produce cancer, whereas the cell's cancer gene does

[30] Irino quoted after Heidelberger, see ref. 24, ref. 349 therein.

[31] D. P. J. Price, 'Inhibition of chemical transformation *in vitro* and tumor induction *in vivo* by inhibition of viral expression,' in 'The Role of Viruses in Human Cancer', ed. G. Giraldo and F. Beth New York, 1980, vol. 1, p. 157

[32] F. Fey, *Arch. Geschwulstforsch.*, 1881, **51**, 611.

[33] J. M. Bishop, *Scientific American*, 1982, **246**, (March), 68.

not? However, it may be assumed that the cellular gene is under control in normal cells, whereas the gene imported by the virus is not. Another explanation put forward is that the imported cancer gene tips the balance in favour of cancer genes within the cell; *i.e.* cancer becomes a dosage problem.

Even in tumour cells induced by chemical carcinogens, 'cancer genes' have been detected. The decisive experiment is very simple. Normal fibroblasts can be transformed *in vitro* by DNA from tumour cells. This transformation is possible even if the tumour cell DNA is cut into pieces. Thus, the tumour-cell DNA contains sequences which are able to make a normal cell neoplastic, and such a sequence might well be a cancer gene.

By genetic engineering techniques with this DNA piece, the capacity to transform normal fibroblasts into tumour cells was multiplied, and the first analyses were made.[34a] These cellular cancer genes, detected by their capacity to transform fibroblasts, seem to be close relatives of the sarcogenes found in tumour viruses. In two examples at least, the bladder carcinoma oncogene is closely related to the Harvey sarcoma virus oncogene. The lung cancer oncogene is the cellular equivalent of the Kirsten sarcoma virus oncogene.[34b]

The task for a chemical carcinogen, however, seems well defined. Chemical carcinogens have to decouple the cancer gene from its normal control mechanisms. They do not have to 'create' a cancer gene, they just have to bring it into operation.

To return to the mechanisms by which chemical carcinogens act, they may activate tumour viruses, but this is inessential as they are not dependent on cancer genes previously installed by tumour viruses. The cancer gene does not have to be imported by tumour viruses, as it is already present within normal cells and is ready to be activated by chemical carcinogens. Chemical carcinogens are not subordinate to tumour viruses.

4 Chemical Carcinogenesis as a Multi-step Process (including some Population Dynamical Remarks)

'A chemical carcinogen hits a cell and transforms it into a tumour cell. This tumour cell then begins to divide a little faster than the surrounding cells. It is then only a question of time until a palpable tumour mass will have accumulated.' This description may be correct in some cases, but in most cases it is not. Chemical carcinogenesis is a multi-step process.

Skin System.—First insights into the multi-step character of the carcinogenesis process came from experiments inducing skin cancer. If a mouse is painted with a sub-threshold dose of a carcinogen (such as DMBA or BP), of course no tumours will arise. If these mice are then painted repeatedly with an extract from croton oil (or pure substances from this source) tumours (mainly papillomas) will arise after a few weeks. Croton oil alone (or the pure substances alone)

[34] (*a*) M. Goldfarb, K. Shimizu, M. Perucho, and M. Wigler, *Nature*, 1982, **296**, 404; (*b*) *New Scientist*, 17 June 1982, p. 772.

produces practically no tumours. Thus, the sum of two non-carcinogenic procedures produces tumours. (For more information see ref. 35.)

The first step in this procedure is usually called initiation, and the second one promotion. Both seem qualitatively different, as initiation is irreversible, but promotion is basically reversible.

In addition to the croton oil factor, many other promotors have been discovered, both natural and synthetic. In addition to the skin system, other systems have been described, such as the colon and the bladder. For the connoisseur, tumour promotion can be resolved into at least two separate steps.[36a]

It is a common belief that, after the treatment with the sub-threshold dose of a carcinogen, so-called latent tumour cells are formed in the basal layer of the epidermis. The only thing necessary to produce a tumour would be the replication of these latent tumour cells. This job could easily be tackled by the promotor, which is well known for its stimulating properties; the promotor stimulates the normal epidermis to a 'thick' epidermis called hyperplastic epidermis.

However, a closer look reveals problems. Cells of the epidermis originate in the basal layer, from which they climb to the layer of so-called differentiated cells, and finally turn into a hornplate. There is a slight complication in this basically simple process. Immediately after cell division, both cells (mother and daughter) remain in the basal cell layer. It is a neighbouring cell which is pushed up indirectly into the layer of differentiated cells.[36b]

Now, let us assume that one of the cells of the basal layer is a latent tumour cell. Then this latent tumour cell also takes part in the dividing/pushing process. All daughter cells of normal and of latent tumour cells will wander through the layers of differentiated cells and finally be turned into a hornplate. Hence, how can a tumour arise in this 'throw-away society'? Even if the latent tumour cell is 'dividing at a slightly higher rate' than the others, all their daughter cells would be finally discarded.

Another mechanism should come into play, when the population of latent tumour cells increases with time. One such mechanism could be the 'increased stickiness' of latent tumour cells to the basal membrane on which the basal cells are situated. If latent tumour cells are a little bit 'stickier' than normal cells, then it will be harder for them to be pushed up by other dividing cells. In the long run, the population within the basal cell layer will shift from less sticky (normal) to stickier (tumour) cells.

This example has been looked at closely because it helps to visualize the problem which arises within a complex framework of cell populations.

A critical remark will end this short examination of skin carcinogenesis. Skin cancer can be produced by simply painting repeatedly small doses of a 'full' carcinogen, without the promotion procedure. It is tempting to assume that this process is also built up of two steps, in other words, that a 'full' carcinogen is both an initiator and a promotor at the same time.

[35] J. D. Scribner and R. Süss *Int. Rev. Exp. Pathol.*, 1978, **18**, 138.
[36] (*a*) G. Fürstenberger, D. L. Berry, B. Sorg, and F. Marks, *Proc. Natl. Acad. Sci. USA*, 1981, **78**, 7722; (*b*) C. S. Potten, and T. D. Allen, *Differentiation*, 1975, **3**, 161.

As has been already mentioned, promotion is reversible, and this is known from spacing experiments. If the croton oil factor is not given twice a week, but, for example, only once in two weeks, the papilloma yields decrease, and when painted every four weeks, no tumours occur.

In the time intervals between croton oil application, regeneration processes can proceed. This does not hold for 'full' carcinogens such as DMBA. If such a carcinogen is painted on the mouse skin with increasing time intervals between the applications, the tumour yields are not reduced, but they may even be increased.[37] This must mean reversible promotion activity is not associated with an active carcinogen.

The skin system led to the definition of different stages during chemical carcinogenesis. However, latent tumour cells have never been identified. This is different from the liver system, where different cell populations are recognisable during chemical carcinogenesis.[38]

Liver System.—Long before a liver tumour (hepatocellular carcinoma) is formed, 'islands' of biochemically changed cells can be seen within the parenchyma. Some of them display a deficiency in specific enzymes, such as glucose-6-phosphatase; some of them are deficient in glycogen, and some show increased glycogen contents. What these cells do not show are signs of tumour cells, such as substantially increased mitotic rates or higher affinities for basophilic dyes. Only much later, new cell populations arise within these islands, possibly giving rise to liver tumours.[39]

It has been suggested that 'toxicity' is a driving force of the chemical carcinogenesis process in the liver. Liver carcinogens are indeed toxic to liver cells, and some of the newly arising cell populations are thought to be resistant to this toxic action. Thus pre-neoplastic cells live without being damaged by these carcinogens, and they seem to have a selective advantage over normal cells.[38]

The idea of a selective process carcinogenesis has been put forward by Warburg.[40] In his view, the chemical carcinogen damages the respiration of normal cells. In a long process, a new cell race is selected which can grow without respiration and the fermenting tumour cell is born. The fermentation theory is somewhat out-dated today, but selection theories, as we see them, still persist.

However, these theories cannot be of general value. In many cases a single application of a carcinogen suffices to bring about cancer. Even in the liver system, where the application of the chemical carcinogen can be stopped, tumours arise although in lower yield. It is hard to see how a chemical carcinogen that is absent can put selective pressure on liver-cell populations.

5 The Winning Cell

Unicellular Origin of Tumours.—Cells of a chemically induced tumour are descendants of one cell only. This has been shown at least for chemically induced tumours of the skin using a rather sophisticated technology.[40]

[37] W. Cramer and R. E. Stowell, *Cancer Res.*, 1941, **1**, 849.
[38] E. Farber, *Adv. Cancer Res.*, 1979, **31**, 125.
[39] P. Bannasch, *Cancer Res.* 1976, **36**, 2555.

First chimeric mice were constructed by amalgamating embryos from two different strains. Each strain had a characteristic variant of a specific enzyme, glucose phosphate isomerase, which is easily analysed by electrophoretic procedures. The chimeric mice were therefore built up from two different sorts of cells, each one of them easily detectable by the enzyme variant.

Analysis of normal tissues of such a chimeric mouse showed always, even in the smallest pieces of tissue, a mixture of cells from both 'parent embryos'. If, however, tissue pieces from tumours were analysed, only one variant of the enzyme could ever be detected.

If a tumour would start, for example from two or more cells, there would be a good chance that in some of the tumours, cells from both embryo parents, *i.e.* from both enzyme variants, would be present. That this was not observed indicates that the tumour originated from a single cell. This conclusion, however, is only valid if the two embryos had mixed perfectly (monodispersially).

It is questionable whether these results are valid for tumour systems other than skin tumours.

Mitosis Increased or Maturation Delayed.—Why do tumour cells compete successfully with normal cells? Do they divide at a faster rate than normal cells? In fact, in some tumours mitotic rate is increased compared with that in normal tissue, and this may be the cause of the increased number of tumour cells finally found in a tumour.

In skin tumours, for example, no increased or only a moderately increased mitotic rate is observed. In these cases, the population of tumour cells is increasing, because of a defective maturation, or in other words, tumour cells in some cases seem to forget to die.[41]

How do tumour cells compete with normal cells, or what makes a cell a tumour cell? At least a formalistic answer can be given, as a tumour cell is a cell which is unco-ordinated with regard to the growth-regulating fields of the organism.

Contact Inhibition.—A possible candidate for such a growth-regulation field is so-called contact inhibition.[42] Cells of a tissue control themselves. Cell contact blocks cell division.

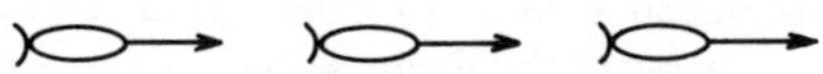

With this model, wound regeneration is easily explained.

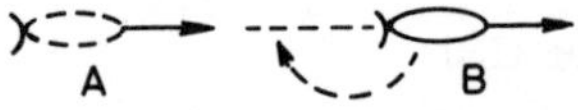

[40] O. Warburg, 'Uber die Ursache des Krebses,' in 'Molekulare Biologie des Malignen Wachstums,' eds. H. Holzer and A. W. Holldorf, Berlin, 1966, p. 1.
[41] P. M. Iannacconne, R. L. Gardner, and H. Harris, *J. Cell Sci.*, 1978, **29**, 249; O. D. Laerum and O. H. Iversen 'Biology of Skin Cancer,' Genf. 1981, p. 129.
[42] G. C. Easty, 'Invasion by Cancer Cells,' in 'The Biology of Cancer,' eds. E. J. Ambrose and F. J. C. Roe, London, 1966, p. 78.

Cell B is no longer inhibited; it divides, but as soon as the wound is closed cell proliferation stops.

Models of tumour cells can be of at least three different types (Figure 1). (a) Tumour cells may have lost their antennae for the growth-regulating signals from a neighbouring cell. They grow despite growth-controlling neighbours.

(b) Tumour cells may have lost their growth-inhibiting signals. In this case, a single tumour cell is still regulated by its neighbours, but as soon as its adjacent cells are tumour cells as well, growth control is no longer possible.

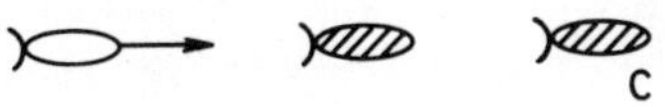

(Tumour cell C is no longer under control.)

(c) Tumour cells may have lost both their antennae and their growth-inhibiting signals.

Contact inhibition is only one possible growth-regulating mechanism; another consists of the so-called chalones.[43]

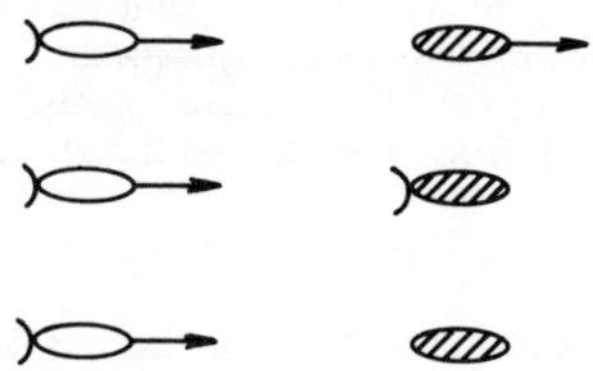

Figure 1 *Three models of turnover cells*

Chalones.—Chalones are tissue-specific inhibitors. For example, in the epidermis the cells of the differentiated cell-layer produce such substances which inhibit the division of the cells belonging to the basal layer. Cell division is possible only when the 'chalone rain' is interrupted for a short period of time. This is the case where the differentiated cell ascends one stage higher to become a hornplate. Then a basal cell divides and pushes an adjacent cell up into the differentiated cell layer. This cell then starts the chalone rain (Figure 2).

From this point of view, a tumour cell is one which maintains cell-division even in the climate of 'chalone rain'. It has discarded its antennae to the growth-inhibiting chalones. Both chalones and contact inhibition function as growth inhibitors. In comparison with tumour cells (*v. supra*), normal cells divide and multiply, but they are regulated by very effective growth inhibitors. This growth inhibition is temporarily released during regeneration and is permanently released in the cancer state.

[43] J. C. Houck and A. M. Attallah, 'Chalones and Cancer,' in 'Cancer', ed. F. F. Becker, vol. 3; F. Marks, 'Chalones,' in 'Biology of Skin Cancer,' eds. O. D. Laerum and O. H. Iversen, Genf., 1981, p. 130.

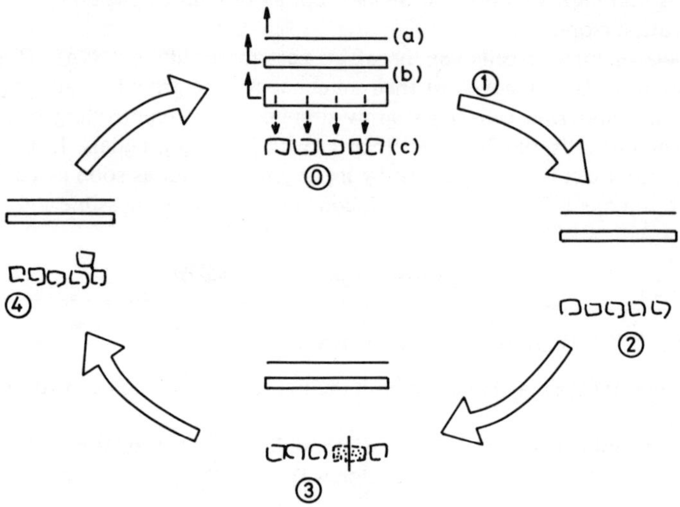

Figure 2 *Cell proliferation cycle in mouse epidermis*

(0) (a) Hornplate; (b) Differentiated Cells; (c) Basal cell layer. A 'chalone rain' coming from the differentiated cells keeps the basal cells from dividing.
(1) Hornplate and differentiated cells move up 'one position' (the hornplate gets lost).
(2) There is 'empty space' above the basal cells and there is therefore no longer a chalone rain.
(3) A basal cell divides.
(4) Pushing up a neighbouring cell into the 'differentiated cell layer'.
(0) The original status is reached again.

However, the release of growth inhibition may not be the only way to bring about cancer. At least some tissue *stimulators* are well known.[44,45]

This short discussion of cellular effects and host factors in chemical carcinogenesis emphasizes rival points of view, and focuses both on important concepts and on the parameters which may be operative.

[44] J. Lobue and M. Potmesil, 'Stimulation,' in 'Cancer,' ed. F. F. Becker, vol. 3.
[45] M. Takashi and S. Iwase, *Nagoya J. Med. Sci.*, 1958, **21**, 153.

Chapter 13 Tissue Specificity

1 Introduction

Tissue specificity, perhaps more than anything else, reveals the response of the mammalian body towards chemical carcinogens (chapter 12). Sometimes, tissue specificity has wide inter-species significance and, for example, vinyl chloride seems to promote liver cancer in all of the mammalian species, including man, which have ever been exposed, but sometimes tissue specificity is combined with species specificity and, for example, β-napthylamine causes bladder cancer in dogs, hamsters, monkeys, and man, but produces hepatomas in mice and is non-carcinogenic to cats, rabbits, and rats.[1,2]

2 The Factors Involved

The reasons for tissue specificity are complex, various factors being determinative in the different biological situations. Thus, in the case of the *N*-nitrosamines in rats, there is an excellent correlation between the organ-specific induction of tumours[3] and the enzymic capacity of the organs concerned to form reactive metabolites[4] (Scheme 1). The tumour incidence increases in the order

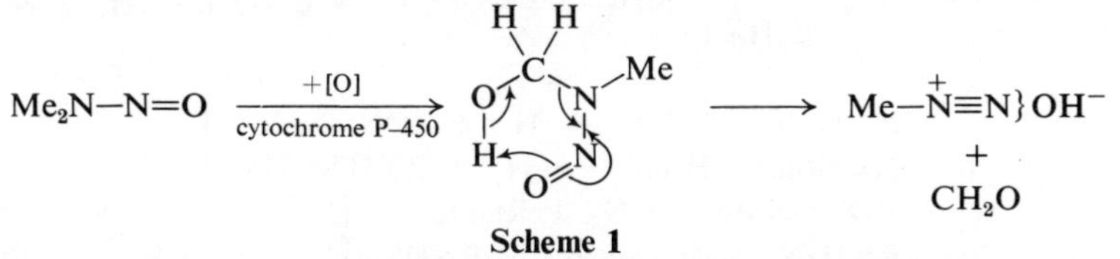

Scheme 1

c.n.s. < bladder < fore-stomach < kidneys < respiratory tract < nasal cavities < oesophagus < liver, and this was paralleled as well by the formation and persistence of O^6-methylguanine in the DNA of those tissues.[5] However, more realistically, it would appear that the balance between the activities of the activating enzyme systems and those of the detoxifying processes would account

[1] D. B. Clayson, in 'Biology of Cancer,' eds. E. J. Ambrose and F. J. C. Roe, Ellis Horwood, Chichester, 2nd edn., 1975, pp. 163—179.

[2] P. Shubik and D. B. Clayson in 'Environmental Pollution and Carcinogenic Risks,' Institut National de la Santé et de la Recherche Médicale Symposia Series Vol. **52** (International Agency for Research on Cancer Scientific Publications no. 13), ed. C. Rosenfeld and W. Davis, Inserm, Paris, 1976, pp. 241—252.

[3] H. S. Druckrey, R. Preussmann, S. Ivankovic, and D. Schmähl, *Z. Krebsforsch.*, 1967, **69**, 103.

[4] R. Montesano and H. Bartsch, *Mutat. Res.*, 1976, **32**, 179.

[5] J. W. Nicoll, P. F. Swann, and A. E. Pegg, *Nature*, 1975, **256**, 261.

for the induction of tumours. Thus, inhibition of the hepatic drug-metabolizing enzymes is paralleled by a lower incidence of liver tumours although, in many circumstances, there is an enhanced incidence of tumours in other parts of the body. Some pharmacological factors, such as the route of administration, alter the kinetics of distribution, which in turn may affect the distribution of tumours in the body. Again, in the final analysis, interaction between cell replication and tissue-specific DNA-repair processes contributes to the expression of carcinogenicity. Thus, in adult rats, the induction of liver tumours by a single dose of *N*-nitroso compound occurs only if the agent is administered 24 h after partial hepatectomy.[6] In comparison with those cases (*v. supra*) where mutagens are produced *de novo* in the target organ(s), 3,3-dimethyl-1-(2,4,6-trichlorophenyl)triazene provides an example where a particular metabolite, [3-methyl-1-(2,4,6-trichlorophenyl)-2-triazeno]methyl β-D-glucuronide,[7] formed

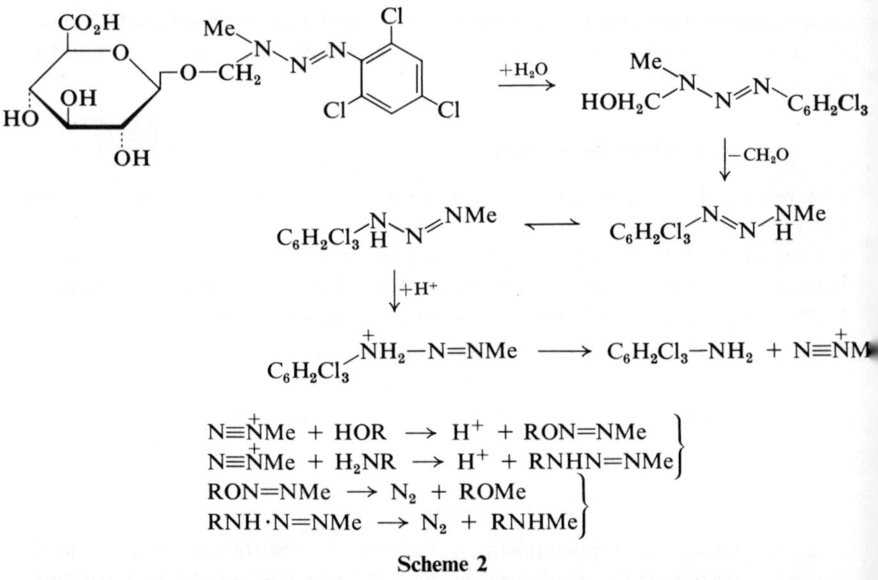

$$\left.\begin{array}{l} N{\equiv}\overset{+}{N}Me + HOR \rightarrow H^+ + RON{=}NMe \\ N{\equiv}\overset{+}{N}Me + H_2NR \rightarrow H^+ + RNHN{=}NMe \end{array}\right\}$$

$$\left.\begin{array}{l} RON{=}NMe \rightarrow N_2 + ROMe \\ RNH{\cdot}N{=}NMe \rightarrow N_2 + RNHMe \end{array}\right\}$$

Scheme 2

in the liver, transports mutagen (Scheme 2) and facilitates its distribution throughout the body. The fact that no tissue fractions have greater enzyme activity for biotransformation into mutagen than those of the liver, although more tumours are formed in some other organs than the liver, supports the foregoing transport mechanism.[8]

[6] V. M. Craddock, in 'Fundamentals in Cancer Prevention,' ed. P. N. Magee, S. Takayama, T. Sugimura, and T. Matsushima, University of Tokyo, 1976, pp. 293—311.
[7] G. F. Kolar and R. Carubelli, *Cancer Lett.*, 1979, **7**, 209.
[8] H. Bartsch, G. P. Margison, C. Malaveille, A. M. Camus, G. Brun, J. M. Margison, G. F. Kolar, and M. Wiessler, *Arch. Toxicol.*, 1977, **39**, 51.

3 Formation of Mutagen *in situ*

1,2-Dimethylhydrazine (*sym*-dimethylhydrazine) is said to afford reactive metabolites by a rather similar mechanism (Scheme 3) to that for cycasin and *N*-nitroso compounds (Scheme 1),[9,10] and the relative amounts of alkylation products

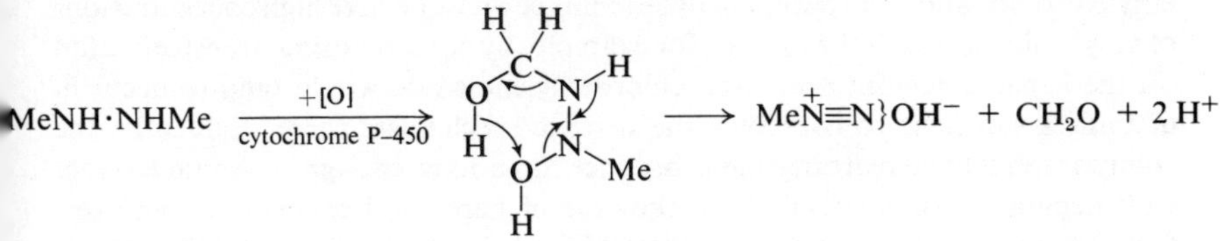

Scheme 3

found in hydrolysates of DNA prepared from the target-organs of rats, which had been treated with the carcinogen, are consistent with this supposition.[11] O^6-Methylguanine was formed in colon and kidney DNA in substantial amounts after the injection of *sym*-dimethylhydrazine, and it remained there for a long time, but O^6-dimethylguanine persisted in greater proportion in the liver DNA throughout the time-course of the animal experiment than in either that of the colon or of the kidneys, which were the principal target organs for the induction of *sym*-dimethylhydrazine tumours.[12,13] Whilst the liver is not a major organ for tumour induction in this case, tumours are formed there, but with a much smaller frequency. This rather suggested that other factors may have been involved, and in this connection, the greater rate of turnover of colon cells than hepatocytes would favour the more extensive O^6-alkylation of the guanine residues in colon DNA than could be measured in an experiment of this kind. On the other hand, the dose (200 mg kg^{-1}) of *sym*-dimethylhydrazine which was used is a high one, and this may have complicated the results, as similar single doses of the corresponding *N*-nitroso compounds (*v. supra*) caused liver cancer, especially where they were administered in conjunction with partial hepatectomy.[14,15]

High sensitivity of the fibroblastic elements tends to interfere with the potential response of parenchymatous (liver)tissue where the carcinogen is administered systemically, and animals often succumb to rapidly growing sarcomas before the specialized tissue has had time to respond.[16] These conclusions were derived from the testing of amino-azo dyes for carcinogenicity,[16] and the case of vinyl chloride liver cancer would appear to be unexceptional. Thus, in the chronic

[9] J. H. Weisburger, *Dis. Colon Rectum*, 1973, **16**, 431.
[10] J. H. Weisburger, in 'Proceedings of the Seventh National Cancer Conference,' J. B. Lippincott, Philadelphia, 1973, pp. 465—473.
[11] K. J. Rogers and A. E. Pegg, *Cancer Res.*, 1977, **37**, 4082.
[12] H. Druckrey, in 'Carcinoma of the Colon and Antecedent Epithelium,' ed. W. J. Burdett, Charles C. Thomas, Springfield, Illinois, 1970, pp. 267—279.
[13] A. Hawkes, R. M. Hicks, J. W. Holsman, and P. N. Magee, *Br. J. Cancer*, 1974, **30**, 429.
[14] V. M. Craddock, *J. Nat. Cancer Inst.*, 1971, **47**, 889.
[15] V. M. Craddock and J. V. Frei, *Br. J. Cancer*, 1974, **30**, 503.
[16] I. Berenblum, 'Carcinogenesis as a Biological Problem,' North-Holland Publishing Company, Amsterdam, 1974, pp. 12, 16.

situation, where administered to experimental animals either by injection or by inhalation, it caused angiosarcoma of the liver.[17–20a] In contrast to hepatic fibroblastic DNA, hepatoctye DNA (in the parenteral administrations) is protected by the high activity of the glutathione–glutathione *S*-epoxide transferase detoxifying enzyme system from attack by the reactive mutagens, chloroethylene oxide and chloroacetaldehyde (chapter 6). But where high concentrations of vinyl chloride reach the liver as, for example, by enteral dosing, transformation (in the hepatocytes) into mutagen chloroethylene oxide would tend to occur in quantities sufficient to overcome the defence mechanism there. Evidently, the chloroacetaldehyde rearrangement product has a long enough $t_{0.5}$ value to react with hepatic fibroblastic DNA, in the case of parenteral exposure,[20b] and this fact seems to link the role of chloroacetaldehyde in vinyl chloride carcinogenesis (*v. supra*) with that of the transport forms of some other carcinogens, which will be described in the present chapter (*v. infra*). Berenblum[16] says that, at lower oral dose-levels, hepatocarcinogens produce mixed sarcomas and hepatomas.

4 Tumour Induction dependent on a Transport Form

Seventy years have elapsed since Leuenberger[21] first predicted that *N*-arylhydroxylamines might be the causative agents for aniline bladder cancer. But, although 2-naphthylhydroxylamine and biphenyl-4-ylhydroxylamine had been prepared already,[22] it took another sixty years before in fact 2-naphthylhydroxylamine was detected in the late urine of dogs, which had been treated chronically with β-naphthylamine.[23] *N*-Hydroxylation occurs in the liver and, in dogs and monkeys and in man, the mutagen is converted straightaway by the hepatic cytosol into the *O*-glucuronide; this is transported to the bladder where it is deconjugated by the lumen epithelial cells, and where the tumour is induced. In mice, which are deficient in UDPGT, the 2-naphthylhydroxylamine, which was synthesized in the liver, gives rise to hepatomas. On the other hand, cats, rabbits, and rats lack the mixed function oxidase for implementing *N*-hydroxylation, and are unaffected by β-naphthylamine.

When an arylhydroxylamine has been formed, it might be activated still further *in vivo*, for example by esterification, as the energy required to remove the elements of acid in order to generate reactive ions is less than that required for the removal of the elements of water from the parent arylhydroxylamine. Thus, sulphation is brought about by soluble liver sulphotransferase systems,

17 C. Maltoni and G. Lefemine, *Atti Accad. Naz. Lincei, Cl. Sci. Fis. Mat. Nat. Rend.*, 1974, [8] **56**, 1.
18 C. Maltoni and G. Lefemine, *Environ. Res.*, 1974, **7**, 387.
19 C. Maltoni, *Environ. Health Perspect.*, 1977, **21**, 1.
20 (*a*) C. Maltoni, Cold Spring Harbor Conf. Cell Proliferation, 1977, **4** (Origins Human Cancer, Book A) pp. 119—146; (*b*) H. Kappus, H. Ottenwälder, and H. M. Bolt, in 'Prevention of Occupational Cancer. International Symposium (Helsinki, April 21—24, 1981),' International Labour Office, Geneva, *Occupational Safety and Health Series*, 1982, **46**, pp. 94—103.
21 S. G. Leuenberger, *Bruns' Beitr. Klin. Chir.*, 1912, **80**, 208.
22 R. Willstätter and H. Kubli, *Ber.*, 1908, **41**, 1936.
23 J. L. Radomski and E. Brill, *Arch. Toxikol.*, 1971, **28**, 159.

and in some cases a deficiency of this enzyme confers resistance to carcinogenesis. On the other hand, sulphation is not the only available mechanism of activation, in which case the absence of this enzyme system from a tissue does not necessarily confer resistance to carcinogenesis. Thus, for example, rat ear-duct and mammary glands have very low sulphotransferase activity, and yet they are tissue-sensitive to fluoren-2-ylacetamide tumours.[24] These tissues may have some other activating enzyme, such as acetyl transferase or peroxidase, which will generate a reactive ester form, or alternatively ring-chain tautomerism[25] may be important (chapter 11). In the case of β-naphthylamine (*v. supra*), esterification seems to be irrelevant to the mechanism of activation. Thus, 2-acetylnaphthalide did not produce tumours in dogs after 2 years' chronic administration, whereas the equivalent dose of the parent β-naphthylamine, administered in just the same way, induced bladder tumours in all of the animals which were exposed.[26] Hence, arylhydroxylamine is likely to be the ultimate carcinogen *per se* in the case of β-naphthylamine, at any rate in dogs. Similarly, whereas rabbits are resistant to fluoren-2-ylacetamide liver cancer, they develop bladder tumours, presumably also through unesterified arylhydroxylamine.

Benzidine is known to be activated *in vivo* through successive acetylation and *N*-hydroxylation.[27] *N*-Acetylbenzidine was transformed by fortified liver microsomes to give *N,N'*-diacetyl-*N*-hydroxybenzidine and *N,N'*-diacetyl-3-hydroxybenzidine, and in the living animal, pre-treatment with 3-methylcholanthrene enhanced both *N*- and 3-hydroxylations. Synthetic *N,N'*-diacetyl-*N*-hydroxybenzidine bound to t-RNA in the presence of liver cytosol: this binding was considered to be catalysed by *N,O*-acyltransferase. In addition, *N,N'*-diacetyl-*N*-hydroxybenzidine was mutagenic in *S. typhimurium* TA1538 strain in the presence of partially purified *N,O*-acyltransferase.[27] Thus, benzidine bladder cancer requires a transport form, presumably the glucuronide derivative of an *N*-hydroxy compound, and this is analogous to β-naphthylamine bladder cancer (*v. supra*).

5 Spill-over Model for Metabolism and Carcinogenicity

Identification in mice, in which 1,1,2-trichloroethylene is both mutagenic and tumourogenic, of the 1,1,2-trichloroethylene metabolites dichloroacetic acid, trichloroacetic acid, and trichloroethanol glucuronide (chapter 6) implied rearrangement of 1,1,2-trichloroethylene oxide into both dichloroacetyl chloride and chloral.[28] The former, by analogy with vinylidene dichloride, the corresponding formation of chloroacetyl chloride,[29] and binding to mouse-kidney DNA,[30,31] is consistent with 1,1,2-trichloroethylene liver cancer in mice.[32–34]

[24] C. C. Irving, D. H. Janss, and L. T. Russell, *Cancer Res.*, 1971, **31**, 387.
[25] G. Lhoest, M. Roberfroid, and M. Mercier, *Biomed. Mass Spectrom.*, 1978, **5**, 38.
[26] G. M. Conzelman and L. E. Flanders, *Proc. West. Pharmacol. Soc.*, 1972, **15**, 96.
[27] K. C. Morton, C. M. King, and K. P. Baetcke, *Cancer Res.*, 1979, **39**, 3107.
[28] D. E. Hathway, *Cancer Lett.*, 1980, **8**, 263.
[29] B. K. Jones and D. E. Hathway, *Br. J. Cancer*, 1978, **37**, 411.
[30] D. E. Hathway, *Environ. Health Perspect.*, 1977, **21**, 55.
[31] B. K. Jones and D. E. Hathway, *Cancer Lett.*, 1978, **5**, 1.
[32] J. W. Lloyd, R. M. Moore, and P. Breslin, *J. Occup. Med.*, 1975, **17**, 603.

The small proportion of dichloroacetic acid in relation to the large one of trichloroacetic acid in the urine of the treated mice agrees with the concept of a spill-over model[28] for a situation where there is a massive excess of epoxide substrate relative to catalytic sites for the usual rearrangement into chloral.[28] Under these circumstances, an alternative metabolic pathway is followed in mice to an extent commensurate with liver-tumour induction.

A spill-over model for 1,1,2-trichloroethylene metabolism and tumourogenicity suggests that such models may have wider applicability, but under physiological conditions, acceptable pathways for foreign compounds *in vivo* belong to a network of kinetically controlled (chapter 7) biochemical and chemical reaction processes. Thus, endogenous methacrylic acid affords acetate and CO_2, and this pathway is followed by the methacrylic acid generated from relatively large doses of exogenous methyl ester.[35] However, if the occurrence of transplacental haemangiomas in the rat pups of dams, which had been treated systemically with methyl methacrylate on days 5, 10, and 15 of gestation,[36] is significant, it may be necessary to evoke a spill-over model for the very high substrate to key enzyme situation. Formation of mutagenic epoxide and a lack of detoxifying epoxide hydratase and glutathione–glutathione *S*-epoxide transferase activity in the foetal livers, at those times in gestation, would be consistent with a rational explanation for this result.[36]

But, even if this is so, only two examples have been instanced where a spill-over mechanism may possibly be involved, so that it appears that the number of cases is limited in which the conditions appertaining to this model are fulfilled. It is pertinent that physiological conditions enforce kinetically controlled biochemical and chemical reaction processes, and that there is no place for biotransformations, however feasible, outside such a system. Nor can spill-over mechanisms be predicted by analogy, and whilst they may apply, under certain special circumstances, to alkyl methacrylate esters (*v. supra*), the case of acrylonitrile c.n.s., zymbal gland, and stomach tumours in rats[37,38] is different. For, as in the case of vinyl chloride (chapter 6), the epoxide is the key intermediate,[39] and acrylonitrile is mutagenic in *S. typhimurium* strains, which are sensitive to base-substitution mutagens.[40] Thus, the expression of carcinogenicity appears to depend on the balance between cytochrome P-450 activity for epoxidation and that of the detoxifying processes presented by epoxide hydratase and glutathione–glutathione *S*-epoxide transferase enzyme systems.

33 'Threshold Limit Values for Chemical Substances and Physical Agents in the Workroom Environment with Intended Changes for 1977,' American Conference of Government Industrial Hygienists, 1978, pp. 40, 41.

34 'Trichloroethylene,' in 'IARC Monographs on the Evaluation of Carcinogenic Risk of Chemicals to Man, Vol. 11, Cadmium, nickel, some epoxides, miscellaneous industrial chemicals and general considerations on volatile anaesthetics,' International Agency for Research on Cancer, Lyon, 1976, pp. 263—276.

35 H. Bratt and D. E. Hathway, *Br. J. Cancer*, 1977, **36**, 114.

36 A. R. Singh, W. H. Lawrence, and J. Autian, *J. Dent. Res.*, 1972, **51**, 1632.

37 J. F. Quast, C. G. Humiston, B. A. Schwetz, J. M. Norris, and P. J. Gehring, 'International Congress on Toxicology,' Toronto, Canada, 1977.

38 *Cah. Notes Docum. Insts. Nata, Secur. Prev. Accid. Travail*, 1979, **94**, 19.

39 P. W. Langvardt, C. L. Putzig, W. H. Braun, and J. D. Young, *J. Toxicol. Environ. Health*, 1980, **6**, 273.

40 C. de Meester, F. Poncelet, M. Roberfroid, and M. Mercier, *Toxicology*, 1978, **11**, 19.

Part VII

Toxicant Allergy

Chapter 14 Antigen Formation and Immunobiological Effects Produced by Foreign Compounds

1 Immune Surveillance System

There is abundant evidence that an immune surveillance system operates in mammals, as follows.

(i) Immunosuppressed animals and human beings are more vulnerable to bacterial, fungal, and virus infections, and to neoplasia, than their normal counterparts.

(ii) Individuals born with immunological dysfunction, for example athymic human subjects, nude mice, *etc*., are extremely susceptible in these ways. Increased susceptibility has been attributed to incomplete development of the immune surveillance system, particularly to the absence of the thymus-dependent lymphocyte (T-cell) component.[1]

(iii) Patients who are being treated with immunosuppressant drugs or radiation to depress the immune surveillance in order to ensure the more adequate retention and sustenance of organ or marrow transplants are more vulnerable to infection and ten thousand times more susceptible to certain tumours.[2,3]

(iv) *Vice versa*, in a high proportion of cancer patients,[4-8] as well as amongst

[1] H. W. Lischner, H. W. Punnett, and A. M. DiGeorge, *Nature*, 1967, **214**, 582.
[2] I. Penn and T. E. Starzl, *Transplant Proc*., 1972, **4**, 732.
[3] R. A. Gatti and R. A. Good, *Cancer*, 1971, **28**, 98.
[4] E. M. Hersh and J. J. Oppenheim, *N. Engl. J. Med*., 1965, **273**, 1012.
[5] T. Han and H. Takita, *N. Engl. J. Med*., 1972, **286**, 606.
[6] W. J. Catalona, W. F. Sample, and P. B. Chretien, *Cancer*, 1973, **31**, 71.
[7] S. H. Golub, T. X. O'Connell, and D. L. Morton, *Cancer Res*., 1974, **34**, 1837.
[8] J. H. Dean, R. Connor, R. B. Herberman, J. L. McCoy, and J. S. Silva, *Int. J. Cancer*, 1977, **20**, 370.

normal members of cancer-prone families,[9,10] impaired immuno-competence has been found. In this connection, rodents bearing genetically compatible, transplantable tumours also show immune dysfunction.[11–14] There may be a casual relationship between immune dysfunction and predisposition towards cancer, but this has never been established. Indeed, some chemical carcinogens may induce neoplasia because of the changed immuno-competence and surveillance that they bring about, although there is no direct evidence for this supposition. On the other hand, the immune depression found in cancer patients and tumour-bearing rodents may result from continuous incompatibility of the immune cells and the neoplastic ones.

(v) The fact that some chemical substances stimulate the immune system and may be used in cancer chemotherapy as immuno-potentiating agents is relevant.

(vi) In addition, still other compounds which are not immunosuppressive *per se* cause hypersensitivity and, for example, some additives in cosmetics, detergents, and soaps might be instanced.

Thus, a general immune surveillance system with a thymus-dependent lymphocyte component seems to confer protection against certain bacterial, fungal, and viral infections and neoplastic cells, against foreign tissue transplants, and against intracellular parasites. Cell-mediated immunity (CMI) involves memory and effector T-cells, macrophages and accessory bursal or bone marrow-dependent lymphocytes (B-cells), and makes up the surveillance (host) parameter. On the other hand, a humoral immune component, which mediates its effect by the B-cells, confers protection through the plasma antibodies. Antibody activity is facilitated in turn by co-factors including the complement proteins. Plasma antibodies protect the host from extracellular and incapsulated bacteria and some viruses.

Depressed antibody immunity and/or depressed CMI, indicative of impaired immuno-competence, occur after exposure to small, but not essentially toxic, amounts of certain chemicals. These include the 2,3,7,8-tetrachlorodibenzo-*p*-dioxin by-product of 2,4,5-trichlorophenol manufacture, heavy metals, Cd, Co, Cr, Ni, Pb, and organometallic compounds such as methylmercuric chloride, polybromo- and polychloro-biphenyls, and pesticides such as carbaryl, carbofuran, DDT, dieldrin, and methyl parathion.

2 Antibodies and the Immune Response

Antibodies or immune globulins appear in the plasma and tissues of a given vertebrate in response to the injection of an antigen, *i.e.* a protein or other

[9] E. T. Creagan and J. F. Fraumeni, *Cancer*, 1973, **32**, 1325.
[10] J. F. Fraumeni, W. Wertelechi, W. A. Blattner, R. D. Jensen, and R. G. Leventhal, *Am. J. Med.*, 1975, **59**, 150.
[11] S. Zolla, *J. Immunol.*, 1972, **108**, 1048.
[12] J. A. Moore and R. E. Faith, *Environ. Health Perspect.*, 1976, **18**, 125.
[13] H. Kirchner, T. M. Chused, R. B. Herberman, H. T. Holden, and D. H. Lavrin, *J. Exp. Med.*, 1974 **139**, 1487.
[14] M. L. Padarathsingh, J. L. McCoy, J. H. Dean, D. D. Lewis, J. W. Northing, and L. W. Law, *J. Nat. Cancer Inst.*, 1977, **58**, 1702.

macromolecule, which is foreign to that species. This reaction, which is known as the immune response, is the basis of the field of immunology. Antibody molecules may combine with the antigen which caused their formation to afford an antigen–antibody complex. Thus, immunity to infection (*v. supra*) may be conferred by injecting very small amounts of certain macromolecular components (antigens) of the causative micro-organism or virus into a human subject. Antibodies are formed, and if the micro-organism gains access subsequently to the blood or lymph of that individual, they will inactivate the micro-organism by combining with its antigenic components. Incidentally, the principle of immunization/vaccination against infection was discovered empirically by an English medical practitioner, Edward Jenner (1749–1823), a century before medicine was in a position to employ it.

Antibodies are highly specific for foreign proteins, which evoke their formation: (i) functionally different proteins from any single species lead to the formation of different antibodies; (ii) homologous proteins of different species are dissimilar immunologically (in the antigen–antibody reaction) as a result of differences in their amino-acid sequences; (iii) antibodies are specific for each vertebrate species, and the resulting specificity reflects phylogenetic relationships.

In human plasma there are four main classes of antibodies of which the IgG globulins are the most abundant and best understood. They have a molecular weight of 150 000, with two identical heavy peptide (H) chains (*M* 50 000) and two identical light peptide (L) chains (*M* 25 000), linked together by disulphide bonds into a macromolecular structure which has two binding sites for the antigen. Each heavy chain contains a covalently bound oligosaccharide residue.

The plasma of a normal human being contains a mixture of many different immunoglobulins, mostly with the foregoing structure pattern. Each type of immunoglobulin combines specifically with a single antigen, and from such a mixture it is impossible to obtain a single molecular species of immunoglobulin for analysis and characterization. However, in *multiple myeloma*, one type of plasma cell multiplies to produce excessive amounts of a single type of immunoglobulin which appears in the blood, and the urine of such patients contains large amounts of another protein, which consists solely of light chains and which is known as a Bence–Jones protein. An individual patient synthesizes a single type of Bence–Jones protein, but no two such patients have identical Bence–Jones proteins. Amino-acid sequencing of Bence–Jones proteins and globulins from different *multiple myeloma* patients shows that the carboxy-terminal one-half (107 amino-acid residues) of the L chain has the same amino-acid sequence in all patients, but the amino-terminal one-half of approximately 107 residues differs in amino-acid sequence from one protein to the next, despite some sequence homology. There are some sequence homologies between the two halves of the L chains. [Similarly, in the H chains from such patients, the amino-terminal segment of 107 residues varies in sequence from one individual to another, but the other 300 residues are constant in sequence.] These results imply: (i) that the variable sequence portions of each L and H chain represent the binding site for the specific antigen; (ii) that successive duplication or repetition of primordial precursor genes appears to code for the immune globulin chain, because there are sequence homologies between the variable and constant halves of L chains and among the four segments of the H chains; each chain is approximately 107 residues in length (but there are no homologies between the variable regions of L chains and of H chains); (iii) sequence studies indicate roughly how many different IgG antibody molecules can be formed theoretically.

Of the 107 residues in the variable-sequence portion of the L chains, 40 differ from one *multiple myeloma* patient to the next; the remainder are invariant. In a chain of 107 residues in which 40 can be occupied by 2 different amino acids, there are 2^{40}, *i.e.* > 10 billion, possible sequences. If each of the 40 variable sites may be occupied by any one of the 20 or so amino acids, then the number of different possible sequences is enormous. As each antibody molecule also has a heavy chain in which many residues may vary as well, it is clear that an exceptionally large number of antibodies may be made by an individual through replacement of the variable amino-acid residues. Such considerations pose the question as to how such an immense number of different antibody molecules can be genetically specified. Is it possible that each individual possesses all the genetic make-up necessary to specify the several billions of different antibodies which might be synthesized theoretically? The present chapter is not the place in which to discuss theories of clonal selection, but to provide relevant information for an understanding of the immunobiological effects of foreign compounds.

3 Antigen Specificity

For students of chemistry at the time of World War II, who extended their reading to include immunochemistry, there were excellent reviews.[15–17] Even at that stage in the development of immunochemistry, two approaches were evident. One, which was concerned with the degradative chemistry of bacterial antigens,* anticipated the elucidation of (bacterial) hapten structure, where a hapten is defined as that specific chemical grouping (of the antigen) to which a single antibody site conforms and with which it reacts. In the other, the chemical basis of antigen specificity was investigated by means of synthetic or conjugated antigens, in which residues of known structure were attached to antigenic proteins, for example serum globulins, and the conjugated antigens were used to raise antibodies in mammals. For the preparation of these conjugated antigens, Landsteiner and Lampl (1917) first coupled aromatic diazonium compounds with the phenolic and imidazole groups of proteins in alkaline solution, and over

* Indeed, immunochemistry might have been seen then as an extension of sugar chemistry, which had made notable advances, *viz.* glycoside synthesis, polysaccharide structural elucidations, and vitamin C degradation and synthesis, during the first four decades of the present century.

[15] K. Landsteiner, 'The Specificity of Serological Reactions,' Charles C. Thomas, Baltimore, 1936.
[16] J. R. Marrack, 'The Chemistry of Antigens and Antibodies,' H.M. Stationery Office, London, 1938.
[17] F. M. Burnet, 'The Production of Antibodies,' Monographs from the Walter and Eliza Hall Institute of Research in Pathology and Medicine, no. 1, Macmillan and Co. Ltd., Melbourne, 1942.

the next two decades, Landsteiner *et al.*[15] exploited this approach most successfully (*v. infra*). In another general method, devised by Clutton, Harington and Mead,[18] a compound with a carboxy group was converted into the acyl azide, which was coupled under mild conditions with a protein. By these means, Clutton, Harington, and Yuill[19] showed that both insulin and gelatin became antigenic when coupled with glucosyltyrosine; the antibodies produced by these antigenic complexes will react with glucosidotyrosyl–globulin. In another study,[20] these authors prepared thyroxyl derivatives of serum globulin and albumin, and of thyroglobulin, and found that immunisation with these complexes produces antisera, which, when injected into rats, protected against the normal physiological effects of exogenously administered thyroglobulin and thyroxine. The interest of this work is evident.

One of the classical experiments in immunochemistry, which still evokes discussion on antibody structure, is that of Landsteiner and van der Scheer.[21] This work relates to antigenic specificity, to antibody heterogeneity, and (by implication) to the lower limit of the size of antibody-binding sites. These authors[21] prepared *sym*-aminoisophthalylglycineleucine (GIL), in which the two amino acids extended outwards in opposite directions from the central aminophenyl residue, as a complex hapten. They made a conjugated antigen by attaching this hapten through a diazo linkage to the washed stroma of horse erythrocytes, and they immunised rabbits with the azostroma. Antisera were obtained, which would precipitate the hapten diazotised and coupled to otherwise unreactive chicken-serum protein.

Landsteiner and van der Scheer[21] prepared two other azostroma, one with *m*-aminobenzoylglycine (G) and the other with *m*-aminobenzoyleucine (L), which they used as insoluble adsorbents for removing antibodies from the test antisera. Both G and L were diazotised and coupled separately to chicken-serum protein, to be used as precipitating antigens in the same way as GIL-serum. Adsorption with G-azostroma removed antibodies which would precipitate with G-azoprotein, but left antibodies which would precipitate with L-azoprotein. Similarly, adsorption with L-azostroma removed antibodies which would precipitate with L-azoprotein, but left antibodies which would precipitate with G-azoprotein. On the other hand, adsorption with a mixture of G- and L-azostroma removed both types of precipitating antibodies simultaneously. Adsorptions with either G- or L-azostroma alone did not affect antibody precipitation with GIL-azoprotein. It was only when adsorption with combined G- and L-azostroma was implemented that the antiserum showed almost entire loss of precipitating capacity with GIL-azoprotein.

The conclusion was drawn[21] that discrete antibodies are formed, which are directed individually towards separate determinants, located rather close together in a (single) low-molecular size substance. Whilst the calculated area (700 Å^2) of an active patch of an anti-GIL antibody surface, which would be

[18] R. F. Clutton, C. R. Harington, and T. H. Mead, *Biochem. J.*, 1937, **31**, 764.
[19] R. F. Clutton, C. R. Harington, and M. E. Yuill, *Biochem. J.*, 1938, **32**, 1111.
[20] R. F. Clutton, C. R. Harington, and M. E. Yuill, *Biochem. J.*, 1938, **32**, 1119.
[21] K. Landsteiner and J. van der Scheer, *J. Exp. Med.*, 1938, **67**, 709.

complementary to the two classes of GIL determinants,[22] defines the upper limit of the size of the combining site for anti-GIL antibodies in Landsteiner and van der Scheer's[21] sera, it is questionable whether this calculation[22] would define the upper limit for antibody-combining sites in general. One-quarter of a century after Landsteiner and van der Scheer's[21] experiments, Levine[23] demonstrated larger combining sites in rabbit antibody than benzylpenicilloyl groups in a Landsteiner–van der Scheer type of experiment. In rabbit sera against benzylpenicilloyl-rabbit normal serum, which was tested with benzylpenicilloyl-polylysine, there were antibodies for the combined benzylpenicilloyl group, the lysine side-chain, and the adjacent peptide of the carrier protein, but none for the end structures. Whilst in this case the active patch of antibody surface far exceeded 700 Å^2, calculations[24] on the basis of serologically active fragments in general infer that an active patch need be only 100—200 Å^2, which would amount to 0.4—0.7% of the total protein surface. As antibody activity may be inhibited by substances which bind with much less than the total active site, the binding of antibody with a small grouping does not mean that the site is necessarily a small one. Clearly, the investigator has little control over the production of antibodies with a particular size of binding site, but a meaningful term of reference would appear to be the smallest upper limit, for example Isliker's[24] 100—200 Å^2.

In experiments designed[25] to separate the anti-G, anti-L, and anti-GIL activities of Landsteiner and van der Scheer's[21] work, and to test the cross-reactivities with G, L and/or GIL, it was found that, whilst a large proportion of the binding energy of hapten and antibody was supplied either by glycine or by leucine, the other amino acid did in fact contribute to a certain extent to the binding energy. The conclusions drawn applied undoubtedly to the sera in question,[25] but not necessarily to those of Landsteiner and van der Scheer[21] on account of heterogeneity in reactivity from one serum to another. Again, the matter of heterogeneity amongst benzylpenicilloyl (BPO) antibodies has been reinvestigated[26] with columns of immunoadsorbents from BPO groups attached to bisdiazotised benzidine-bovine γ-globulin complexes, and using a series of nine different BPO analogues as eluants, applied in different sequences in the various runs. In marked contrast to Levine's[23] results, at least five antibody populations were established.[26] Antibodies were found respectively with a preference for 6-acetylaminopenicilloic acid, for phenylacetic acid, for phenylacetylglycine, for benzylpenicilloic acid, and for benzylpenicilloyl-ε-aminocaproic acid.

Work by Landsteiner and van der Scheer[27] (*cf.* refs. 28 and 29) on the serological specificity of peptides showed that strong reactions involved not only

[22] D. H. Campbell and N. Bulman, *Fortschr. Chem. Org. Naturst.*, 1954, **9**, 443.
[23] B. B. Levine, *J. Exp. Med.*, 1963, **117**, 161.
[24] H. Isliker, *Gazzetta*, 1962, **92**, 850.
[25] V. P. Kreiter and D. Pressman, *Immunochemistry*, 1964, **1**, 151.
[26] T. Atsumi, K. Nishida, Y. Kinoshita, K. Shibata, and Y. Horinchi, *J. Immunol.*, 1967, **99**, 1286.
[27] K. Landsteiner and J. van der Scheer, *J. Exp. Med.*, 1939, **69**, 705.
[28] K. Landsteiner and J. van der Scheer, *J. Exp. Med.*, 1932, **55**, 781.
[29] K. Landsteiner and J. van der Scheer, *J. Exp. Med.*, 1934, **59**, 769.

end groups but other parts of the molecule as well. They coupled the pentapeptides, G_5, G_4L, G_2LG_2, and L_3G_2 to horse azostroma for immunising rabbits and for adsorption, and they coupled them to chicken-serum protein for use as test antigens. Irrespective of the dominance of either carboxy or amino groups, antibodies appeared to be specific for the entire pentapeptide and not for a part of it. The authors[27] suggested that specific combinations which occurred in antigen–antibody reactions, were not of the same kind, *i.e.* that the antibody-binding sites were not always made up of the same elements arranged variously, and that their pentapeptides (*v. supra*) may be insufficiently large to attain the upper limit possible for antibody-site conformation. Similarly, with polyalanines[30] the pentamer was the most inhibitory hapten. From the hexamer upwards in size there was an increasing tendency in this series towards formation of α-helices, but an insufficient tendency to account for the difference in inhibition between pentamer and hexamer. In its extended form, the pentamer was calculated to be $25 \times 11 \times 6.5$ Å^3, and an interhelical, cavity shaped[31] antibody-binding site to encompass the hapten would have an overall surface area of *ca.* 2000 Å^2. Kabat and Berg's[32,33] discovery that α(1→6)linked dextrans were antigenic in man prompted further studies,[34–36] which showed: (i) that the antibody was specific for α(1→6)linked anhydroglucopyranose units such as isomaltose, isomaltotriose, *etc.*, and not for the α(1→4)linked series, for example maltose and maltotetraose, and the β(1→6)linked oligomers such as gentiobiose and β-gentiobiose-β-gentiobiose, and (ii) that isomaltotetraose fitted the antibody-binding site better than the triose, whilst the pentaose had even better binding power, and the hexaose with only slightly superior inhibition seemed to approach an upper limit. Because of heterogeneity, there was a possibility that a heptasaccharide might be marginally better still. As the isomaltohexaose is capable of considerable free rotation about the α(1→6)linkages, a number of shapes would be possible and heterogeneity would be considerable, yet complementarity to the α(1→6)linkages would be maintained. For the extended form, the dimensions of the hexasaccharide would be $34 \times 12 \times 7$ Å^3, and an antibody-binding site to encompass this hapten would present an interhelical cavity[31] of *ca.* 2000 Å^2. Although the surface of such an hypothetical site would be maximal, it would represent only a relatively small part of the total immunoglobulin surface.

In questioning the possibility of a deep and large-surfaced interhelical cavity as an antibody-binding site, Sage *et al.*[30] based their reservation on the fact that the binding of penta-L-alanine depended much more on the uninterrupted sequence of L-alanine residues, irrespective of position, than upon terminal status, which would have been necessary for deep cavity binding. They[30] thought that the probability of a shallow antibody cavity of *ca.* 700 Å^2 was much greater.

30 H. J. Sage, G. F. Deutsch, G. D. Fasman, and L. Levine, *Immunochemistry*, 1964, **1**, 133.
31 F. Karush, *J. Am. Chem. Soc.*, 1956, **78**, 5519.
32 E. A. Kabat and D. Berg, *Ann. N. Y. Acad. Sci*, 1952, **55**, 471.
33 E. A. Kabat and D. Berg, *J. Immunol.*, 1953, **70**, 514.
34 E. A. Kabat, *J. Am. Chem. Soc.*, 1954, **76**, 3709.
35 E. A. Kabat, *J. Immunol.*, 1956, **77**, 377.
36 E. A. Kabat, *J. Immunol.*, 1960, **84**, 82.

In their analysis of the situation, Mage and Kabat[37] had considered that an oversized hapten either would have a statistically greater number of ways of fitting the shallow cavity site than a small hapten or would fold much more easily to a specific conformation commensurate with the surface of the antibody site. The former concept would accommodate better the results of Landsteiner and van der Scheer[27] and of Sage *et al.*,[30] where a folded conformation for small polypeptides is improbable, but either of the possibilities would be compatible with Kabat's[34–36] dextran data and those[38] in which the upper limit of the inhibiting power of the polynucleotides of thymine for anti-DNA was realized by pentathymidylic acid. From one point of view, the assumption of a shallow binding site for pentapeptides, hexasaccharides, and pentanucleotides is consistent with Karush's[31] deep site against a small hapten and the calculated[39] binding-site size for antibody against the β-D-galactoside hapten.

The trouble with the shallow cavity concept of Sage *et al.*[30] was that it did not hold for cases where it seemed apposite. Thus, the capacity of a series of oligoalanines to inhibit the reaction of rabbit anti-poly-L-alanyl ribonuclease with poly-L-alanyl-rabbit serum albumin has been studied.[40] Wherever D-alanine was located at the N-terminus of an oligoalanine chain, the inhibitory effect of the L-peptide sequence was eliminated. On the other hand, the presence of D-alanine at the C-terminus had no effect, the L-alanine peptide sequence remaining fully inhibitory. In this series, the N-terminus was very important. In the Schechter series,[41–43] the most significant finding was that the pentapeptide was not a better inhibitor than a tetrapeptide, and sometimes a tetrapeptide was no better than a tripeptide. This result was true not only for rabbits but also for goats, not only in the γG series but in the γM one as well; the response was identical whether the homologous series consisted of poly-L-alanine, poly-D-alanine, or poly-D-alanine-glycine. What did make a difference was the nature of the residue that was located in the second and third position to the N-terminus, as well as that of the one in the first position. Replacement of alanine by glycine in those positions, but not in the fourth and fifth positions, greatly diminished the inhibitory capacity. Furthermore, if the antisera were prepared against D-Ala-Gly-RNase instead of $(D\text{-Ala})_3$-Gly-RNase, none of the alanine oligomers would be satisfactory; only an inhibitor such as D-Ala-Gly-ε-NH_2 caproate was effective. In order to account for regions of specificity in the side-chains of *Salmonella* polysaccharides, Luderitz, Staub, and Westphal[44] produced figures indicating affinity zones around immunodominant sugars and the participation of adjacent sugar residues. This concept[44] seems to embody the ideas both of Sage *et al.*[30] and of Schechter *et al.*[40–43]

[37] R. Mage and E. A. Kabat, *J. Immunol.*, 1963, **91**, 633.
[38] D. Stollar, L. Levine, H. I. Lehrer, and H. van Vunakis, *Proc. Nat. Acad. Sci., USA*, 1962, **48**, 874.
[39] S. M. Beiser and S. W. Tanenbaum, *Ann. N. Y. Acad. Sci.*, 1963, **103**, 595.
[40] I. Schechter and M. Sela, *Biochim. Biophys. Acta*, 1965, **104**, 298.
[41] I. Schechter, B. Schechter, and M. Sela, *Biochim. Biophys. Acta*, 1966, **127**, 438.
[42] B. Schechter, I. Schechter, and M. Sela, *J. Biol. Chem.*, 1970, **245**, 1438.
[43] B. Schechter, I. Schechter, and M. Sela, *Immunochemistry*, 1970, **7**, 587.
[44] O. Luderitz, A. M. Staub, and O. Westphal, *Bacteriol. Rev.*, 1966, **30**, 192.

The problem was explored further[43] with an immunoadsorbent prepared by reaction of poly-D-alanyl-rabbit serum albumin with bromoacetylcellulose. Rabbit antibodies against poly-D-alanyl-RNase and $(D\text{-Ala})_3$-Gly-RNase respectively were eluted from the immunoadsorbent with eluant containing excess of di-D-alanine, with that containing tetra-D-alanine, and with 0.1 M-acetic acid. Schechter *et al.*[43] found that the first fraction was inhibited by dipeptide ten times more effectively than the second fraction, that the first fraction was inhibited two or three times more effectively by tripeptide than the second fraction, and that both fractions were inhibited to the same extent by tetrapeptide. They[43] concluded either (i) that the first fraction was a mixture of antibodies with combining sites complementary to peptides of different sizes such that a higher proportion of antibody molecules possessed smaller combining sites and the second fraction consisted mainly of antibodies complementary to tetrapeptide, or (ii) that all of the resulting antibodies have combining sites complementary to tetrapeptide, but they are heterogeneous in their capacity to bind dipeptide. In that connection, antibodies complementary to a tetrapeptide would differ in their capacity to interact with dipeptide.

Enough has been said to show that the essentially simple and straightforward biological experiments, which were made in the 1930s, were still being re-investigated forty years later, employing the wide range of oligosaccharide and polypeptide methodology and of chromatography, and that the new and old results were interpreted and reinterpreted in terms of theoretical and physical chemistry. Central to our understanding of immunochemistry is the accommodation of antigenic determinants by antibody-binding sites and this depends in turn on such parameters as affinity, homogeneous binding, and immunogenetics.

The work which has been described raises the question of the energetics and kinetics of the reactions of antibodies with haptens and the virus model. These matters cannot be discussed within the compass of a short chapter devoted to other objectives, and the interested reader is referred to Day's treatise.[45] On the other hand, it is felt that the foregoing treatment of antigen specificity and antibody binding may provide clues as to how small molecular toxicants or their reactive metabolites might be expected to form antigens *in vivo* and to produce the immunobiological effects with which this chapter is concerned (section 4).

4 Effects of Foreign Compounds

Effects of Lead, Cadmium, and Methylmercury.—One method for determining whether low chronic exposure to a toxicant or environmental contaminant may affect the immune response has already been mentioned (section 1) and consists of challenging the treated animals with an LD_{50} dose of bacterium, bacterial toxin, or virus. Thus, mice treated with sub-toxic doses of $Pb(NO_3)_2$ showed greater susceptibility to *Salmonella typhimurium*,[46] encephalomyocarditis

[45] E. D. Day, 'Advanced Immunochemistry,' Williams and Wilkins, Baltimore, 1972.
[46] F. E. Hemphill, M. L. Kaeberle, and W. B. Buck, *Science*, 1971, **172**, 1031.

virus,[47] and to Langat virus.[48] However, responses to Cd^{2+} are known to be complicated (i) by the duration of exposure, and Duffus[49] mentions that the lungs are the target organs for short-term exposure to high levels of atmospheric Cd and the kidneys for long-term exposure to low levels, and (ii) by the route of administration.[50] Thus, a single dose of Cd^{2+} injected i.p. in mice increased formation of antibody, whereas oral administration diminished it.[50] Exposure to Cd^{2+} increased dramatically the susceptibility of rats to an inoculation with bacterial endotoxin,[51] enhanced the mortality of CD-1 mice inoculated with encephalomyocarditis,[47] and killed mice infected naturally with *Hexamita muris*.[52] Both inorganic[47] and organic Hg[53] increased the mortality of mice inoculated with encephalomyocarditis virus. The fact that 1 p.p.m. of $MeHg^+$ produced a significant increase in mortality showed that prolonged exposure to sub-toxic amounts may augment host susceptibility to viral infection.

These substances were immunosuppressive, as circulating concentrations of antibody to infectious agents from animals exposed to Pb^{2+},[54] Cd^{2+},[54] Hg^{2+},[54] and $MeHg^+$ [55] were significantly lower than those in untreated animals. Lead acetate caused a nine-fold decrease in antibody concentration in rabbits which had been exposed to pseudorabies virus, and the low antibody levels in general in animals exposed to metals might explain the known increase in sensitivity to endotoxins and bacterial infections when animals have been exposed to lead. Injection of Cd^{2+} 14 days before assault by an antigen increased antibody synthesis, but injection 7 days before the antigen decreased it.[56] Thus, the type of immune response elicited by some antigens depends on the time of exposure to foreign compounds in relation to antigen stimulation.

The fact that chronic exposure to Pb^{2+} decelerated IgG antibody synthesis[57,58] implied that the memory cell or T-helper cell was affected, as the IgG response would be more dependent than the IgM one (see ref. 62). Cadmium also depressed the IgG antibody response in mice,[59] but $MeHg^+$ suppressed both primary (IgM) and secondary (IgG) responses.[60,61] The greatest decrease in antibody synthesis occurred in animals exposed perinatally to methylmercury.[61]

Fewer rosettes in an erythrocyte–antibody–complement assay were formed by splenic B lymphocytes from mice exposed to Pb^{2+} or Cd^{2+} than B-cells

[47] J. H. Gainer, *Am. J. Vet. Res.*, 1977, **38**, 869.
[48] I. S. Third, G. S. Third, and D. B. Louria, 'Internat. Symp. on Clin. Chem. Toxicol of Metals,' Monte Carlo, March 1977.
[49] J. H. Duffus, 'Environmental Toxicology,' Edward Arnold, London, 1980, p. 9.
[50] L. D. Koller, J. H. Exon, and J. G. Roan, *Proc. Soc. Exp. Biol. Med.*, 1976, **151**, 339.
[51] J. A. Cook, E. O. Hoffman, and N. R. DiLuzio, *Proc. Soc. Exp. Biol. Med.*, 1975, **150**, 741.
[52] J. H. Exon, N. M. Patton, and L. D. Koller, *Arch. Environ. Health*, 1975, **31**, 463.
[53] L. D. Koller, *Am. J. Vet. Res.*, 1975, **36**, 1501.
[54] L. D. Koller, *Am. J. Vet. Res.*, 1973, **34**, 1459.
[55] L. D. Koller, J. H. Exon, and B. Arbogast, *J. Toxicol. Environ. Health*, 1977, **2**, 1115.
[56] R. H. Jones, R. L. Williams, and A. M. Jones, *Proc. Soc. Exp. Biol. Med.*, 1971, **137**, 1231.
[57] M. I. Luster, R. E. Faith, and C. A. Kimmel, *J. Environ. Path. Toxicol.*, 1978, **1**, 397.
[58] L. D. Koller and S. Kovacic, *Nature*, 1974, **250**, 148.
[59] L. D. Koller, J. H. Exon, and J. G. Roan, *Arch. Environ. Health*, 1975, **30**, 598.
[60] L. D. Koller, J. H. Exon, and J. A. Brauner, *Proc. Soc. Exp. Biol. Med.*, 1977, **155**, 602.
[61] G. Otti, M. Fukuda, H. Seto, and H. Yagyu, *Bull. Environ. Contamination Toxicol.*, 1976, **15**, 175.
[62] H. R. Anderson, D. W. Dresser, and H. H. Wortis, *Clin. Exp. Immunol.*, 1974, **16**, 393.

from untreated animals, and Koller and Brauner[63] reasoned that the direct effect of these substances on B-cells might account in part for the suppression by these substances of the humoral immune response. Lead and cadmium stimulated phagocytosis and increased acid phosphatase activity in macrophages,[64] but the increased activity did not mitigate against the prevailing secondary immune suppression that these metals evoke. In any case, macrophages influence the primary immune response more than the secondary one and they may not interfere therefore with the markedly suppressed secondary immune response.[65,66]

Moreover, lymphocyte stimulation of responder cells from CMI mice exposed to Pb^{2+}, Cd^{2+}, or $MeHg^{+}$ for 10 weeks was found to be altered inappreciably in comparison with that evoked from untreated animals.[67]

Hence, lead, cadmium, and methylmercury augment the susceptibility of host mammals to infectious disease, and the synergistic mechanism is due, at least in part, to the immunosuppressive properties of these substances.

Effect of Polychlorinated Biphenyls (PCBs) and Hexachlorobenzene.—Modification of the immune response was evaluated[68] in mice which were administered polychlorinated biphenyl (Aroclor 1242, PCB) or hexachlorobenzene in their diets by critical comparison of antibody formation, endotoxin sensitivity, and resistance to malaria. Antibody synthesis to the sheep antigen RBC was lowered very appreciably in animals that had been treated (167 p.p.m.) with PCB or hexachlorobenzene; untreated mice elicited a two-fold increase in antibody formation compared with the chemically treated animals. Plasma IgA levels were consistently lower in the PCB- and hexachlorobenzene-treated mice than the control values, but IgM was also reduced and this seems to be consistent with a primary splenic response (in contrast to that of the metals, *vide supra*). Morphological changes did not occur, and immunosuppression seems therefore to have resulted from changes in function. Mice showed hypersensitivity towards *Salmonella typhosa* (Gram-negative) endotoxin after dietary administration of PCB (167 p.p.m.) or hexachlorobenzene (1242 p.p.m.), both for 3-week or for 6-week periods. In fact, Aroclor 1016 and 1242 were equally effective in enhancing endotoxin sensitivity when administered in the diet at levels of 5 p.p.m. for 3 weeks. Diminished resistance to a challenge with malaria was shown in addition in mice fed Aroclor 1242 for 3 or 6 weeks and inoculated with *Plasmodium berghei* (NYU-2). Infected mice which had received hexachlorobenzene for periods of 3 or 6 weeks showed huge reductions in survival times (see also refs. 69—72). Impaired host resistance to malaria in animals given

[63] L. D. Koller and J. A. Brauner, *Toxicol. Appl. Pharmacol.*, 1977, **42**, 621.
[64] L. D. Koller and J. G. Roan, *J. Reticuloendothelial Soc.*, 1977, **21**, 7.
[65] R. W. Gillette and M. H. Swanson, *J. Reticuloendothelial Soc.*, 1974, **15**, 31.
[66] L. Treagan, *Chem. Pathol. Pharmacol.*, 1975, **12**, 189.
[67] L. D. Koller, *Drug Chem. Toxicol.*, 1979, **2(1 and 2)**, 99—110.
[68] L. D. Loose, J. B. Silkworth, S. P. Mudzinski, K. A. Pittman, K.-F. Benitz, and W. Mueller, *Drug Chem. Toxicol.*, 1979, **2(1 and 2)**, 111.
[69] M. Friend and D. O. Trainer, *Science*, 1970, **170**, 1314.
[70] J. H. Gainer, *Am. J. Vet. Res.*, 1972, **33**, 2067.
[71] J. H. Gainer and T. W. Pry, *Am. J. Vet. Res.*, 1972, **33**, 2299.
[72] G. A. Fairchild, J. Roan, and J. McCarroll, *Arch. Environ. Health*, 1972, **25**.

PCB or hexachlorobenzene in their diet seems to reflect the immunosuppression incurred by these compounds in the absence of morphological change to the lymphoid macrophages. The impaired immune response in the chemically treated mice, together with the immune suppression which occurs in malarial infection, and which has been shown[73] to be associated with macrophage dysfunction, results in a compromised defence status in animals exposed to these polyhalogeno aromatic compounds and assaulted with the parasite. As macrophages play an important role in defence against protozoa, their function seems to have been impaired by the compounds in question. The fact that mice which received hexachlorobenzene in their diet were more sensitive to the lethal effects of endotoxin and the malarial parasite than those that received PCB seems to be related to the greatly increased levels of hexachlorobenzene, relative to those of PCB, in the lymphoid macrophage tissues, *viz.* the liver, lungs, spleen, and thymus.

In further work,[74] pregnant rats were given diets containing hexachlorobenzene, and dosing was continued throughout lactation and after weaning; the immune system was assessed functionally in the 5-week-old pups which had thus been exposed perinatally. The resistance to *L. monocytogenes* infection was found to be suppressed, as was that to infection with *T. spiralis*, but no effect was observed on allograft rejection or on the mitogenic response of thymus and spleen cells. Hexachlorobenzene enhanced the thymus-dependent antibody response to *T. spiralis* antigen and to tetanus toxoid. No effect was found on the IgM response to *E. coli* lipopolysaccharide, on passive cutaneous anaphylaxis, and on (macrophages) the clearance of carbon particles and *L. monocytogenes*. Hexachlorobenzene treatment caused morphological changes in the lymph nodes, liver, and lungs.

It is concluded that hexachlorobenzene suppresses CMI and enhances humoral immunity.

Effects of 2,3,7,8-Tetrachlorodibenzofuran.—The presence of polychlorinated dibenzofurans in commercial polychlorinated biphenyls was first detected by Vos *et al.*,[75] and they were found subsequently in commercial preparations from various countries as well as in PCB-contaminated rice oil.[76–78] These substances were highly toxic, and the LD_{50} of 2,3,7,8-tetrachlorodibenzofuran in guinea-pigs was 5—10 $\mu g\ kg^{-1}$. Amongst the pathological changes found[79] was thymus (cortex) atrophy. Diminished host resistance to *Salmonella bera* infection

[73] L. D. Loose, J. A. Cook, and N. R. DiLuzio, *Proc. Helminthol.*, 1972, **39**, 484.
[74] J. G. Vos, M. J. van Logten, J. G. Kreeftenberg, P. A. Steerenberg, and W. Kruizinga, *Drug Chem. Toxicol.*, 1979, **2(1 and 2)**, 61.
[75] J. G. Vos, J. H. Koeman, H. L. van der Maas, M. C. ten Noever de Brauw, and R. H. de Vos, *Food Cosmet. Toxicol.*, 1970, **8**, 625.
[76] G. W. Bowes, M. J. Mulvihill, B. R. T. Simoneit, A.-L. Burlingame, and R. W. Risebrough, *Nature*, 1975, **256**, 305.
[77] J. A. G. Roach and I. H. Pomerantz, *Bull. Environ. Contam. Toxicol.*, 1974, **12**, 330.
[78] J. Nagayama, M. Kuratsune, and Y. Masuda, *Bull. Environ. Contam. Toxicol.*, 1976, **15**, 9.
[79] B. N. Gupta, J. G. Vos, J. A. Moore, J. G. Zinkl, and B. C. Bullock, *Environ. Health. Perspect.*, 1973, **6**, 125.

was reported by other workers.[80] A more recent study[81] demonstrated, at high dose levels, depressed hypersensitivity responses, lymphokine production, and lympho-proliferative responses after stimulation with the T-lymphocyte mitogen phytohaemoagglutinin, suggesting suppression of the CMI. That humoral immunity might also be compromised was suggested[81] by lowered lympho-proliferative responses to lipopolysaccharide endotoxin, but serum concentrations of IgG and antibody levels to immunisation with bovine γ-globulin were almost unaltered. Dysfunction of the immune system by 2,3,7,8-tetrachlorodibenzofuran was essentially similar to that evoked by 2,3,7,8-tetrachlorodibenzo-*p*-dioxin (*v. infra*).

Effects of Polybrominated Biphenyls (PBBs).—The interest of this work arises from the accidental contamination in Michigan (1977) of animal feed with Firemaster FF-1 flame retardant containing PBBs, followed by the consequential unwitting contamination of beef, butter, cheese, eggs, milk, and poultry for human consumption, and thus of human beings, in whom PBBs were identified.[82–86] PBBs are clearly lipid-soluble, and they accumulate in the adipose tissues, brain, liver, and thymus of exposed mammals, where they have a long $t_{0.5}$. Because of the toxicity and the apparent lack of metabolism of PBBs in mammals, investigations were implemented to allay suspicion of risk as far as this was possible; the study included some work on the immune response.[87,88] Abnormalities included decreased populations of T-lymphocytes with a simultaneous increase in null cells, *i.e.* lymphocytes with no apparent surface marking and altered (lymphocyte) function. There was no correlation between impaired lymphocyte function and delayed cutaneous hypersensitivity, nor between lymphocyte dysfunction and plasma PBB concentrations, but there was a better correlation between lymphocyte dysfunction and the distribution of PBBs in the white-cell fraction. Again these findings appear to implicate the CMI.

Effects of 2,3,7,8-Tetrachlorodibenzo-*p*-dioxin.—2,3,7,8-Tetrachlorodibenzo-*p*-dioxin is a by-product of 2,4,5-trichlorophenol production, and it contaminates the reaction product.[89] Several studies[90–92] in adult animals and their young have

[80] J. E. Thigpen, R. E. Faith, E. E. McConnell, and J. A. Moore, *Infect. Immunol.*, 1975, **12**, 131.
[81] M. I. Luster, R. E. Faith, and L. D. Lawson, *Drug Chem. Toxicol.*, 1979, **2**, 49.
[82] L. G. Carter, *Science*, 1976, **192**, 240.
[83] A. E. Dunckel, *J. Am. Vet. Med. Assoc.*, 1975, **167**, 838.
[84] T. F. Jackson and F. L. Halbert, *J. Am. Vet. Med. Assoc.*, 1974, **165**, 437.
[85] H. A. Anderson, R. Lilis, and I. J. Selikoff, *Environ. Health Perspect.*, 1978, **23**, 217.
[86] R. Lilis, H. A. Anderson, J. A. Valciukas, S. Freedman, and I. J. Selikoff, *Environ. Health Perspect.*, 1978, **23**, 105.
[87] J. G. Bekesi, J. F. Holland, H. A. Anderson, A. S. Fischbein, W. Prom, M. S. Wolff, and I. J. Selikoff, *Science*, 1978, **199**, 1207.
[88] J. G. Bekesi, J. Roboz, H. A. Anderson, J. P. Roboz, A. S. Fischbein, I. J. Selikoff, and J. F. Holland, *Drug Chem. Toxicol.*, 1979, **2**, 179.
[89] R. R. Woolsen and P. Ensor, *J. Agric. Food Chem.*, 1972, **20**, 351.
[90] R. Kinbrugh, *CRC Crit. Rev. Toxicol.*, 1974, **2**, 445.
[91] R. Faith and J. Moore, *J. Toxicol. Environ. Health.*, 1977, **3**, 451.
[92] J. Vos and J. Moore, *Int. Arch. Allerg. Appl. Immunol.*, 1974, **47**, 777.

shown that this substance has an adverse effect on the thymus and CMI. As this immunosuppression had occurred sometimes in animals, which showed toxic effects,[92] it was prudent for the immune function to be evaluated[93] in the pups of mice that were exposed chronically to sub-toxic amounts. (Sub-toxic levels of exposure for the mothers were defined as ones which did not cause obvious toxic effects in the progeny.) Accordingly, the dams were fed perinatally 2.5 or 5.0 p.p.b. of 2,3,7,8-tetrachlorodibenzo-*p*-dioxin. In this sensitive testing procedure, the pups showed thymus (cortex) atrophy and significantly reduced spleen plaque-forming cell response to anti-sheep erythrocyte, although the antibody levels against this antigen were normal; thus, the CMI appears to be implicated. However, contact sensitivity response was reduced significantly only in the pups fed at the 5 p.p.b. level of exposure, and the blastogenic response of splenic T- and B-lymphocytes to concanavalin-A and *E. coli* lipopolysaccharide was unaffected by perinatal exposure to 2,3,7,8-tetrachlorodibenzo-*p*-dioxin. This was confirmed by the normal appearance of the T- and B-cell dependent areas of spleens from all of these animals. There were no differences in differential white-cell counts between the controls and treated animals, nor in resistance to a challenge with living *Listeria*. It followed that the progeny were more sensitive than the adults to the effects of low 2,3,7,8-tetrachlorodibenzo-*p*-dioxin exposure, and showed thymic atrophy and certain types (CMI) of immunosuppression at levels of exposure insufficient to evoke obvious toxic effects.

Concluding Remarks.—Despite a lack of direct evidence, there is a strong supposition that the immunosuppressive effects (i) of Pb^{2+}, Cd^{2+}, and $MeHg^{+}$ cations are due to their capacity to form ligands with antigenic proteins, and (ii) of the polyhalogenated aromatics and heterocyclics relate to S_N2 reaction between the primary amino groups of antigenic protein and the reactive halogen of these compounds. Supporting evidence for reactivity of such halogen atom(s) derives from the formation, under gentle conditions, of 2,3,7,8-tetrachlorodibenzo-*p*-dioxin (1) from 2 mol equiv. of 2,4,5-trichlorophenol and of the corresponding 2,3,7,8-tetrachlorodibenzofuran (2) from 2,2′,4,4′,5,5′-hexachlorobiphenyl. Predictably, the polyhalogenated aromatics and heterocyclics, assisted

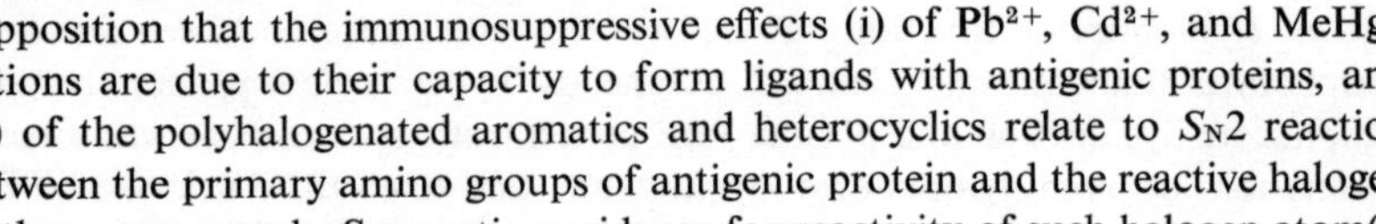

(1)

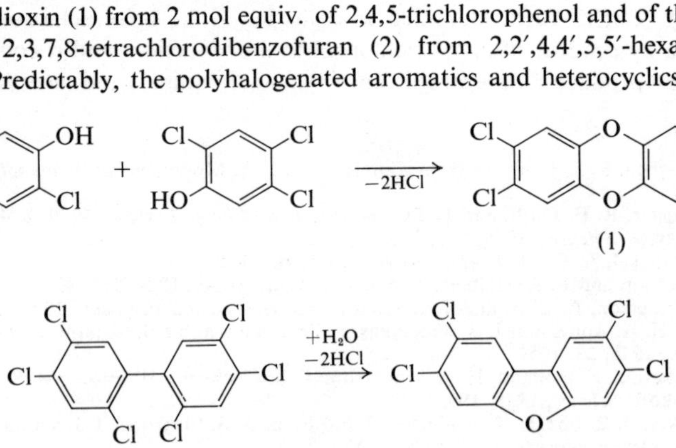

(2)

[93] P. T. Thomas and R. D. Hinsdill, *Drug Chem. Toxicol.*, 1979, **2**, 77.

by their lipid solubility, would be transported across membranes by passive diffusion, in contrast to the known behaviour of the metallic and organometallic cations. This is perfectly consistent with the fact that the polyhalogenated aromatics and heterocyclics accumulate in and affect thymus and lymphocyte function, and modify CMI, and that the metallic and organometallic cations react with serum protein to form antigens, and modify the humoral immunity.

Subject Index